Anti-obesity and Anti-aging Natural Products

Anti-obesity and Anti-aging Natural Products

Guest Editors

Rosario Mare
Vincenzo Musolino

MDPI

Basel • Beijing • Wuhan • Barcelona • Belgrade • Novi Sad • Cluj • Manchester

Guest Editors

Rosario Mare
Department of Medical and Surgical Sciences
University "Magna Græcia" of Catanzaro
Catanzaro
Italy

Vincenzo Musolino
Department of Health Sciences
University "Magna Græcia" of Catanzaro
Catanzaro
Italy

Editorial Office

MDPI AG
Grosspeteranlage 5
4052 Basel, Switzerland

This is a reprint of the Special Issue, published open access by the journal *Pharmaceuticals* (ISSN 1424-8247), freely accessible at: https://www.mdpi.com/journal/pharmaceuticals/special_issues/M48Z81W30B.

For citation purposes, cite each article independently as indicated on the article page online and as indicated below:

Lastname, A.A.; Lastname, B.B. Article Title. *Journal Name* **Year**, *Volume Number*, Page Range.

ISBN 978-3-7258-6802-5 (Hbk)
ISBN 978-3-7258-6803-2 (PDF)
https://doi.org/10.3390/books978-3-7258-6803-2

Contents

About the Editors

Rosario Mare

Rosario Mare is a researcher in Food Science and Applied Dietetic Techniques at the Magna Graecia University of Catanzaro, where he focuses on advancing the understanding of natural bioactive compounds and their applications in metabolic and nutritional health. He earned a master's degree in Pharmacy and a PhD in Life Sciences from the same university, with a research fellowship at the University of Oklahoma Health Sciences Center in the United States. His research interests focus on innovative methods for extracting, purifying, and quantifying bioactive compounds from food matrices, designing customized formulations to protect and deliver natural compounds, and developing functional foods and nutraceuticals for the prevention of metabolic-nutritional diseases. He has co-authored over 30 publications in international scientific journals with significant citations, and his work spans studies on metabolic syndrome, obesity, diabetes, and hepatic steatosis, among other areas. As a Guest Editor for *Pharmaceuticals*, he helps shape the scientific conversation about natural products targeting obesity and aging-related processes by bringing together interdisciplinary insights into molecular mechanisms and health-promoting strategies that leverage natural sources.

Vincenzo Musolino

Vincenzo Musolino is a researcher in Pharmaceutical Biology at the University Magna Graecia of Catanzaro, where he carries out research within the Department of Health Sciences and teaches courses including Plant Biology, Pharmaceutical Botany, and Pharmacognosy of wellness products. He graduated in Industrial Biotechnology from the University of Milano-Bicocca and earned his PhD in Pharmaceutical Sciences at the University Magna Graecia of Catanzaro, including a research period at the Charité in Berlin. His scientific work centers on the botanical, phytochemical, and pharmacognostic study of medicinal plants, focusing on the identification and characterization of bioactive plant complexes and their potential therapeutic applications, optimization of extraction methodologies, and evaluation of biological activities including antioxidant properties and formulation of innovative functional foods through in vitro and in vivo testing. He has co-authored over one hundred scientific publications in international journals with a significant citation record, reflecting his contributions to natural product research and pharmaceutical plant biology. As a Guest Editor for *Pharmaceuticals*, he brings his expertise in natural bioactive compounds and their roles in health and disease to the curation of cutting-edge research on anti-obesity and anti-aging natural products.

Preface

Obesity and aging are two interrelated global health challenges that profoundly impact metabolic function, quality of life, and long-term health outcomes. Traditional pharmacological approaches for managing metabolic disorders and physiological aging have provided important advances, yet issues of efficacy, adverse effects, and long-term sustainability persist. In recent years, a growing body of scientific research has focused on the potential of natural products derived from plants, herbs, and other biological sources to modulate key biological pathways involved in weight regulation, metabolic health, and age-associated decline.

This Reprint brings together a curated collection of high-quality research and authoritative reviews that examine the roles of natural compounds in counteracting obesity and slowing aspects of the aging process. The assembled contributions span mechanistic studies, preclinical investigations, and translational insights into how phytochemicals, antioxidants, botanicals, and bioactive extracts influence metabolic balance, inflammation, oxidative stress, adipose tissue dynamics, and functional resilience. Included work explores diverse subjects such as the impact of specific botanical extracts on lipid metabolism and insulin sensitivity, modulation of gut microbiota, adipocyte biology and thermogenesis, neuroprotective effects, and comprehensive analyses of bioactive compounds in the management of complex metabolic diseases.

This Reprint reflects the current scientific dialogue on natural alternatives and adjuncts to conventional interventions, emphasizing biological plausibility, molecular targets, and therapeutic potential. By highlighting innovative research that bridges natural product chemistry, pharmacology, and metabolic science, it aims to inform researchers, clinicians, and health professionals seeking integrative strategies for improving metabolic health and promoting healthier aging.

Rosario Mare and Vincenzo Musolino

Guest Editors

pharmaceuticals

Article

Zibibbo Grape Seeds' Polyphenolic Profile: Effects on Bone Turnover and Metabolism

Mariagiovanna Settino [1], Samantha Maurotti [1], Luca Tirinato [2], Simona Greco [2], Anna Rita Coppoletta [3], Antonio Cardamone [3], Vincenzo Musolino [4], Tiziana Montalcini [1,5], Arturo Pujia [2,5,*] and Rosario Mare [2,*]

1 Department of Clinical and Experimental Medicine, University "Magna Græcia" of Catanzaro, 88100 Catanzaro, Italy; margiov.settino@gmail.com (M.S.); smaurotti@unicz.it (S.M.); tmontalcini@unicz.it (T.M.)

2 Department of Medical and Surgical Sciences, University "Magna Græcia" of Catanzaro, 88100 Catanzaro, Italy; tirinato@unicz.it (L.T.); simona.greco001@studenti.unicz.it (S.G.)

3 Pharmacology Laboratory, Department of Health Sciences, Institute of Research for Food Safety and Health IRC-FSH, University "Magna Græcia" of Catanzaro, 88100 Catanzaro, Italy; annarita.coppoletta1@gmail.com (A.R.C.); tony.c@outlook.it (A.C.)

4 Laboratory of Pharmaceutical Biology, Department of Health Sciences, Institute of Research for Food Safety & Health IRC-FSH, University "Magna Græcia" of Catanzaro, 88100 Catanzaro, Italy; v.musolino@unicz.it

5 Research Center for the Prevention and Treatment of Metabolic Diseases, University "Magna Græcia" of Catanzaro, 88100 Catanzaro, Italy

* Correspondence: pujia@unicz.it (A.P.); mare@unicz.it (R.M.); Tel.: +39-09613697080 (A.P.); +39-09613964067 (R.M.)

Abstract: Background: The consumption of seeds as food has become increasingly common due to their numerous health benefits. Among these, the seeds of the Zibibbo grape from Pantelleria, a native species of southern Italy, remain largely unexplored and are usually considered waste material from viticulture. Nevertheless, Zibibbo grape seeds may offer health benefits, particularly for the elderly and people with metabolic disorders, due to their potential content of beneficial compounds such as polyphenols. Methods: The Zibibbo grape seeds extract (ZSE) was characterized using UV-visible spectrophotometry and HPLC chromatography. The antioxidant activity of ZSE was measured by different colorimetric assays and Electronic Paramagnetic Resonance (EPR). Additionally, specific in vitro tests were conducted on human osteoblast cell lines (Saos-2 and MG63) aiming to evaluate the ZSE's effects on bone turnover and metabolism. Western blotting was used to assess the impact on specific proteins and pathways related to bone health. Results: The ZSE contained almost ~3 mg/mL of carbohydrates and phenolic compounds, including rutin (~6.4 ppm) and hesperidin (~44.6 ppm). The extracts exhibited an antioxidant activity greater than 90% across all tests performed. Moreover, the Zibibbo seed extracts exerted a significant proliferative effect on the Saos-2 cell human osteoblast-like cell line, also modulating the phosphorylation of specific kinases involved in cell health and metabolism. Conclusions: Zibibbo grape seeds are rich in phenolic compounds, especially flavonoids with strong antioxidant and free radical scavenging properties. ZSE demonstrated beneficial effects on bone metabolism and osteoblast proliferation, suggesting potential for counteracting osteodegenerative conditions like osteoporosis. If confirmed through further studies, Zibibbo grape seed phenolic compounds could serve as an adjunctive therapy for osteoporosis, helping to slow aging and bone degeneration.

Keywords: grape seeds; polyphenols; flavonoids; osteoporosis; bone health

1. Introduction

Following the Mediterranean diet on a daily basis is commonly associated with different benefits to health and pathological status [1]. Among vegetables and plant derivatives, the consumption of fresh or dried seeds is becoming widespread because of the macromolecules they contain. In fact, seeds are usually considered a waste material from fruit processing procedures, but several studies have shown that they contain multiple beneficial molecules such as vitamins, organic acids and polyphenolic compounds, including several flavonoids, which could be useful in various pathological conditions [2]. In particular, several beneficial effects have recently been associated with the consumption of grape seeds and their derivatives, which have been shown to be advantageous in improving gastrointestinal mobility [3], cardiovascular and metabolic diseases [4,5] and even in cancer therapy [6]. Despite the growing interest in grape seeds, there is still a lack of comprehensive studies on certain varieties of grapes, particularly regarding their biochemical diversity and potential health applications. It is well known that the biochemical properties of grapes can vary significantly depending on the botanical species and the climatic conditions [7]. This variability suggests the importance of investigating specific grape varieties to better understand their unique compositions and potential health benefits.

Zibibbo grape is a peculiar grape species, cultivated in some Italian regions and predominant on Pantelleria island [8]. Despite the interest of the scientific community in grape seeds, the Zibibbo grape was mostly, if not exclusively, studied for winemaking [9] or for making raisins [10]. Therefore, the only studies available in the literature concern "passito" wines and the microbiological characteristics of grapes for producing them [11]. As a result, there is a significant gap in the literature regarding the potential health benefits of Zibibbo seeds. In fact, within the literature there is a lack of information about their potential nutritional or medical applications. However, recent scientific evidence demonstrates that grape seeds are also rich in polyphenolic and antioxidant substances, which could play a crucial role in various pathologies related to oxidative stress [12]. In addition, the consumption of seeds has been shown to help mitigate osteodegenerative diseases such as osteoporosis, a frequent condition that occurs in post-menopausal women and during the physiological aging process [13].

This study aims to fill the gap in the literature about Zibibbo seeds by characterizing their bioactive profile, focusing particularly on the polyphenolic compounds and antioxidant properties they contain. Additionally, this study offers an evaluation of antioxidant power using different analytical methods, finally investigating the biocompatibility and safety of Zibibbo seed extracts (ZSEs) on osteoblast-like cell lines, with the goal of exploring their potential benefits through in vitro models. By addressing this knowledge gap, we aim to contribute to the understanding of the unique properties of Zibibbo grape seeds and clarify their potential beneficial effects on bone tissues and the aging processes.

2. Results

2.1. Chemical Analyses

Purified ZSEs were analyzed using an UV-Vis spectrophotometer after being diluted in a 1:200 ratio with the same hydro-alcoholic mixture used for the extraction. All ZSEs showed a main and characteristic peak between 250 nm and 300 nm, with maximum absorbance at λ~280 nm (Figure 1).

Zibibbo seeds extracts were characterized through different analytical approaches. The results for the main macromolecules detected and quantified in the ZSEs are listed and described in Table 1. In detail, according to the Bradford assay, the protein content was ~0.69 $\pm$ 0.02 mg/mL, equivalent to that in bovine serum albumin (EBSA—Table 1). The amounts of carbohydrates contained in the ZSEs were estimated using the sulfuric acid–phenol assay and compared with a stock mixture containing glucose, sucrose and fructose in equal ratio (conc. 6.25–75 ppm). The mean carbohydrates content in the ZSEs was ~3.23 $\pm$ 0.49 mg/mL, equivalent to that in sucrose (SEq—Table 1).

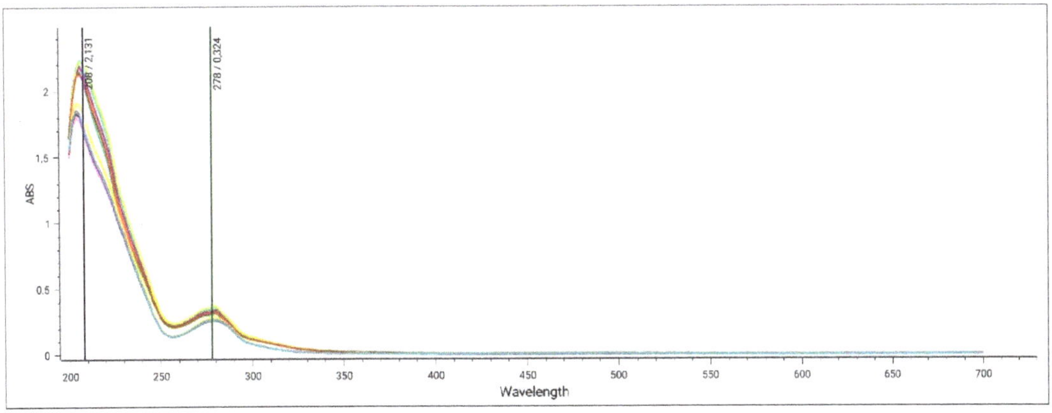

Figure 1. Spectrophotometric analyses of Zibibbo seed extracts (ZSEs) at wavelengths (λ) between 200 nm and 700 nm. Different colors refer to the analysis of different extractions.

A total phenolic content assay provided information about the presence of phenolic compounds and tannin-like molecules in the ZSEs. The reaction with Folin–Ciocalteu's reagent allowed us to detect ~1.575 ± 0.19 mg/mL molecules, equivalent to gallic acid (GAE—Table 1). The application of the sodium nitrite–aluminum chloride assay allowed us to discriminate flavonoids. All samples demonstrated the peculiar and characteristic red color of molecules with a catechinic structure. The spectrophotometric analyses showed a content of ~2.05 ± 0.25 mg/mL, and mean flavonoids content was ~102 ± 12 mg for every gram of seed powder investigated (Table 1).

Table 1. Chemical characterization of Zibibbo seeds extracts (ZSEa) using a UV-Vis spectrophotometer.

Macromolecule	Method	Amount ± SD
Proteins	Bradford Assay	~0.69 ± 0.02 mg/mL EBSA [1]
Carbohydrates	Phenol–Sulfuric Acid	~3.23 ± 0.49 mg/mL SEq [2]
Phenolic Content	Folin–Ciocâlteu Assay	~1.575 ± 0.19 mg/mL GAE [3]
Flavonoids	Nitrite–Aluminum Assay	~ 2.05 ± 0.25 mg/mL [4]

[1] EBSA = equivalent to bovine serum albumin; [2] SEq = equivalent to sucrose; [3] GAE = equivalent to gallic acid; [4] quantified using a flavonoids mixture calibration curve. Data are expressed as mean ± standard deviation (SD).

HPLC analyses confirmed the presence of flavonoids in the extracts and specifically detected and quantified them as a function of the standard molecules available (Figure 2). In detail, the injection peak, which is appreciable in all HPLC analyses, was detectable after ~1 min retention. Rutin and hesperidin signals eluted, respectively, with an R.T. of 7.5 min. and 12.5 min., with the latter having a concentration approximately seven times higher than rutin. In fact, the mean concentrations of rutin and hesperidin in ZSE were approximately ~6.4 ± 0.3 ppm and 44.6 ± 4.5 ppm (Figure 2). Moreover, The HPLC analyses highlighted the presence of a large peak (R.T. ~17 min) attributable to another polyphenolic substance, which is presumably a flavonoid but remains unknown. The increase in absorbance detected after ~23 min is due to the increase in the organic phase in the elution mixture, but it does not represent a peak (Figure 2).

The Zibibbo seed extracts showed strong antioxidant and free-radical scavenging activities, regardless of the technique used (Figure 3). In detail, the interaction with the 2,2-Diphenyl-1-picrylhydrazyl (DPPH) was expressed as percentage of free radicals inhibited (%I). In this case, the ZSEs showed a percentage of antioxidant activity ~82 ± 3% in comparison with a solution of L-ascorbic acid (5 mg/mL) enrolled as a positive control (Figure 3A).

The ABTS assay echoed the DPPH colorimetric assay's results, but provided superior data, finally confirming the ZSEs' antioxidant activity of ~97 ± 1% I (Figure 3B). The use of Electronic Paramagnetic Resonance (EPR) allowed us to assess the free radical scavenging activity of ZSE. L-ascorbic acid (5 mg/mL solution) was also enrolled as positive control in this test. The pure DPPH solution had a spectral area (a.u.) of ∫ = 1754 ± 3. The mixture obtained by adding ascorbic acid had a spectral area of ∫ = 42 ± 2. However, the addition of the Zibibbo seeds extract to the DPPH solution showed spectral area values (∫) between 56 ± 3 and 93 ± 3, finally demonstrating an average free-radical scavenging activity of 95.75% (Figure 3C).

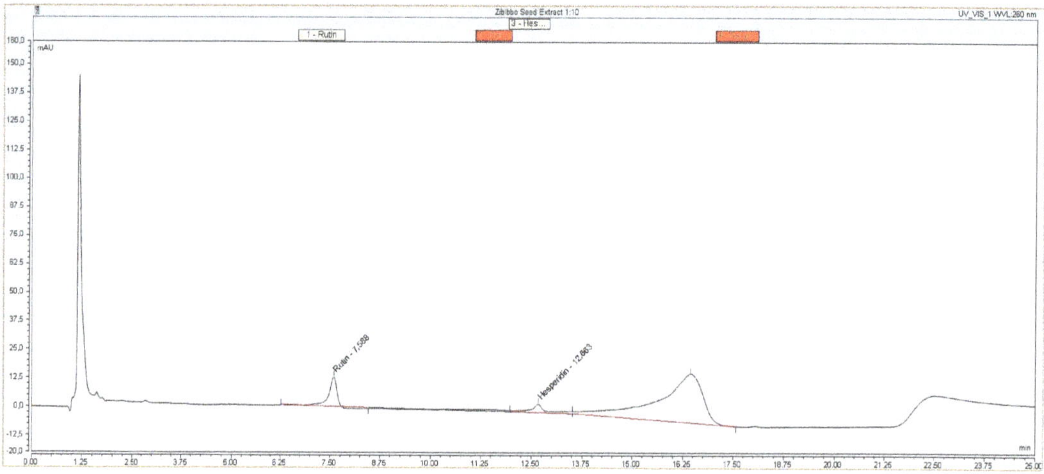

Figure 2. Chromatogram of Zibibbo seed extracts (ZSEs) analyzed by HPLC equipped with a 100 mm reverse-phase C18 column. Acquisition wavelength (λ) was set at 260 nm.

2.2. *Effect of ZSE on Saos-2 Osteoblast In Vitro Model*

We investigated the effects of Zibibbo seed polyphenols on Saos-2 osteoblast cells. Specifically, changes in cell proliferation, ERK1/2 and AKT proteins phosphorylation were examined, as well as the intracellular production of oxygen free radicals, aiming to evaluate ZSEs' influences on bone turnover and metabolism. After 24 h of incubation, the ZSEs showed a statistically significant proliferative effect on a Saos-2 cell line at doses between 5 and 40 μg/mL as well as at a dose of 0.31 μg/mL compared to the control group (Figure 4A). In addition to this, in the Saos-2 cell line, the ZSEs showed a statistically significant proliferative effect at doses greater than 1.25 μg/mL compared to the control group treated with ethanol 70%, finally showing a dose-dependent proliferative effect (Figure 4A).

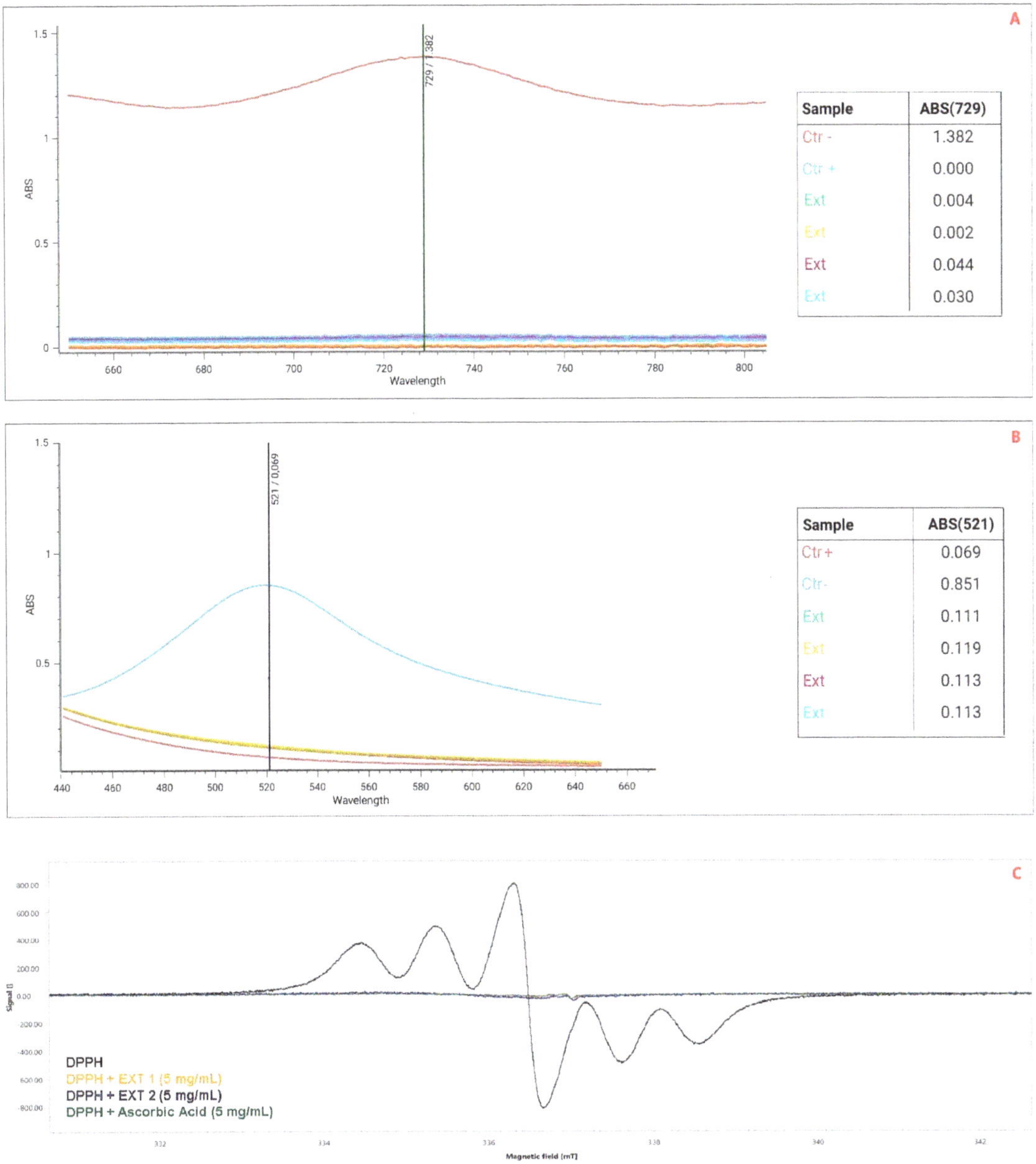

Figure 3. Antioxidant activity of Zibibbo seed extracts (ZSEs) analyzed by ABTS assay (**A**), DPPH assay (**B**) and through Electronic Paramagnetic Resonance (EPR-**C**). CTR+ = positive control; CTR− = negative control; DPPH = 2,2-Diphenyl-1-picrylhydrazyl; EXT = extract.

The effect of the ZSEs on ERK1/2 and AKT phosphorylation was assessed by treating Saos-2 cells with a 10 nM dexamethasone medium containing the ZSEs in concentrations between 2.5 μg/mL and 40 μg/mL (Figure 4B,C). The incubation with ZSEs increased ERK1/2 phosphorylation in a dose-dependent manner compared to the untreated control group ($p = 0.0011$; Figure 4B). In detail, treatment with the ZSEs resulted in a statistically significant increase in p-ERK1/2 at doses of 10 μg/mL, 20 μg/mL ($p < 0.001$) and 40 μg/mL

($p < 0.01$) (Figure 4B). Additionally, on the same cell line, the incubation with ZSE also increased AKT phosphorylation in a dose-dependent manner, compared to the untreated control group ($p < 0.0001$), thus resulting in a statistically significant increase in AKT phosphorylation at doses of 10 µg/mL ($p < 0.05$), 20 µg/mL and 40 µg/mL ($p < 0.0001$) (Figure 4C).

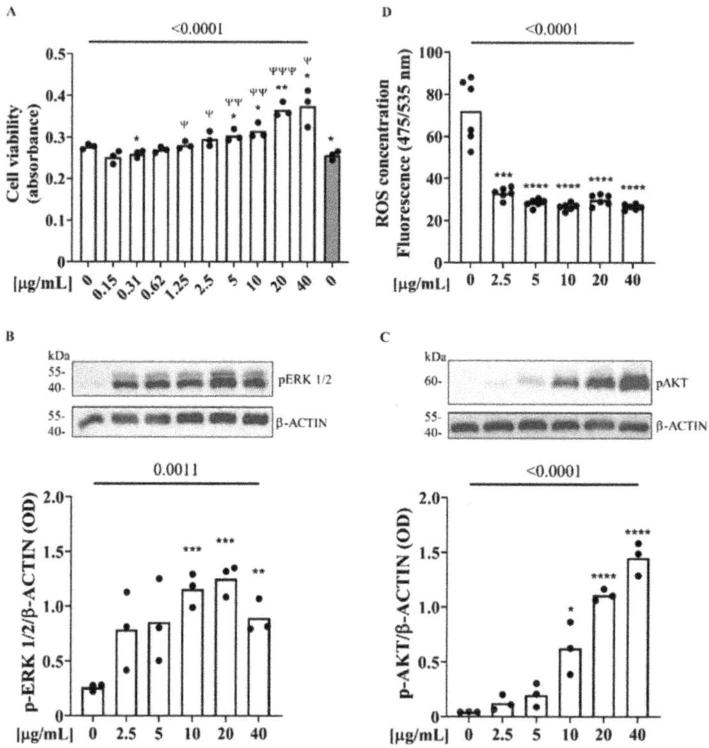

Figure 4. Effect of ZSEs on Saos-2 osteoblast cells' proliferation after 24 hours of treatment (**A**). Variation in ERK1/2 and AKT protein phosphorylation level after 10 min treatment with ZSE ((**B**,**C**), respectively). Cell proteins were analyzed by Western blotting using specific antibodies to detect phosphorylated ERK and AKT, as well as for ß-actin. Evaluation of radical oxygen species released by Saos-2 cells after 45 min treatment with ZSE, according to the ROS Assay Kit [AB113851] (**D**). Data are expressed as mean of independent experiments (three at least) including distribution spots for standard deviation. (* and $^{\Psi}$ $p < 0.05$; ** and $^{\Psi\Psi}$ $p < 0.01$; *** and $^{\Psi\Psi\Psi}$ $p < 0.001$; **** $p < 0.0001$).

Moreover, treatment with ZSEs was shown to significantly reduce the amount of reactive oxygen species (ROS) released from cells regardless of the dose examined; finally, a dose-dependent trend was also shown for this parameter (Figure 4D).

2.3. *Effect of ZSE on MG63 Osteoblast In Vitro Model*

Given that the MG63 cell line is an advantageous model for investigating the early stages of osteoblastic differentiation, we used this cell line to test the ZSEs using same conditions and dosages previously employed for the Saos-2 cells [14].

After 24 h of incubation with MG63 cells, treatment with 10 µg/mL of ZSE showed a significant increase in cell viability compared to the control group and the ethanol-treated control (Figure 5A, $p < 0.05$). On the contrary, the 40 µg/mL dose resulted in a significant reduction in cell viability (Figure 5A, $p < 0.05$). Similarly, the evaluation of pERK1/2 protein expression showed a reduction in the phosphorylated form of the protein at the 10 µg/mL dose, but did not reveal any significant changes at the other doses investigated. On the contrary, treatment with the ZSEs increased AKT phosphorylation in a dose-dependent manner, if compared to the untreated control group (Figure 5C, $p < 0.0001$). This resulted in a statistically significant increase in protein phosphorylation at doses of 10 μg/mL and 40 μg/mL ($p < 0.001$) as well as treatment with 20 μg/mL ($p < 0.01$) (Figure 5C).

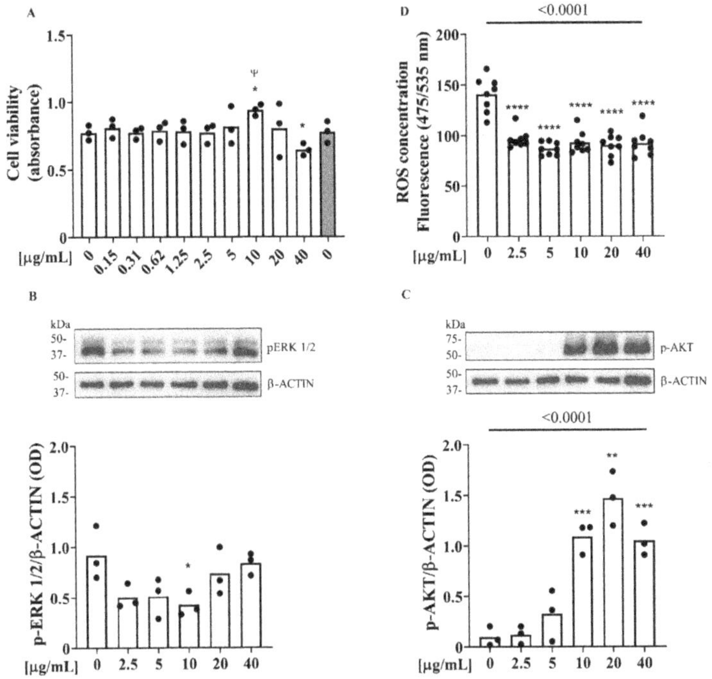

Figure 5. Effect of ZSEs on MG63 osteoblast cells' proliferation after 24 treatment (**A**). Variation in ERK1/2 and AKT protein phosphorylation level after 10 min treatment with ZSEs ((**B**,**C**), respectively). Cell proteins were analyzed by Western blotting using specific antibodies to quantify phosphorylated ERK and AKT, as well as for ß-actin. Evaluation of radical oxygen species released by MG63 cells after 45 min treatment with ZSEs, according to the ROS Assay Kit [AB113851] (**D**). Data are expressed as mean of independent experiments (three at least) including distribution spots for standard deviation (* and $^{\Psi}$ $p < 0.05$; ** $p < 0.01$; *** $p < 0.001$; **** $p < 0.0001$).

Moreover, and similarly to the Saos-2 cells, treatments with ZSEs were able to significantly reduce the number of reactive oxygen species (ROS) released from cells, regardless of the doses examined, and a dose-dependent trend was also shown for this parameter. (Figure 5D, $p < 0.0001$ in all cases).

3. Discussion

Adherence to the Mediterranean diet appears to be the most beneficial approach to pursuing healthy aging. Most of the recognized benefits of the Mediterranean diet are related to the naturally high contents of polyunsaturated fatty acids, vitamins and polyphenolic compounds in the foods. In particular, polyphenols were demonstrated to play a key role in promoting people's health and the prevention of various diseases, such as type 2 diabetes, cardiovascular diseases, obesity and even neurological pathologies. In fact, polyphenols are known to be directly involved in glucose regulation and transportation, as well as in the protection of β-cells from glucose toxicity [15,16]. They also exerted effects on reducing platelet activation and reducing LDL cholesterol [17], on adipocyte oxidation [18] and on psychological and cognitive health, and there were cases in which the consumption of coffee, tea and red wine resulted in a reduction in depressive symptoms and perceived stress [19].

Seeds have long played crucial roles in human nutrition throughout history, but in recent decades, they have captured the attention of the scientific community because of the potential health benefits associated with their regular consumption. In particular, different nutrients, fat-soluble bioactives and polyphenols have been abundantly found in seeds collected from hemp [13], black cumin, chia, flax, perilla, pumpkin, quinoa and sesame, thus conferring them different health benefits that are mainly related to their antioxidant activity, good bioavailability and toxicological safety [20].

Although several research groups have analyzed grape seeds, most of them focused on lipophilic molecules [21].

The Zibibbo seed extracts were analyzed unconditionally and regardless of all the information in the literature concerning grape berries and juice. This approach was necessary and justified by the qualitative and quantitative differences existing between the molecules contained in leaves, fruits and seeds belonging to the same plant species [22]. These differences, in agreement with data described in the literature, did not facilitate the use of a predictive approach regarding the molecules contained in the extract, especially considering this is the first study about Zibibbo seeds available in the literature. The extraction procedure was effective in isolating the hydrophilic compounds present in the Zibibbo seeds, with the extracts containing a substantial number of phenolic compounds besides a small fraction of proteins and carbohydrates. Interestingly, the total carbohydrates content was analogous to the overall phenolic content detected in the extract. This phenomenon may be justified by the fact that most of the phenolic compounds in fruits and vegetables are spontaneously conjugated to a glucidic molecule, particularly D-glucopyranose or rutinose. In agreement with our hypothesis, several studies in the literature confirm that phenolic compounds are predominantly in the glycosylated form [23].

The phenolic fraction was rich in flavonoids and gallic acid-like polyphenols, which overall showed a remarkable antioxidant capacity and strong scavenging activity against free radicals with all in vitro assay proposed in the study. This aligns with findings from the current literature, supporting the notion that the antioxidant and free radical scavenging effects can be attributed to the phenolic compounds, placing specific emphasis on the flavonoids contained within the Zibibbo seed extract (ZSE) [24,25].

The use of the HPLC apparatus allowed the analytical discrimination and quantification of rutin and hesperidin contained in the extracts. Interestingly, one of the phenolic compounds contained in the extract was unidentified due to the absence of the reference standard molecule. Nevertheless, the use of chromatography allowed us to gain more detailed information about the analytical composition of the extract compared to the exclusive use of spectrophotometric analyses, as frequently reported in the literature [26,27]. This represents an advantage of the data described in this study, given the concomitant presence of colorimetric assays aimed at completing the chemical–physical characterization of the extracts.

The chemical composition of the molecules found in the Zibibbo grape seeds is similar to other grape species previously analyzed, and data available in the literature include slight differences related to the diversity between plant species investigated as well as by the differences in cultivation conditions [21,28].

The abundances of the compounds mentioned above in the extract contribute to its efficacy in reducing oxidative stress and neutralizing free radicals, as substantiated by established scientific knowledge [29]. The extracts we obtained from Zibibbo seeds, likely because of their abundance in phenolic compounds, showed a sustained antioxidant effect in vitro and proved to be effective in reducing the reactive oxygen species produced by both the MG63 and Saos-2 cell lines. The oxidative phenomena and the production of free radicals are involved in the aging process and in the onset and worsening of several pathologies including osteoporosis; therefore, the flavonoids contained in Zibibbo seeds could help to contrast these pathological conditions. In support of our hypothesis, ZSE also showed a proliferative effect on Saos-2 osteoblast-like cells and, partially on the MG63 cell line. The difference observed in the cells' proliferation could be due to the different stages of differentiation in the cell lines. In fact, Saos-2 cells are a useful model for studying the later stages of osteoblast differentiation in human cells, while MG63 cells correspond to the early stages [30].

The trends observed in the cell viability tests are consistent with the results obtained for the proteins and pathways we analyzed in both cell lines. In fact, phosphorylated ERK and AKT are protein kinases playing a crucial role in promoting cells' survival and proliferation, also inducing the expression of genes involved in DNA replication and cell division. The results obtained on early differentiated MG63 cells and those made by the osteoblast cell line Saos-2, both suggest the effectiveness of ZSE in promoting bone turnover and opposing to the onset of osteoporosis, a pathological condition typically characterized by a specific reduction in osteoblastic cells in bone tissue [31,32]. The promising results obtained with in vitro cellular models and the antioxidant power demonstrated in laboratory tests suggest that the consumption of Zibibbo grape seeds may contribute to reducing osteodegenerative processes and the onset of osteoporosis.

This study analyzes, for the first time, the effect of flavonoids contained in Zibibbo grape seeds, finally suggesting their direct involvement in bone turnover. These represent the major advantages and innovations of the results obtained, especially considering that most of the studies in the literature are exclusively based on molecules contained in fruits and pulp, such as anthocyanins [33,34].

4. Materials and Methods

4.1. Chemicals and Reagents

Dexamethasone (DEX) and Bradford reagent for protein quantification, as well as Folin–Ciocalteu reagent, phenol, sodium carbonate, gallic acid, 2,2-diphenyl-1-picrylhydrazyl (DPPH), aluminum chloride, sodium nitrite and sodium hydroxide required for spectrophotometric assays, were purchased from Sigma-Aldrich (St. Louis, MO, USA). Gibco (Life technologies, Grand Island, NY, USA) provided Dulbecco Modified Eagle Medium (DMEM) and McCoy's 5A modified medium, fetal bovine serum (FBS), and trypsin-EDTA; penicillin/streptomycin was purchased from Lonza (Basel, Switzerland). The cellular ROS Assay Kit [AB113851] DCFDA/H2DCFDA was provided by Abcam (Abcam Limited, Cambridge, UK). Methanol and all other solvents and reagents were of analytical grade (Carlo Erba, Milan, Italy).

4.2. Seeds Supply, Processing and Extraction

The seeds were obtained from the Zibibbo grape variety, which was purchased from company Agricultural Cooperative Capers Producers SOC. COOP. The company is located in Pantelleria (TP) – Sicily, a volcanic island in the Strait of Sicily characterized by a subtropical Mediterranean climate, with hot, dry and humid summers, as well as mild, frost-free winters. The island benefits from constant sea breezes that moderate daytime summer temperatures, resulting in a relatively stable thermal environment.

The Zibibbo berries were dried naturally by exposing them to sunlight and, once they arrived in the laboratory, each grape was individually opened, and the seeds removed with a scalpel and tweezers. The seeds were washed and dried to deprive them of the adherent pulp, and finally stored in a −80 °C freezer until the next processing step. The grape seeds were crushed manually in a mortar, using liquid nitrogen to ease the process and avoid temperature increases due to friction. The powder thus obtained was subsequently used for the extraction procedure, as previously described by Spigno et al., with slight modifications [35]. In detail, the seed powder was incubated with a hydro-alcoholic solution of ethanol and milliQ® water (Carlo Erba, Milan, Italy) in a 7:3 molar ratio. The ratio between the seed powder and extractive medium was 1:50 weight/volume. The mixture was incubated for 24 h under continuous stirring and a temperature set at 45 °C.

The extract obtained was subsequently purified by two different centrifugation cycles. The first cycle was performed using an Eppendorf 5810R centrifuge set at 2500 rpm and 18 °C for 5 min, while the second one had a duration of 8 min during which the sample was centrifuged at 14,000× *g* by a ThermoFisher Scientific – Fresco 21 apparatus (ThermoFisher Scientific, Rosano, MI, Italy), with the temperature set at 4 °C. Pellets were always disposed of as waste material, while the supernatant was further characterized.

4.3. Chemical Analyses

Zibbibo seed extracts (ZSEs) were analyzed with ThermoScientific-Genesys 150® (ThermoFisher Scientific, Rosano, MI, Italy) before being characterized. All analyses were performed using quartz cuvettes. The instrument was set to scansion mode with a wavelength (λ) range set between 200 nm and 700 nm. The hydro-alcoholic mixture used for extraction procedure was also used as blank and diluent before analyses. ZSE were characterized in terms of the content of proteins, carbohydrates and polyphenols as previously described [13]. In addition to this, we also specifically determined flavonoids contained in the extracts according to a method recently published in the literature [36].

The proteins contained in the ZSEs were quantified using the Bradford solution. In detail, Bradford solution was mixed with milliQ® water in a 1:4 ratio. Then, 2 μL samples were added to the mixture and the absorbance was read at λ = 595 nm. Bovine serum albumin (BSA) with a fixed concentration was used as a standard reference.

The carbohydrate profile of the ZSE was assessed using the phenol-sulfuric acid assay. Briefly, the phenol-sulfuric acid assay involves the incubation of 500 μL of sample with 1.25 mL of concentrated sulfuric acid. After vortexing, 250 μL of an aqueous solution containing phenols (5% *w*/*v*) was added to the sample. The obtained mixture was incubated on ice for 20 min and was finally read using a UV-vis spectrophotometer set at λ = 490 nm. A properly diluted stock solution containing sucrose (conc. 6.25–75 ppm) was used as reference standard.

The total content of polyphenolic molecules (TPC) with a tannin-like structure was evaluated by incubating the sample for 5 min with Folin–Ciocalteu's reagent in a 1:5 ratio. Subsequently, a solution of sodium carbonate was added to the mixture and the absorbance was read at λ = 760 nm. Gallic acid was used as reference standard molecule.

4.4. Evaluation of Antioxidant and Free Radicals Scavenging Activities

The ZSEs were also characterized in terms of antioxidant activity and free radicals scavenging activity using three different approaches. The free radical scavenging activity of the ZSEs was evaluated by incubating the sample with two free radicals, 2,2-Diphenyl-1-picrylhydrazyl (DPPH) and 2,2′-Azino-bis-3-ethylbenzothiazoline-6-sulfonic acid (ABTS), as previously described in the literature [37].

For the DPPH assay, 25 μL of sample were incubated in the dark for 30 min with 0.004% *w/v* radical solution and absorbance detected at λ = 517 nm.

Concerning the ABTS assay, a 2.45 mM solution of potassium persulfate was previously prepared and mixed with a 7 mM aqueous solution of ABTS, followed by an incubation overnight protected from light, with the aim of producing the ABTS radicals. The working solution was obtained by adding milli Q® water at a volume equal to 35 times the ABTS radical mixture. Finally, an appropriately diluted ZSE was mixed with the working solution in a 1:4 ratio and the absorbance was measured at 734 nm after 5 min incubation. In both assays, the variation in radical concentration was detected and quantified by a UV-Vis spectrophotometer, and the percentage of inhibition was calculated using the following equation:

$$I\ (\%) = [(A_0 - A_1)/A_0] \times 100$$

A_0 = absorbance of negative control; A_1 = absorbance of extracts/standards.

The scavenging activity of the ZSE against DPPH radicals was also evaluated through Electronic Paramagnetic Resonance (EPR). The decrease in EPR signal intensity (spectral area) represented the free radical scavenging activity of the extracts. The scavenging activity was finally expressed as the percentage of reduction in curve area ± standard deviation (a.u. − ∫ ± S.D.) Ascorbic acid was used as the reference molecule (5 mg/mL).

4.5. HPLC Analyses

The HPLC apparatus consisted of a ThermoFisher Scientific Vanquish System Base VC-S01-A-02 equipped with a VC-P20-A-01 quaternary pump, a VC-A13-A-02 split sampler, a VC-C10-A-03 column compartment and a VF-D40-A UV/VIS variable wavelength detector (ThermoFisher Scientific, Rosano, MI, Italy). The Chromeleon® software version 7.2 was used for data processing and was purchased from ThermoFisher Scientific (Rosano, MI, Italy). The analytical column was an Acclaim® 120 reverse phase C18 (100 mm 4.6 mm), with a 5 µm particle size. The mobile phase was a H_3PO_4 10 mM aqueous solution/ACN with different ratios during the analysis. The column temperature was 30 °C and the absorbance was acquired at wavelengths of 260 nm and 270 nm. Peak identification was carried out through a comparison of the retention times with those obtained with key molecules representing the main categories of flavonoids (Supplementary Materials). In detail, rutin was used as a model flavanol bearing a catechol ring; hesperidin was used as a flavanone containing a methoxy derivative; and naringin and apigenin were recruited as flavones containing p-hydroxy-phenolic rings in CIS and TRANS positions, respectively (Supplementary Materials). Suitable calibration curves (min conc. 15.625 ppm and max conc. 250 ppm–$r^2 > 0.97$ in all cases) were used for the identification of flavonoids contained in samples. The samples (20 µL) were injected into HPLC apparatus with the total acquisition time set at 25 min.

4.6. Cell Line and Culture Conditions

The Saos-2 and MG63 cell lines were obtained from ATCC (ATCC, Milan, Italy) and were used in this study, respectively, as human osteoblast-like and fibroblast cells lines. Saos-2 cells were maintained in McCoy's 5A (Gibco, Carlsbad, CA, USA) supplemented with 15% fetal bovine serum (Gibco, Carlsbad, CA, USA), while the MG63 cell lines were maintained with DMEM 1×-high glucose (Gibco, Carlsbad, CA, USA) supplemented with 10% fetal bovine serum (Gibco, Carlsbad, CA, USA). Both media were also supplemented with a 1% penicillin–streptomycin solution (PAA, Linz, Austria), to avoid bacteria proliferation. Maintenance conditions were temperature set at 37 °C with 5% CO_2. All cell cultures were harvested using trypsinization and were subcultured twice a week, and both were incubated with dexamethasone 10 nM (Sigma Aldrich, St. Louis, MO, USA), respectively, for 48 and 24 h before treatments to obtain more differentiated cell lines.

4.7. Cell Viability Assay

To evaluate cell viability, Saos-2 and MG63 cells were seeded at a density of 1×10^4 cells/well in 96-well plates. Cells were treated in serum-free medium and incubated with ZSEs at concentrations ranging from 0.15 to 40 µg/mL for 24 h. Cell viability was determined using the 3-(4,5-dimethylthiazol-2- yl)-2,5-diphenyltetrazolium bromide (MTT) assay. Briefly, 10 µL of MTT solution (5 mg/mL) was added to each well and incubated at 37 °C for 2 h. The supernatants were then removed and replaced with 100 µL of DMSO. The absorbance of the obtained solution was measured at a wavelength of 595 nm by a multiplate spectrophotometer (BioTek–800TS microplate reader, Agilent, Santa Clara, CA, USA).

4.8. Western Blotting

To investigate the pathways involved in the bone remodeling process, Saos-2 and MG63 cells were seeded at a density of 4×10^5 cells/well in p60 plates. Cultures were starved with serum-free media for 4 h before treatments. Cells were treated in serum-free medium and incubated with ZSEs at concentration ranging from 2.5 to 40 µg/mL for 10 min. Cells were lysed in Mammalian Protein Extraction Reagent (M-PER) (Pierce, Thermo Fisher Scientific). The medium from the cell cultures was centrifuged using Amicon Ultra Centrifugal Filters (Merck Millipore, Milano, Italy) to concentrate the extracellular proteins. The total amount of proteins was quantified using the Bradford spectrophotometric assay. A Western blot analysis of the proteins extracted from the cell lysates was performed according to standard procedures. The following antibodies were used: rabbit anti-p Extracellular Signal-regulated Kinase (ERK)1/2 (9101), and mouse anti-pAKT(3700), by Cell Signaling Technology (Beverly, MA, USA); from Sigma Aldrich (St. Louis, MO, USA); ß-actin by Abcam (Cambridge, UK).

4.9. Kit ROS DCFDA

The cellular ROS Assay Kit [AB113851] DCFDA/H2DCFDA was used as prescribed by the supplier company. In detail, bone cells (2.5×10^4) were seed on a 96-wells plate and allowed to attach overnight.

The culture media were removed, and cells were washed with 1x buffer provided. Subsequently, cells were stained with DCFDA 25 µM in 1x buffer and incubated for 45 min at 37 °C. Cells were washed again with the 1x buffer and 100 µL of the solution containing the ZSEs was added to each well. After 45 min incubation at 37 °C, the 96-well plate were analyzed using Gloomax Discover (Promega-Promega Italia Srl-Milano). In detail, each well was exited at wavelength 475 nm and signals emitted between 500 and 550 nm were captured. Background noise was subtracted from all signals obtained and the results were expressed as the percentage variation in comparison with the control group.

4.10. Statistical Analysis

All data describe the average of three independent experiments and are expressed as the mean including distribution spots for standard deviation or percentage in weight and volume. Data concerning all physicochemical properties of the extracts were processed using Microsoft® Excel™ (Microsoft office 2016). HPLC and UV/VIS graphs were realized with SigmaPlot 12.0 (Systat Software INC, 2011, Chicago, IL, USA). All data related to the in vitro study were analyzed with the GraphPad Prism 5.0 software using a two-tailed Student's t-test for pairwise comparisons and an ANOVA test to compare the means among three or more groups. Significant differences were assumed to be present at $p < 0.05$. The * symbol was used to compare the data with control group, while $^{\Psi}$ describes statistical significance versus the solvent used for the extracts (ethanol 70% v/v). In detail, we used * and $^{\Psi}$ for $p < 0.05$; ** and $^{\Psi\Psi}$ for $p < 0.01$; *** and $^{\Psi\Psi\Psi}$ $p < 0.001$ and **** $p < 0.0001$.

5. Conclusions

Seeds are an important food source of biomolecules. Zibibbo grape seeds were shown to contain a significant number of phenolic compounds, especially flavonoids, which have strong antioxidant and free radical scavenging properties. Polyphenolic extracts from Zibibbo grape seeds (ZSEs) have been shown to exert beneficial effects on bone metabolism and promote osteoblast proliferation, thus probably helping to counteract and reduce osteodegenerative diseases, such as osteoporosis. The consumption of Zibibbo grape seeds could, therefore, help mitigate the aging process and delay osteodegenerative processes. If confirmed by further analysis, the phenolic compounds in Zibibbo grape seeds could represent a valid adjuvant therapy for treating osteoporosis.

6. Limitations of the Study

Despite the promising results achieved in this work, this study has some limitations. First, the effects potentially deriving from lipophilic molecules usually contained in the seeds were not evaluated. Additionally, more in-depth chemical analyses based on mass spectrometry (LC/MS) could provide a more accurate profile of the extracts. Furthermore, other foods rich in flavonoids, especially rutin and hesperidin, were not considered and compared. Finally, other specific pathways involved in bone metabolism could be evaluated to validate and strengthen the results of this study.

Supplementary Materials: The following supporting information can be downloaded at: https://www.mdpi.com/article/10.3390/ph17111418/s1, Figure S1: Chromatogram of standard flavonoids (rutin, naringin, hesperidin and apigenin) with their molecular structures.

Author Contributions: Conceptualization, R.M. and A.P.; methodology, L.T. and S.M.; software, A.C. and A.R.C.; validation, R.M., L.T., S.M. and V.M.; formal analysis, M.S. and S.G.; investigation, M.S. and S.G.; resources, A.P.; data curation, R.M., L.T., S.M. and V.M.; writing—original draft preparation, R.M.; visualization, V.M.; supervision, T.M.; project administration, R.M., L.T. and S.M.; funding acquisition, T.M. and A.P. All authors have read and agreed to the published version of the manuscript.

Funding: This research received no external funding.

Institutional Review Board Statement: Not applicable.

Informed Consent Statement: Not applicable.

Data Availability Statement: The original contributions presented in the study are included in the article/Supplementary Materials, further inquiries can be directed to the corresponding author.

Acknowledgments: The authors would like to thank the the University "Magna Græcia" of Catanzaro, University Library System (SBA UMG) for providing the English lexical revision service..

Conflicts of Interest: The authors declare no conflicts of interest. Except for the researchers, nobody had a role in the design of the study; in the collection, analyses, or interpretation of data; in the writing of the manuscript; or in the decision to publish the results.

References

1. Gerber, M.; Hoffman, R. The Mediterranean diet: Health, science and society. *Br. J. Nutr.* **2015**, *113*, S4–S10. [CrossRef]
2. Balakrishna, R.; Bjørnerud, T.; Bemanian, M.; Aune, D.; Fadnes, L.T. Consumption of Nuts and Seeds and Health Outcomes Including Cardiovascular, Diabetes and Metabolic Disease, Cancer, and Mortality: An Umbrella Review. *Adv. Nutr.* **2022**, *13*, 2136–2148. [CrossRef] [PubMed]
3. Choi, N.R.; Kim, J.N.; Kwon, M.J.; Lee, J.R.; Kim, S.C.; Lee, M.J.; Choi, W.-G.; Kim, B.J. Grape seed powder increases gastrointestinal motility. *Int. J. Med. Sci.* **2022**, *19*, 941. [CrossRef] [PubMed]
4. Fitzpatrick, D.F.; Bing, B.; Maggi, D.A.; Fleming, R.C.; O'malley, R.M. Vasodilating procyanidins derived from grape seeds. *Ann. N. Y. Acad. Sci.* **2002**, *957*, 78–89. [CrossRef] [PubMed]
5. Feringa, H.H.; Laskey, D.A.; Dickson, J.E.; Coleman, C.I. The effect of grape seed extract on cardiovascular risk markers: A meta-analysis of randomized controlled trials. *J. Am. Diet. Assoc.* **2011**, *111*, 1173–1181. [CrossRef] [PubMed]
6. Iannone, M.; Mare, R.; Paolino, D.; Gagliardi, A.; Froiio, F.; Cosco, D.; Fresta, M. Characterization and in vitro anticancer properties of chitosan-microencapsulated flavan-3-ols-rich grape seed extracts. *Int. J. Biol. Macromol.* **2017**, *104*, 1039–1045. [CrossRef]
7. Tonietto, J.; Carbonneau, A. A multicriteria climatic classification system for grape-growing regions worldwide. *Agric. For. Meteorol.* **2004**, *124*, 81–97. [CrossRef]
8. Corona, G. Cenni storici sullo zibibbo nell'isola di pantelleria. In *Il Ruolo Del Settore Vitivinicolo Nei Processi Di Sviluppo Sostenibile*; Franco Angeli: Milan, Italy, 2007; pp. 372–374.
9. Di Lorenzo, R.; Lo Vetere, R. Aromatic compounds in "Zibibbo" grape, bush and VSP trained in Pantelleria Island. Preliminar results. In Proceedings of the Primo Congresso Internazionale Sulla Viticoltura di Montagna e in Forte Pendenza, Saint Vincent, Italy, 17–18 March 2006; pp. 89–90.
10. Astorino, S.; Di Stefano, R. Composizione di uve passe Zibibbo ottenute con processi di disidratazione diversi. *Enologo-Milano* **2003**, *39*, 99–104.
11. Ciolfi, G.; Catanzaro, P.; D'Agostino, S. Microbiological characteristics and drying and re-hydration of Zibibbo dried grape for the CDO Passito wines production [Controlled Designation of Origin-Sicily]. *Ind. Delle Bevande* **2002**.
12. Mandic, A.I.; Đilas, S.M.; Ćetković, G.S.; Čanadanović-Brunet, J.M.; Tumbas, V.T. Polyphenolic composition and antioxidant activities of grape seed extract. *Int. J. Food Prop.* **2008**, *11*, 713–726. [CrossRef]
13. Maurotti, S.; Mare, R.; Pujia, R.; Ferro, Y.; Mazza, E.; Romeo, S.; Pujia, A.; Montalcini, T. Hemp seeds in post-arthroplasty rehabilitation: A pilot clinical study and an in vitro investigation. *Nutrients* **2021**, *13*, 4330. [CrossRef]
14. Pujia, A.; Russo, C.; Maurotti, S.; Pujia, R.; Mollace, V.; Romeo, S.; Montalcini, T. Bergamot polyphenol fraction exerts effects on bone biology by activating ERK 1/2 and Wnt/β-catenin pathway and regulating bone biomarkers in bone cell cultures. *Nutrients* **2018**, *10*, 1305. [CrossRef] [PubMed]
15. Prasad, C.; Davis, K.E.; Imrhan, V.; Juma, S.; Vijayagopal, P. Advanced glycation end products and risks for chronic diseases: Intervening through lifestyle modification. *Am. J. Lifestyle Med.* **2019**, *13*, 384–404. [CrossRef] [PubMed]
16. Addepalli, V.; Suryavanshi, S.V. Catechin attenuates diabetic autonomic neuropathy in streptozotocin induced diabetic rats. *Biomed. Pharmacother.* **2018**, *108*, 1517–1523. [CrossRef] [PubMed]

17. Vaisman, N.; Niv, E. Daily consumption of red grape cell powder in a dietary dose improves cardiovascular parameters: A double blind, placebo-controlled, randomized study. *Int. J. Food Sci. Nutr.* **2015**, *66*, 342–349. [CrossRef] [PubMed]
18. Boccellino, M.; D'Angelo, S. Anti-obesity effects of polyphenol intake: Current status and future possibilities. *Int. J. Mol. Sci.* **2020**, *21*, 5642. [CrossRef]
19. Micek, A.; Jurek, J.; Owczarek, M.; Guerrera, I.; Torrisi, S.A.; Castellano, S.; Grosso, G.; Alshatwi, A.A.; Godos, J. Polyphenol-rich beverages and mental health outcomes. *Antioxidants* **2023**, *12*, 272. [CrossRef]
20. Alasalvar, C.; Chang, S.K.; Bolling, B.; Oh, W.Y.; Shahidi, F. Specialty seeds: Nutrients, bioactives, bioavailability, and health benefits: A comprehensive review. *Compr. Rev. Food Sci. Food Saf.* **2021**, *20*, 2382–2427. [CrossRef]
21. Zarev, Y.; Marinov, L.; Momekova, D.; Ionkova, I. Exploring phytochemical composition and in vivo anti-inflammatory potential of grape seed oil from an alternative source after traditional fermentation processes: Implications for phytotherapy. *Plants* **2023**, *12*, 2795. [CrossRef]
22. Dussert, S.; Guerin, C.; Andersson, M.; Joët, T.; Tranbarger, T.J.; Pizot, M.; Sarah, G.; Omore, A.; Durand-Gasselin, T.; Morcillo, F. Comparative transcriptome analysis of three oil palm fruit and seed tissues that differ in oil content and fatty acid composition. *Plant Physiol.* **2013**, *162*, 1337–1358. [CrossRef]
23. Xiao, J.; Muzashvili, T.S.; Georgiev, M.I. Advances in the biotechnological glycosylation of valuable flavonoids. *Biotechnol. Adv.* **2014**, *32*, 1145–1156. [CrossRef] [PubMed]
24. Pietta, P.-G. Flavonoids as antioxidants. *J. Nat. Prod.* **2000**, *63*, 1035–1042. [CrossRef] [PubMed]
25. Masuoka, N.; Matsuda, M.; Kubo, I. Characterisation of the antioxidant activity of flavonoids. *Food Chem.* **2012**, *131*, 541–545. [CrossRef]
26. Ispiryan, A.; Atkociuniene, V.; Makstutiene, N.; Sarkinas, A.; Salaseviciene, A.; Urbonaviciene, D.; Viskelis, J.; Pakeltiene, R.; Raudone, L. Correlation between Antimicrobial Activity Values and Total Phenolic Content/Antioxidant Activity in *Rubus idaeus* L. *Plants* **2024**, *13*, 504. [CrossRef] [PubMed]
27. Du, J.; Li, X.; Liu, N.; Wang, Y.; Li, Y.; Jia, Y.; An, X.; Qi, J. Improving the quality of Glycyrrhiza stems and leaves through solid-state fermentation: Flavonoid content, antioxidant activity, metabolic profile, and release mechanism. *Chem. Biol. Technol. Agric.* **2024**, *11*, 105. [CrossRef]
28. Karagecili, H.; İzol, E.; Kirecci, E.; Gulcin, İ. Determination of antioxidant, anti-alzheimer, antidiabetic, antiglaucoma and antimicrobial effects of zivzik pomegranate (*Punica granatum*)—A chemical profiling by LC-MS/MS. *Life* **2023**, *13*, 735. [CrossRef]
29. Cotelle, N. Role of flavonoids in oxidative stress. *Curr. Top. Med. Chem.* **2001**, *1*, 569–590. [CrossRef]
30. Maiuolo, J.; Carresi, C.; Gliozzi, M.; Musolino, V.; Scarano, F.; Coppoletta, A.R.; Guarnieri, L.; Nucera, S.; Scicchitano, M.; Bosco, F. Effects of bergamot polyphenols on mitochondrial dysfunction and sarcoplasmic reticulum stress in diabetic cardiomyopathy. *Nutrients* **2021**, *13*, 2476. [CrossRef]
31. Weinstein, R.S.; Manolagas, S.C. Apoptosis and osteoporosis. *Am. J. Med.* **2000**, *108*, 153–164. [CrossRef]
32. Marie, P.J.; Kassem, M. Osteoblasts in osteoporosis: Past, emerging, and future anabolic targets. *Eur. J. Endocrinol.* **2011**, *165*, 1–10. [CrossRef]
33. Quek, Y.Y.; Cheng, L.J.; Ng, Y.X.; Hey, H.W.D.; Wu, X.V. Effectiveness of anthocyanin-rich foods on bone remodeling biomarkers of middle-aged and older adults at risk of osteoporosis: A systematic review, meta-analysis, and meta-regression. *Nutr. Rev.* **2024**, *82*, 1187–1207. [CrossRef] [PubMed]
34. Novita, N.; Pudyani, P.S.; Alhasyimi, A.A.; Suparwitri, S. Effect of anthocyanin to post-orthodontic treatment: A review. *Indones. J. Orthod. (InJO)* **2024**, *1*, 1–8.
35. Spigno, G.; Tramelli, L.; De Faveri, D.M. Effects of extraction time, temperature and solvent on concentration and antioxidant activity of grape marc phenolics. *J. Food Eng.* **2007**, *81*, 200–208. [CrossRef]
36. Mare, R.; Pujia, R.; Maurotti, S.; Greco, S.; Cardamone, A.; Coppoletta, A.R.; Bonacci, S.; Procopio, A.; Pujia, A. Assessment of Mediterranean Citrus Peel Flavonoids and Their Antioxidant Capacity Using an Innovative UV-Vis Spectrophotometric Approach. *Plants* **2023**, *12*, 4046. [CrossRef]
37. Patitucci, F.; Motta, M.F.; Dattilo, M.; Malivindi, R.; Leonetti, A.E.; Pezzi, G.; Prete, S.; Mileti, O.; Gabriele, D.; Parisi, O.I. 3D-Printed Alginate/Pectin-Based Patches Loaded with Olive Leaf Extracts for Wound Healing Applications: Development, Characterization and In Vitro Evaluation of Biological Properties. *Pharmaceutics* **2024**, *16*, 99. [CrossRef]

pharmaceuticals

MDPI

Article

Bixin Combined with Metformin Ameliorates Insulin Resistance and Antioxidant Defenses in Obese Mice

Camila Graça Pinheiro [1], Bruno Pereira Motta [1], Juliana Oriel Oliveira [1], Felipe Nunes Cardoso [1], Ingrid Delbone Figueiredo [1], Rachel Temperani Amaral Machado [2], Patrícia Bento da Silva [2], Marlus Chorilli [2], Iguatemy Lourenço Brunetti [1] and Amanda Martins Baviera [1,*]

[1] Department of Clinical Analysis, School of Pharmaceutical Sciences, São Paulo State University (UNESP), Araraquara 14800-903, SP, Brazil; camila.pinheiro@unesp.br (C.G.P.); motta.bp@gmail.com (B.P.M.); juliana.oriel@gmail.com (J.O.O.); felipe.n.cardoso@unesp.br (F.N.C.); ingrid.delbone@unesp.br (I.D.F.); iguatemy.brunetti@unesp.br (I.L.B.)

[2] Department of Drugs and Medicines, School of Pharmaceutical Sciences, São Paulo State University (UNESP), Araraquara 14800-903, SP, Brazil; racheltemperani@gmail.com (R.T.A.M.); patrbent@gmail.com (P.B.d.S.); marlus.chorilli@unesp.br (M.C.)

* Correspondence: amanda.baviera@unesp.br; Tel.: +55-16-3301-5717

Abstract: Bixin ($C_{25}H_{30}O_4$; 394.51 g/mol) is the main apocarotenoid found in annatto seeds. It has a 25-carbon open chain structure with a methyl ester group and carboxylic acid. Bixin increases the expression of antioxidant enzymes, which may be interesting for counteracting oxidative stress. This study investigated whether bixin-rich annatto extract combined with metformin was able to improve the disturbances observed in high-fat diet (HFD)-induced obesity in mice, with an emphasis on markers of oxidative damage and antioxidant defenses. HFD-fed mice were treated for 8 weeks with metformin (50 mg/kg) plus bixin-rich annatto extract (5.5 and 11 mg/kg). This study assessed glucose tolerance, insulin sensitivity, lipid profile and paraoxonase 1 (PON-1) activity in plasma, fluorescent AGEs (advanced glycation end products), TBARSs (thiobarbituric acid-reactive substances), and the activities of superoxide dismutase (SOD), catalase (CAT), and glutathione peroxidase (GSH-Px) in the liver and kidneys. Treatment with bixin plus metformin decreased body weight gain, improved insulin sensitivity, and decreased AGEs and TBARSs in the plasma, liver, and kidneys. Bixin plus metformin increased the activities of PON-1, SOD, CAT, and GSH-Px. Bixin combined with metformin improved the endogenous antioxidant defenses in the obese mice, showing that this combined therapy may have the potential to contrast the metabolic complications resulting from oxidative stress.

Keywords: carotenoids; advanced glycation end products; glycoxidative stress; antioxidant enzymes; natural bioactives

1. Introduction

Obesity and overweight are highly prevalent clinical conditions and act as risk factors for the development of type 2 diabetes mellitus (T2DM). These conditions trigger cellular processes responsible for the development of insulin resistance, culminating in chronic hyperglycemia typical of DM [1]. On the other hand, chronic hyperglycemia contributes to the establishment of glycoxidative stress, which is responsible for tissue damage, induced by the glycation of macromolecules and the excessive production of advanced glycation end products (AGEs) and reactive oxygen species (ROS) [2]. Therefore, the adoption of therapeutic regimens that can reduce both glycemia and glycoxidative stress becomes important, aiming to mitigate the complications of these metabolic diseases [3].

Metformin is the most used drug for the treatment of T2DM, as it acts efficiently in glycemic control, mainly through the inhibition of hepatic gluconeogenesis [4]. However, despite its good efficiency in controlling glycemia, metformin therapy can cause important adverse effects, which are responsible for treatment abandonment in up to 10% of cases [5].

Furthermore, the glycemic control achieved with the use of metformin is not able to prevent the development of long-term complications of T2DM given its mechanisms related to metabolic memory, which is defined as the persistence of complications caused by hyperglycemia even after the achievement of glycemic control due to several detrimental changes triggered by AGEs and ROS [6].

Bioactive compounds of natural origin become interesting in the search for complementary options to the traditional therapy for T2DM, as many of them have antioxidant and antiglycation activities. Among these interesting natural bioactive compounds are carotenoids. Carotenoids have a chemical structure that allows the accommodation of unpaired electrons from radical species, which makes them potent antioxidants. Bixin ($C_{25}H_{30}O_4$; 394.51 g/mol) is the main apocarotenoid (70–80%) constituent of seeds from annatto (*Bixa orellana* L.), which grows in tropical countries from Central and South America to India, Indonesia, and East Africa. Annatto is widely used in popular cuisine as a condiment. Bixin has a 25-carbon open chain structure with double bonds and contains a methyl ester group and carboxylic acid. It is a carotenoid pigment with reddish-orange tonality. Bixin and annatto extracts are known for their antioxidant properties and beneficial effects on the prevention and treatment of various diseases [7,8]. Bixin can interact with important transcription factors to promote effective cellular responses in controlling lipid metabolism and combating oxidative stress, including peroxisome proliferator-activated receptor γ (PPARγ) and nuclear factor erythroid 2-related factor 2 (NRF-2) [9,10].

It seems interesting to explore combined therapy strategies based on the use of a traditional antidiabetic drug (such as metformin) and a natural bioactive compound (such as bixin), aiming to achieve responses related to glycemic control and mitigating the mechanisms associated with metabolic memory and glycoxidative stress. However, both metformin and bixin have low bioavailability [11,12], which makes it difficult to promote their pharmacological effects in vivo. This situation can be overcome by incorporating bixin into pharmaceutical delivery systems, including nanostructured lipid systems, which allow greater interaction with the aqueous environment and biological membranes, increasing absorption and reducing the need for high doses of drugs during oral administration [13,14].

The proposal of this study was to investigate the impacts of a bixin-rich annatto extract, alone or co-administered with metformin and delivered in a nanostructured lipid system, on physiometabolic parameters, glycoxidative stress biomarkers, and antioxidant defenses in an in vivo model system of obesity and insulin resistance.

2. Results

2.1. Physiological and Biochemical Parameters

From the fifth week of the experiment, the mice fed an HFD showed a significant increase in their body weight gain in comparison with the corresponding values of the C group. From the 12th week, the HFD-fed mice belonging to the M, B1, B2, MB1, and MB2 groups had low body weight gain in comparison with the mice from the H group (Figure 1).

As expected, the H mice exhibited decreased food intake, accompanied by increased energy intake. Treatments with bixin-rich annatto extract and metformin, alone or in combination, were not able to promote changes in either the food or energy intake of the HFD-fed mice until the end of the treatments (Figure 2).

There were significant increases in the weights of the epididymal white adipose tissues of the H and V mice in relation to these corresponding values for the C mice. This finding, together with the increase in body weight gain, indicates that the production of an in vivo model system of obesity occurred in the mice fed an HFD. Treatments of the HFD-fed mice with metformin or bixin-rich annatto extract (both doses), alone or in combination, decreased the weights of their epididymal white adipose tissues in comparison with the corresponding values for the H mice (Table 1). Treatments with metformin or 5.5 and 11 mg/kg bixin-rich annatto extract, alone or in combination, also decreased the weights of their brown adipose tissues in comparison with the values from the C group (Table 1). The weights of the livers of the mice treated with metformin + 5.5 mg/kg bixin-rich extract also decreased when compared with the values found in the mice from the H group (Table 1).

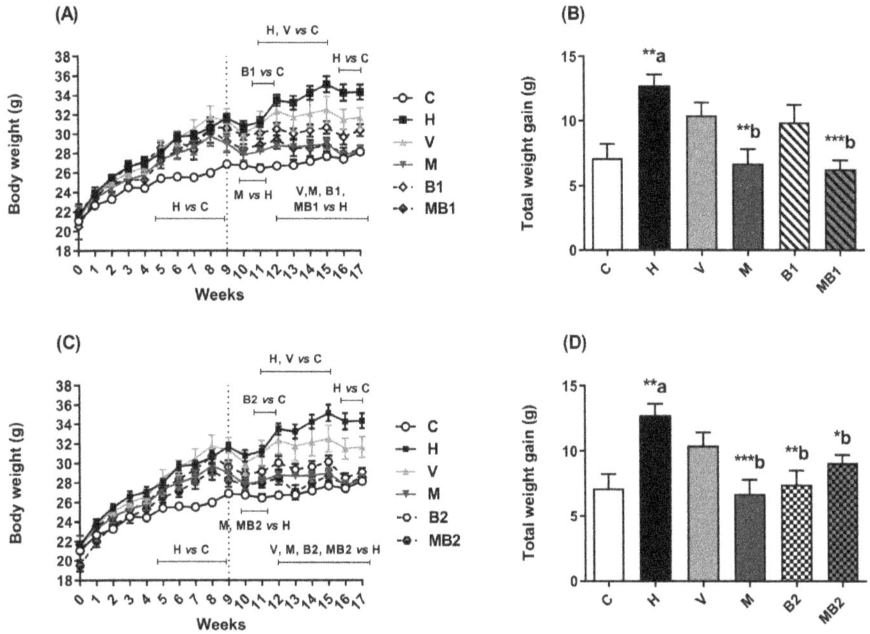

Figure 1. Body weight of HFD-fed mice treated for 8 weeks with metformin and/or 5.5 and 11 mg/kg bixin-rich annatto extract. Evolution of body weight (**A**,**B**) and total weight gain from week 0 to week 17 (**C**,**D**). Results are expressed as mean ± standard error. C: mice fed control diet; H: mice fed HFD; V: mice fed HFD and treated with vehicle; M: mice fed HFD and treated with 50 mg/kg metformin; B1: mice fed HFD and treated with 5.5 mg/kg bixin-rich extract; MB1: mice fed HFD and treated with 50 mg/kg metformin + 5.5 mg/kg bixin-rich extract; B2: mice fed HFD and treated with 11 mg/kg bixin-rich extract; MB2: mice fed HFD and treated with 50 mg/kg metformin + 11 mg/kg bixin-rich extract. Differences between groups were considered significant at * $p < 0.05$, ** $p < 0.01$, and *** $p < 0.001$. a, differences from C; b, differences from H.

Table 1. Weights of tissues (mg/mm of tibia) of HFD-fed mice treated for 8 weeks with metformin and/or 5.5 and 11 mg/kg bixin-rich annatto extract.

Groups	C	H	V	M	B1	B2	MB1	MB2
Liver	59.5 ± 1.0	64.1 ± 1.9	58.3 ± 2.2	57.4 ± 1.8	57.2 ± 1.6	57.5 ± 1.8	55.0 ± 1.8 [b]	57.9 ± 2.2
Kidneys	9.2 ± 0.6	10.4 ± 0.7	9.7 ± 0.7	9.1 ± 0.6	9.4 ± 0.8	9.7 ± 0.7	9.1 ± 0.4	6.7 ± 0.3
Heart	7.0 ± 0.2	7.4 ± 0.1	7.1 ± 0.2	7.1 ± 0.2	7.3 ± 0.2	7.1 ± 0.2	7.1 ± 0.2	7.1 ± 0.2
Muscles (gastrocnemius)	8.1 ± 0.1	8.4 ± 0.2	8.1 ± 0.1	8.1 ± 0.1	8.1 ± 0.1	8.2 ± 0.1	8.1 ± 0.1	8.1 ± 0.1
WAT (epididymal)	26.7 ± 1.5	66.4 ± 5.3 [a]	54.6 ± 3.8 [a,b]	41.2 ± 5.0 [b]	37.4 ± 2.9 [b]	43.3 ± 4.0 [b]	44.2 ± 4.8 [a,b]	42.1 ± 3.2 [b]
BAT (interscapular)	4.1 ± 0.2	3.8 ± 0.3	3.5 ± 0.2	3.0 ± 0.2 [a]	2.9 ± 0.1 [a]	3.2 ± 0.2 [a]	3.2 ± 0.2 [a]	3.1 ± 0.2 [a]

Results are expressed as mean ± standard error. C: mice fed control diet; H: mice fed HFD; V: mice fed HFD and treated with vehicle; M: mice fed HFD and treated with 50 mg/kg metformin; B1: mice fed HFD and treated with 5.5 mg/kg bixin-rich extract; MB1: mice fed HFD and treated with 50 mg/kg metformin + 5.5 mg/kg bixin-rich extract; B2: mice fed HFD and treated with 11 mg/kg bixin-rich extract; MB2: mice fed HFD and treated with 50 mg/kg metformin + 11 mg/kg bixin-rich extract. Differences between groups were considered significant at $p < 0.05$. a, differences from C; b, differences from H.

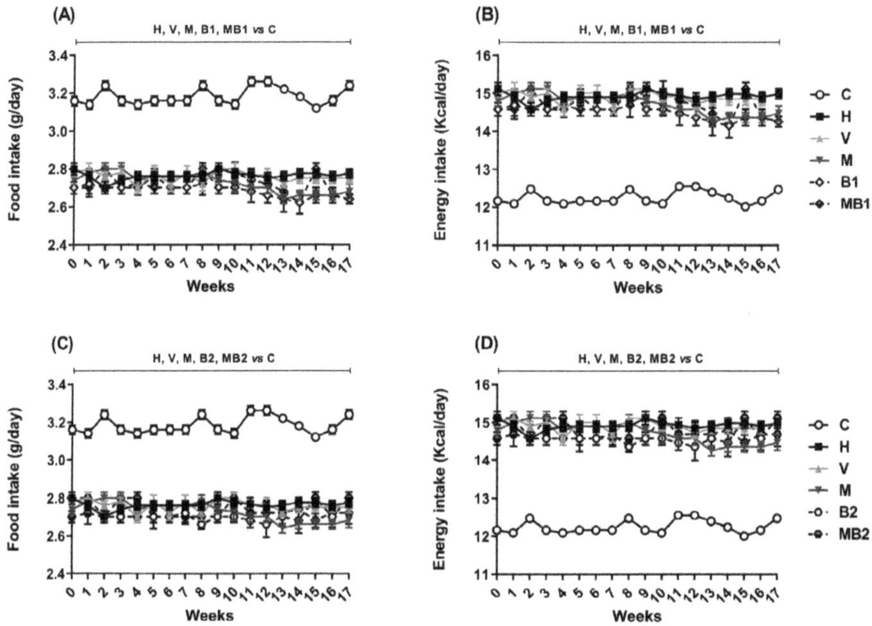

Figure 2. Food and energy intake of HFD-fed mice treated for 8 weeks with metformin and/or 5.5 and 11 mg/kg bixin-rich annatto extract. Food intake (**A**,**C**) and energy intake (**B**,**D**). Results are expressed as mean ± standard error. C: mice fed control diet; H: mice fed HFD; V: mice fed HFD and treated with vehicle; M: mice fed HFD and treated with 50 mg/kg metformin; B1: mice fed HFD and treated with 5.5 mg/kg bixin-rich extract; MB1: mice fed HFD and treated with 50 mg/kg metformin + 5.5 mg/kg bixin-rich extract; B2: mice fed HFD and treated with 11 mg/kg bixin-rich extract; MB2: mice fed HFD and treated with 50 mg/kg metformin + 11 mg/kg bixin-rich extract. Differences between groups were considered significant at $p < 0.05$.

No significant differences were observed in the weights of the kidneys, hearts, or gastrocnemius skeletal muscles between the experimental groups studied (Table 1).

The mice from the H and V groups had high plasma levels of total cholesterol and high-density lipoprotein cholesterol (HDL-cholesterol) and low levels of triglycerides when compared to the values found in the mice from the C group. The mice from the M, B1, B2, MB1, and MB2 groups had low levels of triglycerides when compared to the mice from the C group, without differences in comparison to the values found in the mice from the H and V groups. The plasma levels of cholesterol were significantly decreased in the mice from the M, B1, B2, MB1, and MB2 groups in comparison to the values of the H group, while the HDL-cholesterol levels were decreased in the mice from the M, MB1, and MB2 groups when compared to the corresponding values of the H group (Table 2).

Table 2. Plasma levels of biochemical markers in plasma of HFD-fed mice treated for 8 weeks with metformin and/or 5.5 and 11 mg/kg bixin-rich annatto extract.

Groups	C	H	V	M	B1	B2	MB1	MB2
Triglycerides (mg/dL)	53.4 ± 7.1	41.3 ± 8.4 [a]	41.6 ± 5.5 [a]	38.6 ± 10.1 [a]	38.1 ± 8.0 [a]	39.8 ± 5.3 [a]	39.4 ± 10.5 [a]	39.5 ± 6.2 [a]
Total Cholesterol (mg/dL)	98.3 ± 3.3	135.6 ± 15.8 [a]	131.2 ± 19.4 [a]	107.3 ± 14.1 [b]	113.3 ± 9.6 [b]	112.3 ± 14.1 [b]	108.5 ± 8.7 [b]	116.0 ± 9.4 [b]

Table 2. *Cont.*

Groups	C	H	V	M	B1	B2	MB1	MB2
HDL-Cholesterol (mg/dL)	79.3 ± 2.5	108.3 ± 15.1 [a]	99.8 ± 7.5 [a]	89.7 ± 14.4 [b]	94.2 ± 2.8	94.0 ± 8.3	90.1 ± 6.6 [b]	90.8 ± 12.2 [b]
Creatinine (mg/dL)	0.16 ± 0.003	0.15 ± 0.002	0.16 ± 0.004	0.15 ± 0.003	0.16 ± 0.011	0.16 ± 0.003	0.16 ± 0.003	0.15 ± 0.003
Uric Acid (mg/dL)	0.4 ± 0.02	0.4 ± 0.02	0.3 ± 0.03	0.3 ± 0.03	0.4 ± 0.09	0.4 ± 0.04	0.4 ± 0.04	0.4 ± 0.07
Albumin (g/dL)	2.1 ± 0.02	2.1 ± 0.03	2.1 ± 0.03	2.1 ± 0.04	2.1 ± 0.03	2.1 ± 0.02	2.1 ± 0.03	2.1 ± 0.03
ALT (U/L)	24.8 ± 2.3	28.4 ± 4.4	27.3 ± 2.4	21.4 ± 2.4	24.4 ± 1.6	21.5 ± 3.1	24.1 ± 2.5	23.0 ± 4.0

Results are expressed as mean ± standard error. C: mice fed control diet; H: mice fed HFD; V: mice fed HFD and treated with vehicle; M: mice fed HFD and treated with 50 mg/kg metformin; B1: mice fed HFD and treated with 5.5 mg/kg bixin-rich extract; MB1: mice fed HFD and treated with 50 mg/kg metformin + 5.5 mg/kg bixin-rich extract; B2: mice fed HFD and treated with 11 mg/kg bixin-rich extract; MB2: mice fed HFD and treated with 50 mg/kg metformin + 11 mg/kg bixin-rich extract. Differences between groups were considered significant at $p < 0.05$. a, differences from C; b, differences from H.

No changes were observed in the plasma levels of creatinine, uric acid, albumin, or ALT among the groups (Table 2).

2.2. Glucose Tolerance and Insulin Sensitivity

In the oral glucose tolerance test (OGTT), 15 min after glucose overload, the mice from the H and V groups had higher glycemic peaks than the values found in the mice from the C group. After 120 min, the mice from the H and V groups continued to have elevated glycemic values when compared to the corresponding values for the C group (Figure 3A,C). Therefore, glucose intolerance occurred in the mice from the H and V groups (Figure 3B,D).

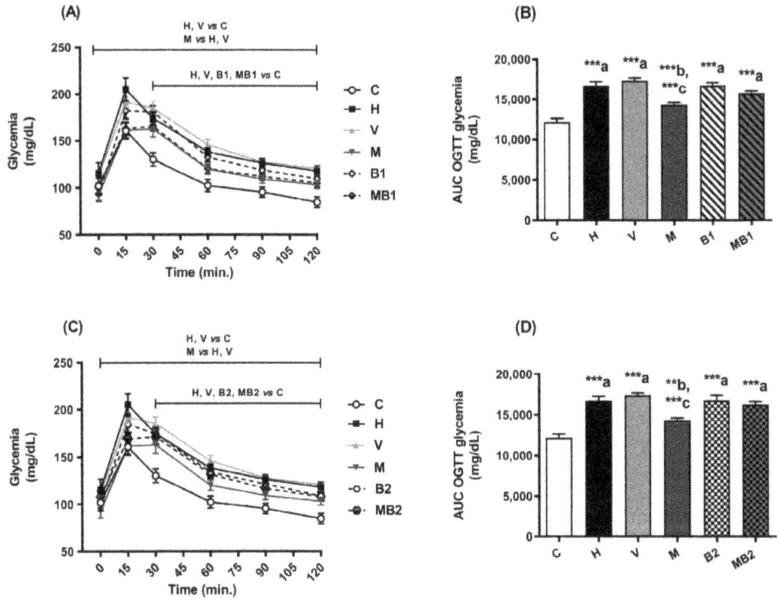

Figure 3. Glucose tolerance of HFD-fed mice treated for 8 weeks with metformin and/or 5.5 and 11 mg/kg bixin-rich annatto extract. Oral glucose tolerance test (OGTT) (**A**,**C**) and AUC of OGTT (**B**,**D**). Results are expressed as mean ± standard error. AUC: area under the curve; C: mice

fed control diet; H: mice fed HFD; V: mice fed HFD and treated with vehicle; M: mice fed HFD and treated with 50 mg/kg metformin; B1: mice fed HFD and treated with 5.5 mg/kg bixin-rich extract; MB1: mice fed HFD and treated with 50 mg/kg metformin + 5.5 mg/kg bixin-rich extract; B2: mice fed HFD and treated with 11 mg/kg bixin-rich extract; MB2: mice fed HFD and treated with 50 mg/kg metformin + 11 mg/kg bixin-rich extract. Differences between groups were considered significant at ** $p < 0.01$ and *** $p < 0.001$. a, differences from C; b, differences from H; c, differences from V.

The HFD-mice treated with metformin showed improvements in their glucose tolerance (Figure 3B,D). The mice from the M group exhibited low fasting glycemia, a minor glycemic peak after the glucose overload, and low glycemia levels after 120 min in the OGTT when compared to the corresponding values in the H and V groups (Figure 3A,C). Treatment with the bixin-rich annatto extract, alone or in combination with metformin, did not improve the glucose tolerance of the HFD-fed mice (Figure 3).

In the insulin tolerance test (ITT), after the administration of insulin, the mice from the H and V groups showed high glycemia levels throughout the monitoring period in comparison with the corresponding values for the C mice (Figure 4A,C). This finding supports the decreased insulin sensitivity in the mice from the H and V groups (Figure 3B,D).

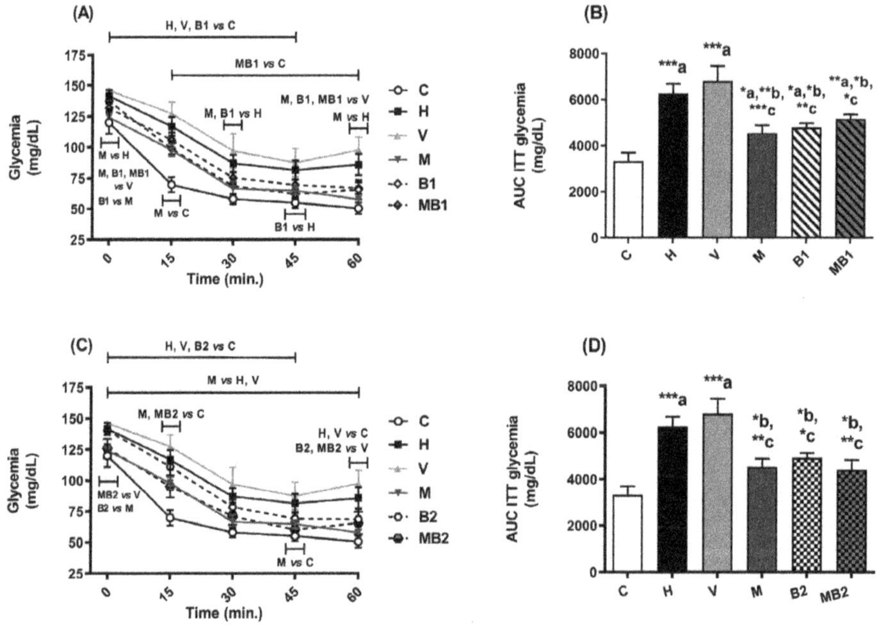

Figure 4. Insulin sensitivity of HFD-fed mice treated for 8 weeks with metformin and/or 5.5 and 11 mg/kg bixin-rich annatto extract. Insulin tolerance test (ITT) (**A**,**C**) and AUC of ITT (**B**,**D**). Results are expressed as mean ± standard error. AUC: area under the curve; C: mice fed control diet; H: mice fed HFD; V: mice fed HFD and treated with vehicle; M: mice fed HFD and treated with 50 mg/kg metformin; B1: mice fed HFD and treated with 5.5 mg/kg bixin-rich extract; MB1: mice fed HFD and treated with 50 mg/kg metformin + 5.5 mg/kg bixin-rich extract; B2: mice fed HFD and treated with 11 mg/kg bixin-rich extract; MB2: mice fed HFD and treated with 50 mg/kg metformin + 11 mg/kg bixin-rich extract. Differences between groups were considered significant at * $p < 0.05$, ** $p < 0.01$, and *** $p < 0.001$. a, differences from P; b, differences from H; c, differences from V.

Treatment with metformin or bixin-rich annatto extract (5.5 and 11 mg/kg) alone was able to improve the insulin sensitivity in the HFD-fed mice (Figure 4). The combined therapies between metformin and bixin-rich annatto extract, at both doses tested, improved insulin sensitivity as efficiently as the treatments with the bioactives alone, which suggests that the combined therapies maintained the beneficial effects of the isolated therapies on the insulin sensitivity of the HFD-fed mice.

2.3. Biomarkers of Glycoxidative Stress and Antioxidant Defenses in Plasma

The mice from the H group showed significantly high plasma levels of fluorescent AGEs (Figure 5A) and TBARSs (Figure 5B) when compared to the corresponding values for the C group. The V group also had high plasma levels of AGEs (Figure 5A) and TBARSs (Figure 5B) at similar values to those for the H group. Therefore, the establishment of glycoxidative stress in the H and V groups occurred as a probable consequence of glucose intolerance and chronic hyperglycemia.

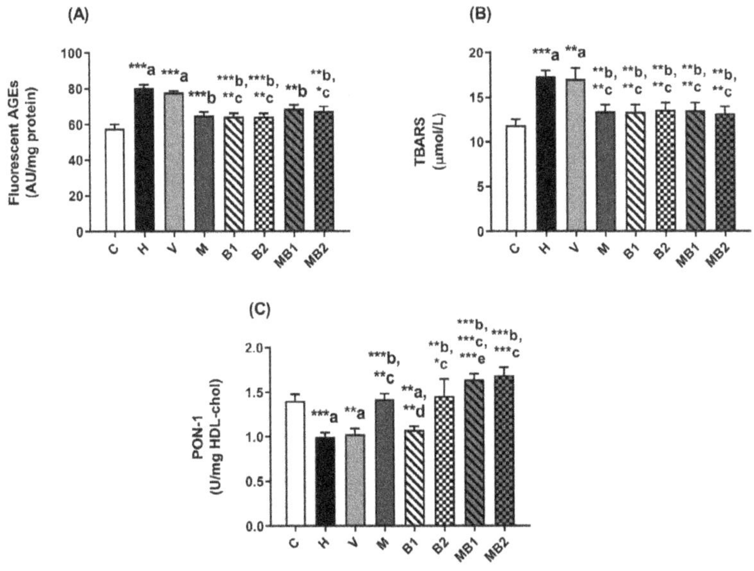

Figure 5. Biomarkers of glycoxidative damage and antioxidant defenses in plasma of HFD-fed mice treated for 8 weeks with metformin and/or 5.5 and 11 mg/kg bixin-rich annatto extract. Fluorescent AGEs (**A**), TBARSs (**B**), and activity of PON-1 (**C**). Results are expressed as mean ± standard error. C: mice fed control diet; H: mice fed HFD; V: mice fed HFD and treated with vehicle; M: mice fed HFD and treated with 50 mg/kg metformin; B1: mice fed HFD and treated with 5.5 mg/kg bixin-rich extract; MB1: mice fed HFD and treated with 50 mg/kg metformin + 5.5 mg/kg bixin-rich extract; B2: mice fed HFD and treated with 11 mg/kg bixin-rich extract; MB2: mice fed HFD and treated with 50 mg/kg metformin + 11 mg/kg bixin-rich extract. Differences between groups were considered significant at * $p < 0.05$, ** $p < 0.01$, and *** $p < 0.001$. a, differences from P; b, differences from H; c, differences from V; d, differences from M; e, differences from B1.

There were significant decreases in the levels of fluorescent AGEs (Figure 5A) and TBARSs (Figure 5B) in the plasma of the M, B1, MB1, B2, and MB2 mice when compared to the corresponding values found in the H mice, without differences between treatments, suggesting that metformin and 5.5 and 11 mg/kg bixin-rich annatto extract decreased glycoxidative stress in the plasma of the HFD-fed mice.

The activity of the antioxidant enzyme paraoxonase-1 (PON-1) in the plasma of the H and V mice was significantly lower than values found in the C mice (Figure 5C).

Treatment with the lower dose (5.5 mg/kg) of bixin-rich annatto extract was not able to improve PON-1 activity. On the other hand, the HFD-fed mice treated with metformin or with bixin-rich annatto extract at the higher dose (11 mg/kg) recovered in their PON-1 activity, the levels of which were similar to those of the C group. About the combined therapies, treatment with metformin + 11 mg/kg bixin-rich annatto extract increased PON-1 activity in a similar way to the isolated therapies. On the other hand, the increase in PON-1 activity observed in the HFD-fed mice treated with metformin + 5.5 mg/kg bixin-rich annatto extract was higher than that based on the effects of bixin alone, suggesting that the combined therapy had an additive effect on triggering endogenous antioxidant defenses (Figure 5C).

2.4. Biomarkers of Glycoxidative Stress and Antioxidant Defenses in the Liver

The levels of fluorescent AGEs (Figure 6A) and TBARSs (Figure 6B) in the livers of the HFD-fed mice from the H and V groups were higher than the values found in the C group. In parallel, the activities of the antioxidant enzymes SOD (Figure 6C), CAT (Figure 6D), and GSH-Px (Figure 6E) were decreased in the H and V mice. These findings support the establishment of oxidative stress in the livers of mice fed an HFD.

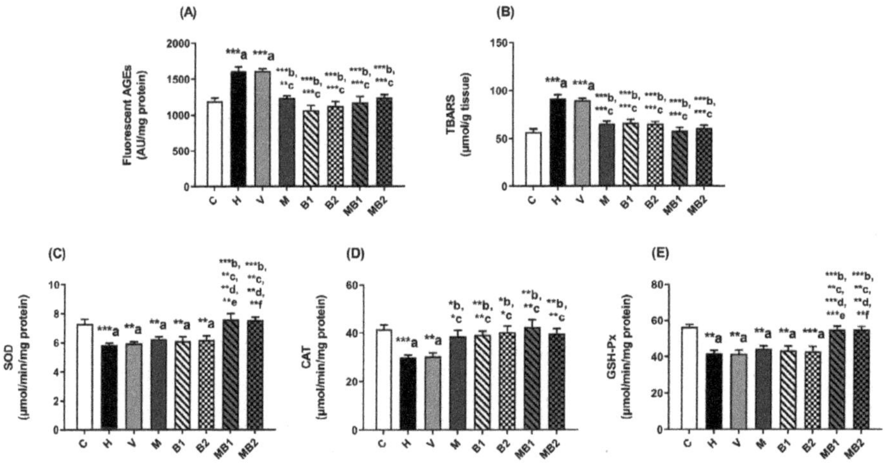

Figure 6. Biomarkers of glycoxidative damage and antioxidant defenses in livers of HFD-fed mice treated for 8 weeks with metformin and/or 5.5 and 11 mg/kg bixin-rich annatto extract. Fluorescent AGEs (**A**), TBARSs (**B**), and activities of SOD (**C**), CAT (**D**), and GSH-Px (**E**). Results are expressed as mean ± standard error. C: mice fed control diet; H: mice fed HFD; V: mice fed HFD and treated with vehicle; M: mice fed HFD and treated with 50 mg/kg metformin; B1: mice fed HFD and treated with 5.5 mg/kg bixin-rich extract; MB1: mice fed HFD and treated with 50 mg/kg metformin + 5.5 mg/kg bixin-rich extract; B2: mice fed HFD and treated with 11 mg/kg bixin-rich extract; MB2: mice fed HFD and treated with 50 mg/kg metformin + 11 mg/kg bixin-rich extract. Differences between groups were considered significant at * $p < 0.05$, ** $p < 0.01$ and *** $p < 0.001$. a, differences from P; b, differences from H; c, differences from V; d, differences from M; e, differences from B1; f, differences from B2.

The treatments with metformin and bixin-rich annatto extract (5.5 and 11 mg/kg), alone or in combination, significantly decreased the hepatic levels of AGEs (Figure 6A) and TBARSs (Figure 6B) in comparison with the values found in the H and V mice. In addition, the treatments with metformin and bixin-rich annatto extract at both doses, alone or in combination, increased the activity of CAT in the livers of the HFD-fed mice (Figure 6D). Conversely, when metformin and bixin-rich annatto extract (5.5 and 11 mg/kg) were administered alone, these bioactives did not improve the activities of SOD (Figure 6C) or GSH-Px (Figure 6E). On the other hand, the HFD-fed mice treated with metformin + bixin-rich annatto extract, at both doses, had notable increases in their activities of SOD (Figure 6C) and GSH-Px (Figure 6E), suggesting that the combined therapy had synergistic effects on triggering endogenous antioxidant defenses in the livers of these HFD-fed mice.

2.5. Biomarkers of Glycoxidative Stress and Antioxidant Defenses in the Kidneys

As well as their plasma and livers, the onset of oxidative stress was also observed in the kidneys of the HFD-fed mice. Increased levels of fluorescent AGEs (Figure 7A) and TBARSs (Figure 7B) were found in the kidneys of the HFD-fed mice from the H and V groups, whose values were higher than those in the C group. In addition, the activities of the antioxidant enzymes SOD (Figure 7C) and CAT (Figure 7D) were decreased in the kidneys of the H and V mice.

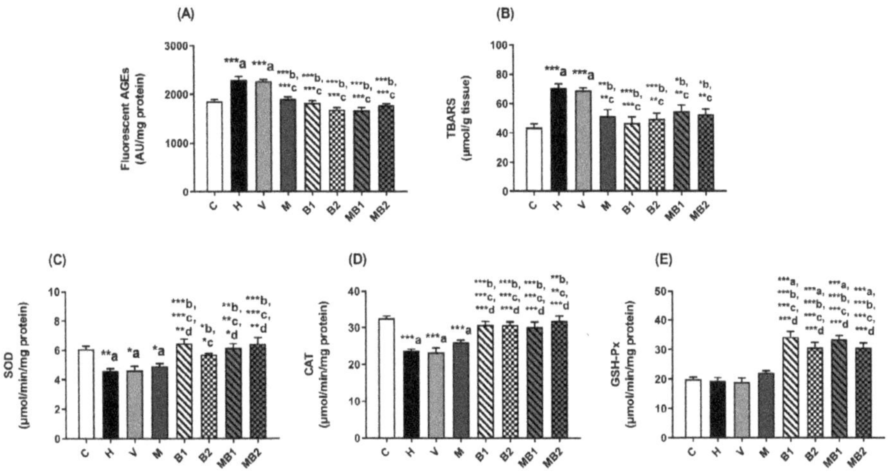

Figure 7. Biomarkers of glycoxidative damage and antioxidant defenses in kidneys of HFD-fed mice treated for 8 weeks with metformin and/or 5.5 and 11 mg/kg bixin-rich annatto extract. Fluorescent AGEs (**A**), TBARSs (**B**), and activities of SOD (**C**), CAT (**D**), and GSH-Px (**E**). Results are expressed as mean ± standard error. C: mice fed control diet; H: mice fed HFD; V: mice fed HFD and treated with vehicle; M: mice fed HFD and treated with 50 mg/kg metformin; B1: mice fed HFD and treated with 5.5 mg/kg bixin-rich extract; MB1: mice fed HFD and treated with 50 mg/kg metformin + 5.5 mg/kg bixin-rich extract; B2: mice fed HFD and treated with 11 mg/kg bixin-rich extract; MB2: mice fed HFD and treated with 50 mg/kg metformin + 11 mg/kg bixin-rich extract. Differences between groups were considered significant at * $p < 0.05$, ** $p < 0.01$, and *** $p < 0.001$. a, differences from P; b, differences from H; c, differences from V; d, differences from M.

The levels of AGEs (Figure 7A) and TBARSs (Figure 7B) were significantly decreased in the kidneys of the mice treated with metformin and bixin-rich annatto extract (5.5 and 11 mg/kg), alone or in combination, when compared with the values found in the H and V mice. However, it is interesting to note that metformin did not improve the activities of the antioxidant enzymes SOD (Figure 7C), CAT (Figure 7D), or GSH-Px (Figure 7E).

Bixin-rich annatto extract, at both doses, alone or in combination with metformin, caused significant increases in the activities of SOD (Figure 7C), CAT (Figure 7D), and GSH-Px (Figure 7E) in the kidneys of the mice fed an HFD, whose effects were greater than those of metformin and maintained the antioxidant responses of bixin-rich annatto extract, which reinforces that the combined therapy had beneficial effects on triggering their endogenous antioxidant defenses.

3. Discussion

The present study provides evidence regarding the effects of a therapeutic strategy based on combining metformin and a bixin-rich annatto extract to combat metabolic disturbances. The main beneficial effects promoted by this combined therapy were the following: (i) bixin-rich annatto extract + metformin had antiobesogenic effects; (ii) bixin-rich annatto extract + metformin improved the insulin sensitivity of the HFD-fed mice; and (iii) bixin-rich annatto extract + metformin had the ability to trigger their endogenous antioxidant machinery.

The increase in the body weight gain and the accumulation of fat in the white adipose tissues of the mice maintained on an HFD occurred as expected in this in vivo model system of obesity. Before the beginning of the treatments (from week 1 to week 8), the HFD-fed mice showed higher body weight values than the corresponding values in the mice fed the control (C) diet, denoting the production of obesity. After the beginning of the treatments with metformin or bixin-rich annatto extract at 5.5 and 11 mg/kg, alone or in combination, the HFD-fed mice had decreases in their body weight gain when compared to untreated the HFD-fed mice (the H group). Furthermore, metformin and/or bixin-rich annatto extract partially prevented fat accumulation in their white adipose tissues. Therefore, an antiobesogenic effect can be attributed to the treatments with metformin and bixin-rich annatto extract, alone or in combination, without changes in food or energy intake. Previously, a study by Gutierrez and Romero [15] observed that the treatment of HFD-fed mice with bixin at doses of 5 and 10 mg/kg for 14 weeks also decreased their body weight gain without decreasing their food intake.

The establishment of obesity favors an increase in the concentrations of free fatty acids and circulating triglycerides, as well as hyperglycemia due to the development of insulin resistance, which is related to lipotoxicity, occurring in animals with obesity [16,17]. These changes favor, at least in part, an increase in the levels of ROS in the intracellular environment and subsequent mitochondrial dysfunction, with losses in β-oxidation and increases in the production of fatty acid radicals in the mitochondrial matrix, leading to events such as the uncoupling of electron transport chains, increased production of superoxide radical anions, and the establishment of oxidative stress [18].

Excess free fatty acids in the cytoplasm serve as a source of precursors for the synthesis of molecules such as diacylglycerol and ceramides, which participate in the development of insulin resistance, culminating in the inhibition of the translocation of vesicles containing the glucose transporter type 4 (GLUT 4) to the plasma membrane of myocytes and adipocytes, thus reducing glucose uptake and contributing to an increase in blood glucose levels [19]. This process is directly related to the results of the OGTT and ITT assays, which point to the establishment of glucose intolerance and insulin resistance, respectively, in the mice from the H and V groups.

The mice from the H and V groups had increased fasting glycemia levels in relation to the values of the mice fed the C diet. The mice fed an HFD and treated with metformin and bixin-rich annatto extract, alone or combination, had better glycemic control when compared to the mice from the H group. Therefore, there is favorable potential for these treatments since metformin + bixin-rich annatto extract improved insulin sensitivity in the animals with obesity.

Glucose intolerance and chronic hyperglycemia contribute to the onset of glycoxidative stress, characterized by an exacerbation of the generation of AGEs in tissues where the uptake of glucose occurs in a non-insulin-dependent manner, including the liver and kidneys [20]. The antihyperglycemic effects of metformin and bixin-rich annatto extract may have contributed to the decrease observed in the levels of fluorescent AGEs in the livers and kidneys of the mice fed an HFD, where the effects of the treatments were most evident. It is known that AGEs are capable of activating signaling pathways that culminate in the activation of kinases such as IKKβ (inhibitory kappa B kinase beta) and JNK (c-Jun N-terminal kinase), both related to the inhibitory phosphorylation of IRS-1 (insulin receptor substrate 1), leading to reduced insulin sensitivity. Apocarotenoids, including bixin, are capable of inhibiting the signaling pathways that activate IKKβ and JNK, contributing to the restoration of insulin sensitivity, which may be related to improvements in insulin sensitivity [21,22]. On the other hand, there are studies showing that the antihyperglycemic activity of bixin may be associated with its ability to reduce carbohydrate absorption via the inhibition of the enzymes α-glucosidase and α-amylase [15]. Additionally, the possibility that bixin may have improved the pancreatic function in the mice fed an HFD cannot be ruled out. Although there are no studies on the effects of bixin or other carotenoids acting as inhibitors of dipeptidyl peptidase-4 (DPP-4), there is growing evidence on bioactives from natural sources having antidiabetic activity via DPP-4 inhibition [23,24]. Furthermore, there is great encouragement of studies on bioactives of a natural origin that act as DPP-4 inhibitors since they possess significant antioxidant properties and their use may be an effective strategy for overcoming oxidative stress in pancreatic β-cells and other important tissues, in parallel to treating diabetes [25]. In this sense, considering the promising results of this study regarding the significant potential of bixin to trigger endogenous antioxidant defenses, this set of information greatly encourages future studies on the mechanism of the antihyperglycemic activity of bixin and its relation to the inhibition of DPP-4.

Metformin has low bioavailability, reaching an absorption rate between 40 and 60% of the administered dose (peak plasma concentration). This is explained by metformin being in its protonated form at a physiological pH, which makes it difficult for it to diffuse through biological membranes. In this context, metformin depends on membrane transporters to enter cells and promote its pharmacological effects [26]. Thus, it is necessary to administer high doses of metformin, and consequently, this increases the chances of adverse effects occurring. The use of a nanostructured lipid system makes it possible to overcome the problem of the low bioavailability of metformin since encapsulation allows greater absorption of the metformin carried in the structure of the vesicles that form the nanostructured system [27]. It can be assumed that once it is incorporated into a nanoemulsion, metformin does not primarily require the process to be mediated by the transporters present in enterocytes to access the cellular environment. Consequently, a low dose of metformin would be required to obtain its therapeutic effect.

The mice fed an HFD and treated with metformin showed low fasting glycemia values, improvements in their glucose tolerance, and increased insulin sensitivity when treated with a dose of 50 mg/kg of the drug, a lower dose than those used in studies with the same in vivo model system of obesity but without the use of a nanostructured lipid system [28,29].

A nanostructured lipid system can also be used to deliver bixin due to this system's ability to increase the absorption of this apocarotenoid, also carried in the micelle's structure and integrated into the lipid portion of the vesicle. Due to the amphipathic nature of the nanostructured lipid system, the interaction of bixin with the aqueous medium can be facilitated, increasing its absorption [30,31]. This conformation allows more efficient delivery of bixin, enabling its more evident antioxidant potential in the plasma, liver, and kidneys, as well as promoting improvements in insulin sensitivity.

After offering an HFD for 17 weeks, increases in the plasma levels of total cholesterol and HDL-cholesterol and a decrease in the levels of triglycerides were observed, reproducing previous findings of our laboratory [32]. This decrease in the plasma levels of triglycerides may be related to an increase in the tissue's accumulation of this lipid promoted by the onset of obesity, observed mainly in the increases in the weight of the white adipose tissues of the animals maintained on the HFD.

The enzyme PON-1 is associated with HDL in plasma, and its activity is related to the protection of this lipoprotein and others, including low-density lipoprotein (LDL), from oxidation [33]. The PON-1 activity was significantly decreased in the plasma of the H and V mice. It is known that in a scenario of hyperglycemia, a decrease in PON-1 activity may be related to the occurrence of the glycation of this enzyme [34,35], which may explain, at least in part, the low PON-1 activity in the plasma of the mice from the H and V groups. In a previous study from our laboratory, we observed that treatment with 5.5 mg/kg of bixin-rich annatto extract for 50 days was also able to increase the PON-1 activity in the plasma of streptozotocin-induced diabetic rats. [36]. The increased PON-1 activities in the plasma of the HFD-fed mice treated with metformin, bixin-rich annatto extract at the highest dose, and combinations of metformin + bixin-rich annatto extract (the MB1 and MB2 groups) may be related to improvements observed in their glycemic control, culminating in less glycation of this enzyme [37].

The enzymes analyzed in this study are part of the first-line antioxidant defenses. Superoxide dismutase (SOD) is the first enzyme in ROS detoxification and the most powerful antioxidant enzyme in the cellular environment. Its activity consists of the dismutation of two superoxide radical anion molecules into hydrogen peroxide and molecular oxygen, thus reducing the damage potential of this reactive species. Catalase (CAT) acts on hydrogen peroxide molecules, reducing them into water and molecular oxygen and using iron and manganese ions as cofactors. The enzyme glutathione peroxidase (GSH-Px) acts on hydrogen peroxide, reducing it into water, but also catalyzes the reduction of lipoperoxides into their corresponding alcohols, mainly in the mitochondria [38,39].

Carotenoids and apocarotenoids, including bixin, are involved in the modulating pathways that activate NRF-2, a transcription factor that acts as a positive regulator of responses to oxidative stress [40]. Therefore, when activating NRF-2, there may be an increase in the expression of these first-line antioxidant enzymes [40,41], which may explain the results found in this study for the three antioxidant enzymes analyzed in the livers and kidneys of the HFD-fed mice treated with bixin-rich annatto extract. Previously, Assis and collaborators [36] also found increases in the activities of SOD and CAT in the livers of streptozotocin-induced diabetic rats treated with 5.5 mg/kg of bixin-rich annatto extract for 50 days.

With increases in the activities of antioxidant enzymes in the mice fed an HFD and treated with metformin or bixin-rich annatto extract, a decrease in the oxidative stress induced by obesity is expected. This was observed in the analysis of their TBARS levels. The animals treated with metformin or bixin-rich annatto extract, alone or in combination, showed significant decreases in the levels of TBARSs in their livers and kidneys. A similar result was found by Ma et al. [9], with a reduction in the levels of malondialdehyde, a biomarker of lipoperoxidation, and an increase in the activities of antioxidant enzymes in the kidneys of the mice through a mechanism dependent on NRF-2 activation in a CCl4-induced kidney inflammation model. Bixin and other carotenoids have important mechanisms of action in regulating inflammatory responses, modulating NF-kB activity and adipocyte differentiation. Carotenoids are involved in the activation of important components, including PPARγ, which is related to the activation of lipogenesis pathways [42]. The activation of PPARγ is fundamental to the differentiation of adipocytes, increasing the hydrolysis rates of the triglycerides present in lipoproteins via the activation of lipoprotein lipase; concomitantly, PPARγ promotes an increase in the transcription of genes involved in the uptake of fatty acids, including the fatty acid transport protein (FATP) and the fatty acid translocase (FAT/CD36) [43].

The activation of PPARγ can lead to a recovery in the lipid storage capacity of the adipose tissues via preservation of adipocytic function, contributing to increased insulin sensitivity [44]. In addition, the present study showed the antiobesogenic potential of both metformin and bixin-rich annatto extract, whether administered alone or in combination. In parallel, these treatments caused improvements in insulin sensitivity. These improvements may be related, at least in part, to the effects of bixin on PPARγ activation in the white adipose tissues. Since bixin is capable of activating PPARγ, its beneficial effects related to antiobesogenic potential and insulin sensitivity restoration may be a consequence of improvements in adipocyte function in a pathway that is not dependent on the dose administered to the animals.

4. Materials and Methods

4.1. Preparation of the Nanostructured Lipid System

The nanostructured lipid system had the following composition: oil phase: sunflower oil (5%); surfactant mixture: Brij O20/soy phosphatidylcholine—2:1 (10%); and aqueous phase: phosphate buffer (pH of 7.4) (85%). Bixin-rich annatto extract and metformin, alone or in combination, were incorporated into the oil phase and the surfactant mixture. Next, the aqueous phase was added, and the mixtures were sonicated with a rod sonicator (Q500 of QSonica®®, Newtown, CT, USA) in an ice bath (25 min at 30 s intervals every minute). The formulations containing the bioactives were centrifuged (11,180× *g* for 15 min) [45].

The formulations based on the nanostructured lipid system contained 1.1 or 2.2 mg/mL bixin-rich annatto extract and/or 10 mg/mL metformin, allowing them to reach final doses of 5.5 or 11 mg/kg bixin-rich annatto extract and/or 50 mg/kg metformin, respectively, alone or in combination.

4.2. Animal Model—Induction of Obesity/Insulin Resistance and Experiment Conclusion

C57BL-6J male mice with body weight values of 21 ± 0.17 g (4 weeks old) were obtained from Anilab (Animais de Laboratório, Criação e Comércio LTDA, Paulínia, Brazil). The mice were housed in polypropylene cages (two animals per cage) and maintained under a light/dark cycle (12 h) and controlled conditions of humidity (55 ± 5%) and temperature (23 ± 1 °C) at the Bioterium of the Department of Clinical Analysis (FCF/UNESP). During the acclimation period (2 weeks), a standard chow diet (Presence Nutrição Animal, Paulínia, São Paulo, Brazil) and water were offered to the mice ad libitum. Next, the mice were fed with a control diet (C; 3.85 kcal/g; 4% lipids) or with a high-fat diet (HFD; 5.40 kcal/g; 35% lipids) (Pragsoluções Biociências Serviços e Comércio Ltd., Jaú, Brazil) (Table S1 in the Supplementary Materials). The HFD enabled the development of obesity and insulin resistance.

The mice were divided into eight groups (n = 12 per group; total of 96 mice): the C group (non-obese mice fed a C diet), the H group (obese, HFD-fed mice), the V group (HFD-fed mice treated with a vehicle—the nanostructured lipid system), the M group (HFD-fed mice treated with 50 mg/kg metformin), the B1 group (HFD-fed mice treated with 5.5 mg/kg bixin-rich annatto extract), the MB1 group (HFD-fed mice treated with 50 mg/kg metformin + 5.5 mg/kg bixin-rich annatto extract), the B2 group (HFD-fed mice treated with 11 mg/kg bixin-rich annatto extract), and the MB2 group (HFD-fed mice treated with 50 mg/kg metformin + 11 mg/kg bixin-rich annatto extract). To allocate the animals into the experimental groups, stratified randomization was used. In addition, standardization of the median body weight values across the groups was applied to composing the experimental groups containing the HFD-fed mice. The inclusion criteria for the groups containing the HFD-fed mice were the animals having body weight values of approximately 30 g before the beginning of the treatments. The exclusion criteria for groups containing the HFD-fed mice were low body weight gain values.

All the treatments were administered orogastrically (gavage). Annato extract powder rich in bixin (*Bixa orellana* L., 60% bixin, Lichnoflora Pesquisa e Desenvolvimento em Produtos Naturais Ltd., Ribeirão Preto, Brazil) and metformin (99.56% metformin hydrochloride, Abhilash Chemicals and Pharmaceuticals, Madurai, India) were incorporated into a nanostructured lipid system. The doses of bixin-rich annatto extract (5.5 and 11 mg/kg) were chosen based on our previous study [36], and the dose of metformin (50 mg/kg) was based on studies performed in mice under experimental models of obesity/insulin resistance and treated with metformin [28,29], and we reduced the dose of the drug since it was administered in a nanostructured lipid system. The experiment was performed for 17 weeks; the mice were treated for the last 8 weeks via daily gavage (5 μL/g animal) between 08:00 and 09:00 h from the 9th to the 17th weeks. The mice from the V group received the vehicle (the nanostructured lipid system without metformin or bixin-rich annatto extract) via daily gavage (5 μL/g animal). Finally, to mimic the oral treatments, the mice from the C and H groups received water by gavage.

Their body weight and food intake were monitored weekly throughout the experimental period. By multiplying their food intake values (g) by the energy values (kcal) provided for the diets, the energy intake values were obtained. The oral glucose tolerance test (OGTT) was performed at week 15 (which corresponded to 6 weeks of treatments). In 12 h-fasted mice, the OGTT was performed at 11:00 a.m. after gavage with 1 g/kg glucose

(glucose overload). Their glycemia levels were monitored before (0 min) and after (15, 30, 60, 90, and 120 min) the glucose overload. A drop of peripheral blood was obtained from the mice's tails to determine their glycemia levels, which were measured by a glucometer (Abbott Diabetes Care Ltd., São Paulo, Brazil) [46]. The insulin tolerance test (ITT) was performed at week 16 (which corresponded to 7 weeks of treatments). In 2 h-fasted mice, the ITT was performed at 01:00 p.m. with an intraperitoneal injection of insulin (0.4 UI/kg). Their glycemia levels were monitored before (0 min) and after (15, 30, 45, and 60 min) the administration of insulin [46].

At week 17 (which corresponded to 8 weeks of treatments), the mice were fasted for 6 h and anesthetized by intraperitoneal administration of xylazine–ketamine (16 mg/kg xylazine–90 mg/kg ketamine). Next, the mice were euthanized by exsanguination via cardiac puncture under anesthesia, and blood samples were collected into heparinized tubes and then centrifuged (700× *g* for 10 min at 25 °C) to obtain plasma samples. Their livers, kidneys, hearts, gastrocnemius skeletal muscles, epididymal white adipose tissues, and interscapular brown adipose tissues were removed, weighed, snap-frozen in liquid nitrogen, and frozen (−80 °C).

All the experimental procedures were previously approved by the Committee for Ethics in Animal Experimentation at the School of Pharmaceutical Sciences, UNESP (CEUA/FCF/CAr n° 19/2019).

4.3. Analysis of Plasma Biochemical Markers

Their plasma levels of glucose, total cholesterol, high-density lipoprotein cholesterol (HDL-cholesterol), triglycerides, albumin, alanine aminotransferase (ALT), creatinine, and uric acid were measured using commercial kits (Labtest Diagnostica SA, Lagoa Santa, Brazil).

4.4. Analysis of Glycoxidative Stress Biomarkers

In the plasma and livers, fluorescent AGEs were measured using 1.2 M chloroform, 0.12 M trichloroacetic acid, and 0.1 M sodium hydroxide (plasma) or 2.4 M chloroform (liver homogenates) [47]. In the kidney homogenates, fluorescent AGEs were measured using 0.1 M sodium hydroxide [48]. Next, the tubes containing these samples were vigorously shaken, and then the tubes were maintained at 10 ± 2 °C for 30 min, followed by centrifugation (10,000× *g* for 10 min at 10 °C). Tissue supernatants were used to measure the fluorescence intensity relative to the AGEs, with excitation and emission wavelengths of 370 nm and 440 nm, respectively, in a microplate multi-mode reader with the split set at 16 nm (Synergy H1TM, BioTek Instruments Inc., Winooski, VT, USA). The results were expressed as arbitrary units (AU) of fluorescence per milligram of protein.

Deproteinized tissue samples (plasma, livers, and kidneys) were used to determine the lipid peroxidation products via a thiobarbituric acid (TBA) assay [49]. The thiobarbituric acid-reactive substances (TBARSs), including malondialdehyde, were measured via spectrofluorescence (with excitation and emission wavelengths of 510 nm and 553 nm, respectively) in the plasma and via spectrophotometry (535 nm) in the livers and kidneys. The results were expressed in terms of μmol/L (plasma) and μmol/g tissue (livers and kidneys).

4.5. Analysis of Endogenous Antioxidant Defenses

The livers and kidneys were used to determine the activities of superoxide dismutase (SOD), catalase (CAT), and glutathione peroxidase (GSH-Px), and the plasma samples were used to determine the activity of paraoxonase 1 (PON-1), according to standardized methods.

Sample preparations: The livers and kidneys (0.1 g) were prepared in 1 mL sodium phosphate buffer (10 mmol/L, pH 7.4) at 4 °C. The homogenates were then centrifuged at 10,000× *g* for 10 min at 4 °C. The activities of SOD, CAT, and GSH-Px were measured in the liver and kidney supernatants.

The SOD activity was measured by monitoring the inhibition of the reduction of nitroblue tetrazolium (NBT). Xanthine oxidase catalyzes xanthine's oxidation, and superoxide anion radical ($O_2^{\bullet-}$) molecules are produced, which reduce NBT into a formazan. The SOD present in the sample catalyzes the dismutation of $O_2^{\bullet-}$, inhibiting the reduction of NBT, which is monitored at 550 nm. The results were expressed in terms of U/mg protein. One SOD unit is defined as the amount of the enzyme required to inhibit the rate of NBT reduction by 50% [50].

The CAT activity was monitored by the consumption of hydrogen peroxide (H_2O_2) at 230 nm. The results were expressed in terms of μmol of H_2O_2 consumed/min/mg protein [51].

The GSH-Px activity was determined by monitoring the oxidation of the reduced form of nicotinamide adenine dinucleotide phosphate (NADPH) into NADP+. GSH-Px catalyzes the oxidation of the reduced form of glutathione (GSH) in the presence of H_2O_2. Glutathione in its oxidized form (GSSG) is reduced into GSH by glutathione reductase (GSH-Rd), with the concomitant oxidation of NADPH into NADP+, monitored at 340 nm. The results were expressed in terms of μmol of NADPH oxidized/min/mg protein [52].

The activity of PON-1 in the plasma was measured by monitoring p-nitrophenol at 405 nm, which is released after paraoxon's hydrolysis by PON-1 [36]. The results were expressed in terms of U/mg HDL-cholesterol (unit = μmoL paraoxon hydrolyzed/min).

The protein levels in the tissue samples were determined according to Lowry et al. [53] to correct the results for SOD, CAT, GSH-Px, and fluorescent AGEs.

4.6. Statistical Analysis

The data are expressed as mean ± standard error of mean (SEM). To compare the intergroup differences, one-way analysis of variance followed by the Student–Newman–Keuls test was used. To compare the intragroup changes in the body weight values relative to week 0, a paired Student's t-test was used. The data were considered statistically different at $p < 0.05$ (*), $p < 0.01$ (**), and $p < 0.001$ (***). Statistical analyses were performed using GraphPad Prism 6.01 (GraphPad Software, San Diego, CA, USA).

5. Conclusions

Combining current medicines with bioactives of a natural origin might be an interesting therapeutic strategy to attenuate or even prevent the complications occurring in obesity and diabetes mellitus. In this regard, the present study showed that metformin combined with bixin-rich annatto extract had antiobesogenic effects and decreased the cholesterol levels and improved the insulin sensitivity in mice fed a high-fat diet, which represents the maintenance of metformin's effects and bixin's effects when they are administered alone. In addition, metformin + bixin-rich annatto extract triggered cytoprotective mechanisms that counteracted the harmful impacts of oxidative stress by increasing their endogenous antioxidant defenses. To the best of our knowledge, by targeting not only obesity, hyperglycemia, and insulin resistance but also hypercholesterolemia and oxidative stress, this study provides the first evidence of a therapeutic strategy based on the combination of bixin and metformin for combating the complications of metabolic disturbances resulting from oxidative stress.

Supplementary Materials: The following supporting information can be downloaded at https://www.mdpi.com/article/10.3390/ph17091202/s1. Table S1: Compositions of control diet (C) and high-fat diet (HFD).

Author Contributions: Conceptualization, M.C., I.L.B. and A.M.B.; methodology, C.G.P., B.P.M., J.O.O., I.D.F., R.T.A.M. and P.B.d.S.; formal analysis, C.G.P., B.P.M., J.O.O. and F.N.C.; investigation, C.G.P., B.P.M., J.O.O., I.D.F., R.T.A.M. and P.B.d.S.; resources, M.C., I.L.B. and A.M.B.; data curation, C.G.P.; writing—original draft preparation, C.G.P., F.N.C. and A.M.B.; writing—review and editing, A.M.B.; visualization, C.G.P., B.P.M. and F.N.C.; supervision, A.M.B.; project administration, A.M.B.; funding acquisition, A.M.B. All authors have read and agreed to the published version of the manuscript.

Funding: This research was funded by Fundação de Amparo a Pesquisa do Estado de São Paulo (FAPESP, 98/09152-6) and Conselho Nacional de Desenvolvimento Científico e Tecnológico (CNPq, 303963/2020-4).

Institutional Review Board Statement: This study was performed according to the national (Brazilian College of Animal Experimentation—COBEA) and institutional (Committee for Ethics in Animal Experimentation of the School of Pharmaceutical Sciences, UNESP, Araraquara) rules for animal experiments. The treatments and protocols used in this study were approved by the Committee for Ethics in Animal Experimentation from the School of Pharmaceutical Sciences, UNESP, Araraquara (CEUA/FCF/CAr nº 19/2019).

Informed Consent Statement: Not applicable.

Data Availability Statement: The datasets generated during and/or analyzed during the current study are available from the corresponding author on reasonable request.

Conflicts of Interest: The authors declare no conflicts of interest.

Abbreviations

AGEs: advanced glycation end products; ALT: alanine aminotransferase; AUC: area under the curve; B1: mice fed an HFD and treated with 5.5 mg/kg bixin-rich annatto extract; B2: mice fed an HFD and treated with 11 mg/kg bixin-rich annatto extract; C: control diet or mice fed the control diet; CAT: catalase; DM: diabetes mellitus; DPP-4: dipeptidyl peptidase-4; FAT/CD36: fatty acid translocase; FATP: fatty acid transport protein; GLUT 4: glucose transporter type 4; GSH: glutathione, reduced form; GSH-Px: glutathione peroxidase; GSH-Rd: glutathione reductase; GSSG: glutathione, oxidized form; H: mice fed a high-fat diet; H_2O_2: hydrogen peroxide; HDL: high-density lipoprotein; HFD: high-fat diet; IKKβ: inhibitory kappa B kinase beta; ITT: insulin tolerance test; IRS-1: insulin receptor substrate 1; JNK: c-Jun N-terminal kinase; LDL: low-density lipoprotein; M: mice fed an HFD and treated with 50 mg/kg metformin; MB1: mice fed an HFD and treated with 50 mg/kg metformin + 5.5 mg/kg bixin-rich annatto extract; MB2: mice fed an HFD and treated with 50 mg/kg metformin + 11 mg/kg bixin-rich annatto extract; NADP+: nicotinamide adenine dinucleotide phosphate, oxidized form; NADPH: nicotinamide adenine dinucleotide phosphate, reduced form; NBT: nitroblue tetrazolium; NRF-2: nuclear factor erythroid 2-related factor 2; $O_2^{\bullet-}$: superoxide anion radical; OGTT: oral glucose tolerance test; PON-1: paraoxonase 1; PPARγ: peroxisome proliferator-activated receptor gamma; ROS: reactive oxygen species; SOD: superoxide dismutase; T2DM: type 2 diabetes mellitus; TBA: thiobarbituric acid; TBARS: thiobarbituric acid reactive substance; V: mice fed an HFD and treated with the vehicle.

References

1. Obri, A.; Serra, D.; Herrero, L.; Mera, P. The Role of Epigenetics in the Development of Obesity. *Biochem. Pharmacol.* **2020**, *177*, 113973. [CrossRef]
2. Ott, C.; Jacobs, K.; Haucke, E.; Navarrete Santos, A.; Grune, T.; Simm, A. Role of Advanced Glycation End Products in Cellular Signaling. *Redox Biol.* **2014**, *2*, 411–429. [CrossRef]
3. Iacobini, C.; Vitale, M.; Pesce, C.; Pugliese, G.; Menini, S. Diabetic Complications and Oxidative Stress: A 20-Year Voyage Back in Time and Back to the Future. *Antioxidants* **2021**, *10*, 727. [CrossRef]
4. Adak, T.; Samadi, A.; Ünal, A.Z.; Sabuncuoğlu, S. A Reappraisal on Metformin. *Regul. Toxicol. Pharmacol.* **2018**, *92*, 324–332. [CrossRef]
5. Nasri, H.; Rafieian-Kopaei, M. Metformin: Current knowledge. *J. Res. Med. Sci.* **2014**, *19*, 658–664, Erratum in: *J. Res. Med. Sci.* **2024**, *29*, 6. [CrossRef]
6. Testa, R.; Bonfigli, A.R.; Prattichizzo, F.; La Sala, L.; De Nigris, V.; Ceriello, A. The "Metabolic Memory" Theory and the Early Treatment of Hyperglycemia in Prevention of Diabetic Complications. *Nutrients* **2017**, *9*, 437. [CrossRef]
7. Enayati, A.; Assadpour, E.; Jafari, S.M. Bixin—Properties and Applications. In *Handbook of Food Bioactive Ingredients*; Jafari, S.M., Rashidinejad, A., Simal-Gandara, J., Eds.; Springer: Cham, Switzerland, 2023. [CrossRef]
8. Vilar, D.A.; Vilar, M.S.; de Lima e Moura, T.F.; Raffin, F.N.; de Oliveira, M.R.; Franco, C.F.; de Athayde-Filho, P.F.; Diniz, M.F.; Barbosa-Filho, J.M. Traditional uses, chemical constituents, and biological activities of *Bixa orellana* L.: A review. *Sci. World J.* **2014**, *2014*, 857292. [CrossRef]

9. Ma, J.Q.; Zhang, Y.J.; Tian, Z.K.; Liu, C.M. Bixin Attenuates Carbon Tetrachloride Induced Oxidative Stress, Inflammation and Fibrosis in Kidney by Regulating the Nrf2/TLR4/MyD88 and PPAR-γ/TGF-B1/Smad3 Pathway. *Int. Immunopharmacol.* **2021**, *90*, 107117. [CrossRef]
10. Roohbakhsh, A.; Karimi, G.; Iranshahi, M. Carotenoids in the Treatment of Diabetes Mellitus and Its Complications: A Mechanistic Review. *Biomed. Pharmacother.* **2017**, *91*, 31–42. [CrossRef]
11. Foretz, M.; Guigas, B.; Viollet, B. Metformin: Update on mechanisms of action and repurposing potential. *Nat. Rev. Endocrinol.* **2023**, *19*, 460–476. [CrossRef]
12. Shahid-ul-Islam; Rather, L.J.; Mohammad, F. Phytochemistry, Biological Activities and Potential of Annatto in Natural Colorant Production for Industrial Applications—A Review. *J. Adv. Res.* **2016**, *7*, 499–514. [CrossRef]
13. Dima, C.; Assadpour, E.; Dima, S.; Jafari, S.M. Bioactive-Loaded Nanocarriers for Functional Foods: From Designing to Bioavailability. *Curr. Opin. Food Sci.* **2020**, *33*, 21–29. [CrossRef]
14. Salvi, V.R.; Pawar, P. Nanostructured Lipid Carriers (NLC) System: A Novel Drug Targeting Carrier. *J. Drug Deliv. Sci. Technol.* **2019**, *51*, 255–267. [CrossRef]
15. Gutierrez, R.M.; Romero, R.V. Effects of bixin in high-fat diet-fed-induced fatty liver in C57BL/6J mice. *Asian Pac. J. Trop. Biomed.* **2016**, *6*, 1015–1021. [CrossRef]
16. Lytrivi, M.; Castell, A.L.; Poitout, V.; Cnop, M. Recent Insights into Mechanisms of β-Cell Lipo- and Glucolipotoxicity in Type 2 Diabetes. *J. Mol. Biol.* **2020**, *432*, 1514–1534. [CrossRef]
17. Zhou, K.; Yee, S.W.; Seiser, E.L.; Van Leeuwen, N.; Tavendale, R.; Bennett, A.J.; Groves, C.J.; Coleman, R.L.; Van Der Heijden, A.A.; Beulens, J.W.; et al. Variation in the Glucose Transporter Gene SLC2A2 Is Associated with Glycemic Response to Metformin. *Nat. Genet.* **2016**, *48*, 1055–1059. [CrossRef]
18. Meex, R.C.R.; Watt, M.J. Hepatokines: Linking Nonalcoholic Fatty Liver Disease and Insulin Resistance. *Nat. Rev. Endocrinol.* **2017**, *13*, 509–520. [CrossRef]
19. Benador, I.Y.; Veliova, M.; Liesa, M.; Shirihai, O.S. Mitochondria Bound to Lipid Droplets: Where Mitochondrial Dynamics Regulate Lipid Storage and Utilization. *Cell Metab.* **2019**, *29*, 827–835. [CrossRef]
20. González, P.; Lozano, P.; Ros, G.; Solano, F. Hyperglycemia and Oxidative Stress: An Integral, Updated and Critical Overview of Their Metabolic Interconnections. *Int. J. Mol. Sci.* **2023**, *24*, 9352. [CrossRef]
21. Roehrs, M.; Conte, L.; da Silva, D.T.; Duarte, T.; Maurer, L.H.; de Carvalho, J.A.M.; Moresco, R.N.; Somacal, S.; Emanuelli, T. Annatto Carotenoids Attenuate Oxidative Stress and Inflammatory Response after High-Calorie Meal in Healthy Subjects. *Food Res. Int.* **2017**, *100*, 771–779. [CrossRef]
22. Roehrs, M.; Figueiredo, C.G.; Zanchi, M.M.; Bochi, G.V.; Moresco, R.N.; Quatrin, A.; Somacal, S.; Conte, L.; Emanuelli, T. Bixin and Norbixin Have Opposite Effects on Glycemia, Lipidemia, and Oxidative Stress in Streptozotocin-Induced Diabetic Rats. *Int. J. Endocrinol.* **2014**, *2014*, 839095. [CrossRef] [PubMed]
23. Shaikh, S.; Lee, E.J.; Ahmad, K.; Ahmad, S.S.; Lim, J.H.; Choi, I. A Comprehensive Review and Perspective on Natural Sources as Dipeptidyl Peptidase-4 Inhibitors for Management of Diabetes. *Pharmaceuticals* **2021**, *14*, 591. [CrossRef]
24. Chhabria, S.; Mathur, S.; Vadakan, S.; Sahoo, D.K.; Mishra, P.; Paital, B. A review on phytochemical and pharmacological facets of tropical ethnomedicinal plants as reformed DPP-IV inhibitors to regulate incretin activity. *Front. Endocrinol.* **2022**, *13*, 1027237. [CrossRef]
25. Singh, A.K.; Yadav, D.; Sharma, N.; Jin, J.O. Dipeptidyl Peptidase (DPP)-IV Inhibitors with Antioxidant Potential Isolated from Natural Sources: A Novel Approach for the Management of Diabetes. *Pharmaceuticals* **2021**, *14*, 586. [CrossRef]
26. Tulipano, G. Integrated or Independent Actions of Metformin in Target Tissues Underlying Its Current Use and New Possible Applications in the Endocrine and Metabolic Disorder Area. *Int. J. Mol. Sci.* **2021**, *22*, 13068. [CrossRef]
27. Kenechukwu, F.C.; Isaac, G.T.; Nnamani, D.O.; Momoh, M.A.; Attama, A.A. Enhanced circulation longevity and pharmacodynamics of metformin from surface-modified nanostructured lipid carriers based on solidified reverse micellar solutions. *Heliyon* **2022**, *8*, e09100. [CrossRef]
28. Guo, W.R.; Liu, J.; Cheng, L.D.; Liu, Z.Y.; Zheng, X.B.; Liang, H.; Xu, F. Metformin Alleviates Steatohepatitis in Diet-Induced Obese Mice in a SIRT1-Dependent Way. *Front. Pharmacol.* **2021**, *12*, 704112. [CrossRef]
29. Zhou, Z.Y.; Ren, L.W.; Zhan, P.; Yang, H.Y.; Chai, D.D.; Yu, Z.W. Metformin exerts glucose-lowering action in high-fat fed mice via attenuating endotoxemia and enhancing insulin signaling. *Acta Pharmacol. Sin.* **2016**, *37*, 1063–1075. [CrossRef] [PubMed]
30. Rostamabadi, H.; Falsafi, S.R.; Jafari, S.M. Nanoencapsulation of Carotenoids within Lipid-Based Nanocarriers. *J. Control. Release* **2019**, *298*, 38–67. [CrossRef] [PubMed]
31. Enayati, A.; Rezaei, A.; Falsafi, S.R.; Rostamabadi, H.; Malekjani, N.; Akhavan-Mahdavi, S.; Kharazmi, M.S.; Jafari, S.M. Bixin-loaded colloidal nanodelivery systems, techniques and applications. *Food Chem.* **2023**, *412*, 135479. [CrossRef]
32. Costa, M.C.; Lima, T.F.O.; Arcaro, C.A.; Inacio, M.D.; Batista-Duharte, A.; Carlos, I.Z.; Spolidorio, L.C.; Assis, R.P.; Brunetti, I.L.; Baviera, A.M. Trigonelline and Curcumin Alone, but Not in Combination, Counteract Oxidative Stress and Inflammation and Increase Glycation Product Detoxification in the Liver and Kidney of Mice with High-Fat Diet-Induced Obesity. *J. Nutr. Biochem.* **2020**, *76*, 108303. [CrossRef]
33. Koren-Gluzer, M.; Aviram, M.; Meilin, E.; Hayek, T. The Antioxidant HDL-Associated Paraoxonase-1 (PON1) Attenuates Diabetes Development and Stimulates β-Cell Insulin Release. *Atherosclerosis* **2011**, *219*, 510–518. [CrossRef] [PubMed]

34. Shokri, Y.; Variji, A.; Nosrati, M.; Khonakdar-tarsi, A.; Kianmehr, A.; Kashi, Z.; Bahar, A.; Bagheri, A.; Mahrooz, A. Importance of Paraoxonase 1 (PON1) as an Antioxidant and Antiatherogenic Enzyme in the Cardiovascular Complications of Type 2 Diabetes: Genotypic and Phenotypic Evaluation. *Diabetes Res. Clin. Pract.* **2020**, *1*, 108067. [CrossRef] [PubMed]
35. Chistiakov, D.A.; Melnichenko, A.A.; Orekhov, A.N.; Bobryshev, Y.V. Paraoxonase and Atherosclerosis-Related Cardiovascular Diseases. *Biochimie* **2017**, *132*, 19–27. [CrossRef]
36. Assis, R.P.; Arcaro, C.A.; Gutierres, V.O.; Oliveira, J.O.; Costa, P.I.; Baviera, A.M.; Brunetti, I.L. Combined Effects of Curcumin and Lycopene or Bixin in Yoghurt on Inhibition of LDL Oxidation and Increases in HDL and Paraoxonase Levels in Streptozotocin-Diabetic Rats. *Int. J. Mol. Sci.* **2017**, *18*, 332. [CrossRef]
37. Koren-Gluzer, M.; Aviram, M.; Hayek, T. Paraoxonasel (PON1) Reduces Insulin Resistance in Mice Fed a High-Fat Diet, and Promotes GLUT4 Overexpression in Myocytes, via the IRS-1/Akt Pathway. *Atherosclerosis* **2013**, *229*, 71–78. [CrossRef]
38. Ighodaro, O.M.; Akinloye, O.A. First Line Defence Antioxidants-Superoxide Dismutase (SOD), Catalase (CAT) and Glutathione Peroxidase (GPX): Their Fundamental Role in the Entire Antioxidant Defence Grid. *Alex. J. Med.* **2018**, *54*, 287–293. [CrossRef]
39. Pisoschi, A.M.; Pop, A.; Iordache, F.; Stanca, L.; Predoi, G.; Serban, A.I. Oxidative Stress Mitigation by Antioxidants—An Overview on Their Chemistry and Influences on Health Status. *Eur. J. Med. Chem.* **2021**, *209*, 112891. [CrossRef] [PubMed]
40. Xue, L.; Zhang, H.; Zhang, J.; Li, B.; Zhang, Z.; Tao, S. Bixin Protects against Particle-Induced Long-Term Lung Injury in an NRF2-Dependent Manner. *Toxicol. Res.* **2018**, *7*, 258–270. [CrossRef]
41. Xu, Z.; Kong, X.Q. Bixin Ameliorates High Fat Diet-Induced Cardiac Injury in Mice through Inflammation and Oxidative Stress Suppression. *Biomed. Pharmacother.* **2017**, *89*, 991–1004. [CrossRef]
42. Luisa-Bonet, M.; Canas, J.A.; Ribot, J.; Palou, A. Carotenoids and Their Conversion Products in the Control of Adipocyte Function, Adiposity and Obesity. *Arch. Biochem. Biophys.* **2015**, *572*, 112–125. [CrossRef] [PubMed]
43. Echeverría, F.; Ortiz, M.; Valenzuela, R.; Videla, L.A. Long-Chain Polyunsaturated Fatty Acids Regulation of PPARs, Signaling: Relationship to Tissue Development and Aging. *Prostaglandins Leukot. Essent. Fat. Acids* **2016**, *114*, 28–34. [CrossRef] [PubMed]
44. Murphy, G.J.; Holder, J.C. PPAR-γ Agonists: Therapeutic Role in Diabetes, Inflammation and Cancer. *Trends Pharmacol. Sci.* **2000**, *21*, 469–474. [CrossRef]
45. de Freitas, E.S.; da Silva, P.B.; Chorilli, M.; Batista, A.A.; de Oliveira Lopes, E.; da Silva, M.M.; Leite, C.Q.; Pavan, F.R. Nanostructured lipid systems as a strategy to improve the in vitro cytotoxicity of ruthenium(II) compounds. *Molecules* **2014**, *19*, 5999–6008. [CrossRef]
46. Motta, B.P.; Pinheiro, C.G.; Figueiredo, I.D.; Cardoso, F.N.; Oliveira, J.O.; Machado, R.T.A.; da Silva, P.B.; Chorilli, M.; Brunetti, I.L.; Baviera, A.M. Combined Effects of Lycopene and Metformin on Decreasing Oxidative Stress by Triggering Endogenous Antioxidant Defenses in Diet-Induced Obese Mice. *Molecules* **2022**, *27*, 8503. [CrossRef]
47. Zilin, S.; Naifeng, L.; Bicheng, L.; Jiping, W. The determination of AGE-peptides by flow injection assay, a practical marker of diabetic nephropathy. *Clin. Chim. Acta* **2001**, *313*, 69–75. [CrossRef]
48. Pokupec, R.; Kalauz, M.; Turk, N.; Turk, Z. Advanced glycation endproducts in human diabetic and non-diabetic cataractous lenses. Graefe's Arch. *Clin. Exp. Ophthalmol.* **2003**, *241*, 378–384. [CrossRef]
49. Kohn, H.I.; Liversedge, M. On a new aerobic metabolite whose production by brain is inhibited by apomorphine, emetine, ergotamine, epinephrine, and menadione. *J. Pharmacol. Exp. Ther.* **1944**, *82*, 292–300.
50. Beauchamp, C.; Fridovich, I. Superoxide dismutase: Improved assays and an assay applicable to acrylamide gels. *Anal. Biochem.* **1971**, *44*, 276–287. [CrossRef]
51. Beers, R.F., Jr.; Sizer, I.W. A spectrophotometric method of measuring the breakdown of hydrogen peroxide by catalase. *J. Biol. Chem.* **1952**, *195*, 133–140. [CrossRef]
52. Rush, J.W.; Sandiford, S.D. Plasma glutathione peroxidase in healthy young adults: Influence of gender and physical activity. *Clin. Biochem.* **2003**, *36*, 345–351. [CrossRef] [PubMed]
53. Lowry, O.H.; Rosebrough, N.J.; Farr, A.L.; Randall, R.J. Protein measurement with the Folin phenol reagent. *J. Biol. Chem.* **1951**, *193*, 265–275. [CrossRef] [PubMed]

pharmaceuticals

MDPI

Article

Docosatrienoic Acid Inhibits Melanogenesis Partly through Suppressing the Intracellular MITF/Tyrosinase Axis

Kyoung Mi Moon [1,†], Min-Kyeong Lee [1,2,†], Su-Yeon Park [1], Jaeseong Seo [1], Ah-reum Kim [1] and Bonggi Lee [1,3,4,*]

1 Department of Food Science and Nutrition, Pukyong National University, Busan 48513, Republic of Korea; omkksm@pknu.ac.kr (K.M.M.); lmk1905@korea.kr (M.-K.L.); suzan@pukyong.ac.kr (S.-Y.P.); syj5528@pukyong.ac.kr (J.S.); kimar0107@pukyong.ac.kr (A.-r.K.)

2 Biotechnology Research Division, National Institute of Fisheries Science, Busan 48513, Republic of Korea

3 Department of Smart Green Technology Engineering, Pukyong National University, Busan 48513, Republic of Korea

4 Marine Integrated Biomedical Technology Center, The National Key Research Institutes, Pukyong National University, Busan 48513, Republic of Korea

* Correspondence: bong3257@pknu.ac.kr; Tel.: +82-51-629-5852

† These authors contributed equally to this work.

Abstract: Melanogenesis, essential for skin photoprotection and pigmentation, can lead to disorders like melasma and hyperpigmentation, which are challenging to treat and affect quality of life. Docosatrienoic acid (DTA), a polyunsaturated omega-3 fatty acid, has been identified as a potential regulator of skin aging. This study investigates DTA's effects on melanogenesis and its underlying molecular mechanisms using in silico and in vitro analyses. SwissSimilarity analysis revealed that DTA shares close structural similarities with known anti-melanogenic lipids, suggesting it may inhibit melanogenesis in similar manners. Our results demonstrated that DTA reduces melanin content and intracellular tyrosinase activity in B16F10 cells, significantly downregulating the mRNA expression of *tyrosinase*, *TRP-1*, and *TRP-2* by inhibiting MITF translocation to the nucleus. While DTA exhibited mild inhibitory effects on mushroom tyrosinase activity and antioxidant properties at higher concentrations, direct inhibition of tyrosinase is likely not the primary mechanism, as the observed anti-melanogenic effects occurred at much lower concentrations compared to those required for direct tyrosinase inhibition. Together, DTA-mediated modulation of MITF and tyrosinase mRNA expression offers a novel approach to treating hyperpigmentation. DTA's potential extends into the cosmetic industry, enhancing product stability, functionality, and aesthetics. Further research is needed to explore DTA's broader applications in skincare and cosmetic formulations.

Keywords: melanogenesis; docosatrienoic acid; fatty acid; skin aging

1. Introduction

Melanogenesis, while essential for protecting the skin from ultraviolet (UV) radiation and contributing to skin and hair pigmentation, can have several harmful effects under certain conditions. Disorders like melasma and post-inflammatory hyperpigmentation result in dark, discolored patches on the skin, which are often challenging to treat and affect individuals' quality of life. Excessive UV exposure linked to melanogenesis can lead to skin cancers, including melanoma, by causing DNA damage in melanocytes. Additionally, chronic UV exposure also results in age-related pigmentation such as lentigines and contributes to photoaging, characterized by uneven skin tone and an aged appearance [1,2]. Furthermore, visible pigmentation disorders can significantly impact self-esteem and mental health, leading to emotional distress [3].

In addition to these risks, genetic disorders related to melanin production, such as albinism, which involves a lack of melanin, make individuals highly susceptible to sunburn and skin cancers, while vitiligo leads to depigmented patches on the skin, causing psychological and social effects. These issues underscore that, although melanogenesis is crucial for photoprotection, its dysregulation can lead to various skin disorders and increased cancer risk, highlighting the need for effective treatments and preventive measures [1,2,4].

Recent research has further elucidated the complex roles that melanin plays beyond mere photoprotection. For example, melanin is now understood to be involved in the modulation of immune responses, neuroprotection, and the regulation of reactive oxygen species (ROS) [5]. These findings underscore the importance of maintaining balanced melanin production, as both overproduction and underproduction can lead to significant physiological consequences.

Melanogenesis is a complex process that occurs within specialized organelles called melanosomes in melanocytes and involves multiple enzymatic reactions. The key enzyme, tyrosinase, catalyzes the conversion of tyrosine to dopaquinone, initiating melanin synthesis [1,6]. This process is tightly regulated by various factors, including tyrosinase-related proteins (TYRP1 and TYRP2), the microphthalmia-associated transcription factor (MITF), and multiple signaling pathways. MITF is particularly significant as it regulates the expression of essential melanogenic enzymes and proteins, thus controlling melanin production [7]. Understanding and regulating these molecular mechanisms is essential for developing therapeutic interventions for pigmentation disorders such as vitiligo, melasma, and hyperpigmentation.

Ultraviolet (UV) radiation, particularly UVB, is a primary environmental factor that induces melanin production. However, UV radiation's effects extend beyond melanin production; it also interacts with the neuroendocrine and immune systems, influencing overall human physiology. This intricate interplay, known as "photo-neuro-immuno-endocrinology", reflects the complex regulatory mechanisms by which UV radiation affects the body, brain, and immune system [8]. These interactions highlight the importance of understanding UV radiation's broader impacts when considering the regulation of melanogenesis.

Melanogenesis is a complex process influenced by various factors, including recent research highlighting the significant role of fatty acids in modulating this process. Fatty acids are known for their functions in energy metabolism and cellular signaling, and they are also recognized for their impact on melanin production [9,10]. These lipids, classified by their chain length and degree of unsaturation, exhibit distinct effects on melanogenesis. Saturated fatty acids, such as palmitic acid, have been shown to stimulate melanin production, whereas polyunsaturated fatty acids, like linoleic acid, have inhibitory effects on this process [11]. The interaction between fatty acids and melanogenesis has important implications in fields such as dermatology, cosmetology, and oncology [12–14]. Insights gained from studying these interactions may lead to novel therapeutic strategies for addressing pigmentation disorders and melanoma.

Docosatrienoic acid (DTA), also known as 22:3(n-3), is a polyunsaturated omega-3 fatty acid with a long carbon chain comprising 22 carbon atoms and three cis double bonds. These double bonds are typically located at the 7th, 10th, and 13th carbon positions from the omega end, contributing to the molecule's flexibility and fluidity in biological membranes. This structural configuration may allow DTA to play a crucial role in maintaining cell membrane integrity and enhancing membrane fluidity [15,16]. However, despite its potential significance, the biological functions of this lipid have not been thoroughly investigated. In this study, we examined whether this fatty acid regulates melanogenesis and explored its underlying molecular mechanisms. To achieve this, we conducted both in silico and in vitro analyses to investigate the anti-melanogenic properties of DTA.

2. Results

2.1. Structural and Functional Analysis of Docosatrienoic Acid (DTA)

SwissSimilarity is a powerful web-based tool designed to facilitate the rapid screening of extensive libraries, including drugs, bioactive small molecules, commercially available compounds, and an ultra-large collection of virtual compounds that can be readily synthesized from commercially available reagents. It enables efficient identification of potential bioactive compounds using molecular fingerprints and both superpositional and fast non-superpositional 3D shape similarity approaches. These methods allow to compare and identify similar compounds quickly, aiding in drug discovery, molecular mechanism studies, and lead compound optimization [17].

Although previous research indicated that DTA accumulates in human fibroblast phospholipids when cultured in a basal nutrient medium (MCDB 110) with reduced fetal bovine serum levels (0.4%) [18], the role of this lipid in skin aging is not well understood. To explore its potential functions in the skin, we used SwissSimilarity to compare DTA with structurally similar lipids. The analysis revealed that DTA shares a high similarity with several lipids: dihomo-gamma-linolenic acid (similarity score 0.999), alpha-linolenic acid (0.999), linoleic acid (0.999), gamma-linolenic acid (0.998), cis-vaccenic acid (0.997), oleic acid (0.997), gondoic acid (0.997), ethanolamine oleate (0.997), arachidonic acid (0.996), alpha-hydroxylinoleic acid (0.996), and palmitoleic acid (0.995) (Figure 1). Of these lipids, palmitoleic acid, alpha-linolenic acid, and linoleic acid [10] exhibited anti-melanogenic properties (Figure 1) [19]. Although found in minimal amounts in mammalian tissues, dihomo-gamma-linolenic acid and its metabolites are increasingly recognized as crucial mediators of inflammation, potentially playing important roles in specific disease conditions including obesity, type 2 diabetes, cardiovascular diseases, hepatic diseases, cancers, gastrointestinal diseases, arthritis, bronchial asthma, and atopic dermatitis [20]. Given the structural similarity of DTA to these lipids, we hypothesized that it might also inhibit melanogenesis. To test this hypothesis, we conducted a series of in vitro and cell-free experiments to evaluate the potential anti-melanogenic effects of DTA.

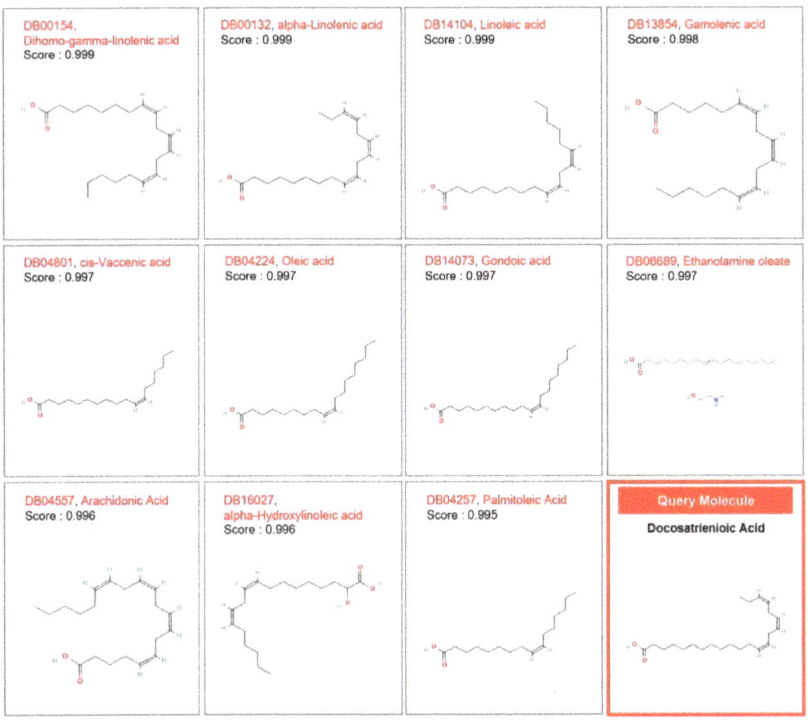

Figure 1. Structural analysis of docosatrienoic acid (DTA) using SwissSimilarity. SwissSimilarity was used to compare docosatrienoic acid (DTA) with structurally similar lipids to predict its potential

functions in the skin. SwissSimilarity enables the rapid analysis of extensive libraries, including drugs, bioactive small molecules, commercially available compounds, and an immense collection of virtual compounds that can be easily synthesized from commercially accessible reagents. The virtual screening process utilizes molecular fingerprints, as well as both super positional and non-super positional 3D shape similarity methods. The chemical structure images for the similar lipids were obtained from PubChem.

2.2. Effects of DTA on Melanogenesis and Tyrosinase Activity in B16F10 Cells

To investigate the effects of DTA on melanogenesis, we first evaluated cytotoxicity in various skin cell lines, including B16F10 cells and HS68 cells. DTA showed no toxicity in B16F10 cells up to 15 μM, whereas toxicity was observed at 100 μM in HS68 cells (Figure 2a,b). Based on these findings, we proceeded to assess melanin content in B16F10 cells. Initially, cells were pre-treated with 1 μM and 5 μM DTA, followed by induction of melanin synthesis using α-MSH for 6 days, starting one hour post-pre-treatment. Results indicated that melanin content increased by 250% with 500 nM α-MSH compared to the control, followed by a concentration-dependent decrease (Figure 2c). Notably, treatment with 5 μM DTA reduced melanin content by up to 150% compared to that of the α-MSH treated group (Figure 2c).

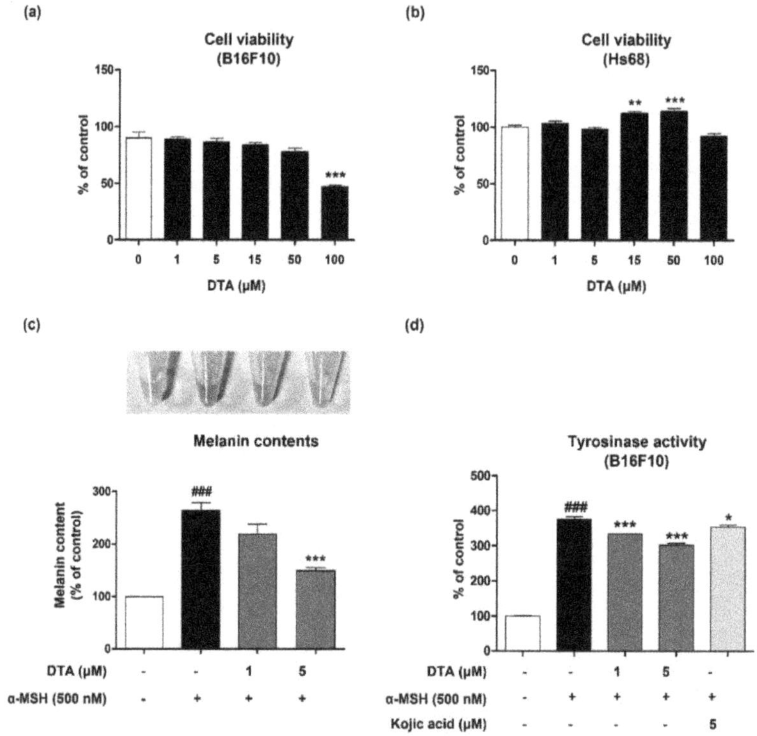

Figure 2. Effects of DTA on melanogenesis in α-MSH-induced B16F10 melanoma cells. Cell cytotoxicity was assessed in (**a**) B16F10 and (**b**) HS68 cells treated with various concentrations of DTA (1–100 μM) for 24 h (n = 4/group). (**c**) Intracellular melanin content and (**d**) tyrosinase activity were measured in B16F10 cells pretreated with various concentrations of DTA (1, 5 μM) and kojic acid (5 μM) for 1 h, followed by stimulation with α-MSH (500 nM) for 6 days (n = 4/group). Results are presented as mean ± SEM. ### $p < 0.001$ compared with the non-treated control group and * $p < 0.05$, ** $p < 0.01$, *** $p < 0.001$ compared with the α-MSH-treated group.

Furthermore, to explore the anti-melanogenic effects and mechanism of DTA, intracellular tyrosinase activity was examined. Tyrosinase activity, which had increased approximately 400% with α-MSH treatment, decreased in a dose-dependent manner with DTA treatment, showing a more pronounced reduction compared to the known anti-melanogenic positive control, kojic acid (Figure 2d). Like the results observed for melanin content, treatment with 5 μM DTA significantly reduced intracellular tyrosinase activity (Figure 2d).

2.3. Analysis of the Inhibitory Effects of DTA on Melanogenesis-Related Gene Expression

To evaluate the impact of DTA on the expression of genes involved in melanogenesis, we measured the mRNA levels of key enzymes such as *TRP-1*, *TRP-2*, and tyrosinase using real-time PCR analysis. Treatment of B16F10 cells with α-MSH significantly increased the mRNA expression levels of *TRP-1*, *TRP-2*, and *tyrosinase* (Figure 3). However, compared to the control group treated only with α-MSH, the DTA-treated group showed a dose-dependent and significant downregulation of these genes (Figure 3).

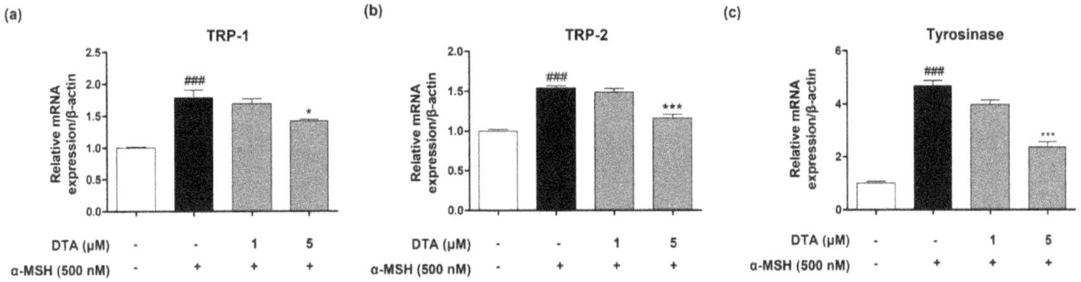

Figure 3. Effects of DTA on the expression of melanogenesis–related genes in B16F10 cells. Real-time PCR analysis of mRNA levels of (**a**) *TRP-1*, (**b**) *TRP-2*, and (**c**) *tyrosinase* in B16F10 cells treated with α-MSH and various concentrations of DTA (1 and 5 μM). The results show a significant downregulation of these genes in a dose-dependent manner with DTA treatment. Results are presented as mean ± standard error of the mean (SEM). ### $p < 0.001$ compared with the non-treated control group, and * $p < 0.05$ and *** $p < 0.001$ compared with the α-MSH-treated group.

MITF is a transcription factor for *TRP-1*, *TRP-2*, and tyrosinase, playing a crucial role in melanin production. Therefore, we used immunofluorescence staining to determine whether DTA treatment inhibits the translocation of MITF to the nucleus in B16F10 cells. The results showed that treatment with α-MSH alone showed abundant MITF in the nucleus (Figure 4). In contrast, in the DTA-treated group, the translocation of MITF was inhibited in a dose-dependent manner compared to the group treated only with α-MSH (Figure 4). These results suggest that DTA effectively inhibits the expression of genes essential for melanin synthesis, at least partially, by preventing the translocation of the key transcription factor MITF to the nucleus, highlighting its potential as a melanogenesis regulator.

2.4. Antioxidant Activity and Tyrosinase Binding Affinity of DTA

Tyrosinase is one of the most important enzymes involved in melanin production. Based on the observed anti-melanogenic effects of DTA in the previous figures, we evaluated whether DTA directly affects tyrosinase activity. Using a cell-free system with mushroom tyrosinase, we treated the enzyme with various concentrations of DTA (5–60 μM) and observed a slight inhibition of tyrosinase activity only at a concentration of 60 μM (Figure 5a).

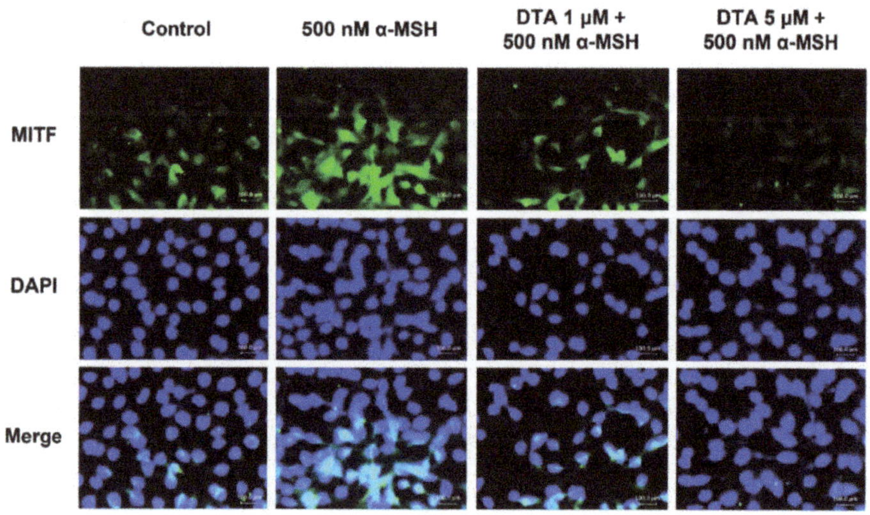

Figure 4. Effects of DTA on MITF nuclear translocation. To evaluate the inhibitory effect of DTA on the nuclear translocation of MITF, immunofluorescence analysis was conducted. B16F10 cells were treated with DTA and observed using fluorescent microscopy. MITF was detected using an anti-MITF monoclonal antibody, followed by an FSD™-conjugated secondary antibody. This analysis shows the localization of MITF and illustrates the impact of DTA on MITF nuclear translocation.

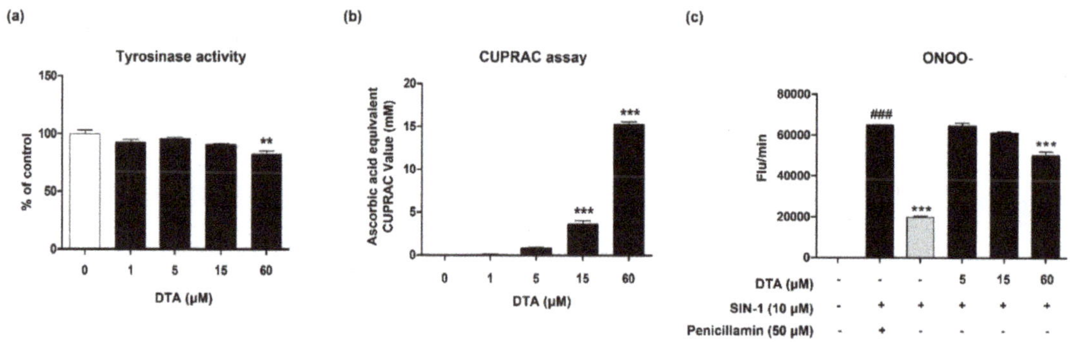

Figure 5. Tyrosinase and antioxidant activities of DTA in a cell−free system. (**a**) Tyrosinase inhibition effect of DTA measured using mushroom tyrosinase. (**b**) Copper ion reduction capacity of DTA determined by CUPRAC analysis, compared to ascorbic acid as a reference. (**c**) Peroxynitrite analysis using DHR123. Data are presented as mean ± standard error of the mean (SEM) (n = 3). Results were analyzed using one-way ANOVA followed by Dunnett's test. ** $p < 0.01$ and *** $p < 0.001$ are compared with the control group in (**a**) and (**b**), ### $p < 0.001$ is compared with the non-treated control group in (**c**), and *** $p < 0.001$ is compared with the α-MSH-treated group in (**c**).

Oxidative stress can induce melanin production, and antioxidants can inhibit melanin synthesis by reducing oxidative stress. Therefore, in this study, we investigated the antioxidant effects of DTA using the CUPRAC assay and peroxynitrite ($ONOO^-$) assay. The results showed that DTA increased the reducing power in the CUPRAC assay at concentrations of 15 μM and 60 μM (Figure 5b). Additionally, SIN-1-induced ONOO- levels were slightly reduced at 60 μM DTA (Figure 5c). Specifically, at higher concentrations (60 μM), DTA demonstrated both an inhibitory effect on mushroom tyrosinase activity and antioxidant activity.

2.5. Protein Docking Simulation of DTA with Tyrosinase

Given the previous results showing that DTA inhibits tyrosinase activity, we conducted docking studies to understand how DTA binds to and deactivates tyrosinase. We compared the docking scores of kojic acid and arbutin to DTA. The predicted binding affinities (docking scores) between tyrosinase and kojic acid, arbutin, and DTA were −5.7, −5.3 kcal/mol, and −5.7 kcal/mol, respectively (Figure 6a,c,e). To better understand their binding modes with tyrosinase, we employed LigandScout 4.4.8 software for binding mode analysis. Kojic acid demonstrated three hydrogen bond acceptor (HBA) interactions and three hydrogen bond donor (HBD) interactions, stabilizing the ligand within the tyrosinase binding site by both accepting and donating hydrogen bonds with surrounding residues (Figure 6b). Arbutin displayed a complex interaction profile with tyrosinase, including seven HBA interactions, five HBD interactions, one hydrophobic (H) interaction, and one aromatic (AR) interaction, contributing to various stabilizing effects within the binding site (Figure 6d). DTA may exhibit two HBA interactions and one negatively charged interaction (NI), potentially enhancing its binding affinity through electrostatic attraction with positively charged residues in the protein (Figure 6f).

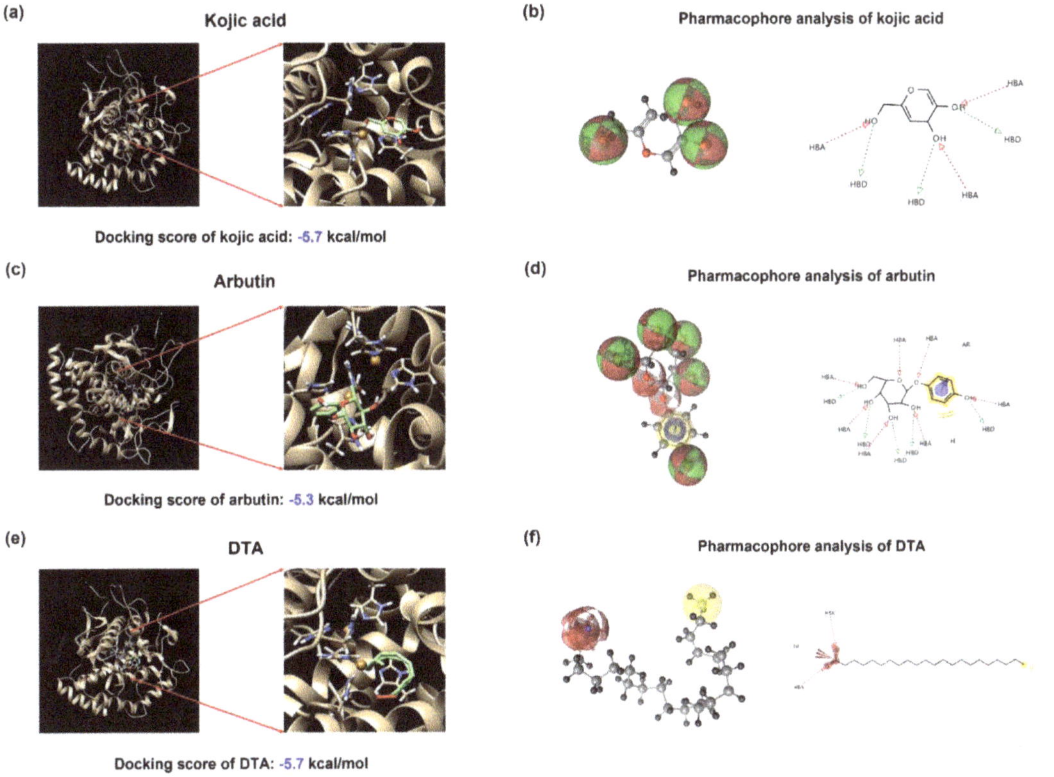

Figure 6. Computational docking analysis of tyrosinase with kojic acid, arbutin, and DTA. Binding affinity analysis between tyrosinase (PDB ID: 2Y9X) and various compounds computational structure prediction for docking simulation between mushroom tyrosinase and various compounds, including (**a**) kojic acid, (**c**) arbutin, and (**e**) dodecanoic acid (DTA). The ligand binding abilities were predicted using AutoDock Vina 1.1.2 software. The indicated boxes show the enlarged images of the binding sites within the tyrosinase structure. The docking scores were: kojic acid (−5.7 kcal/mol), arbutin (−5.3 kcal/mol), and DTA (−5.7 kcal/mol). Pharmacophore analysis was performed to analyze the binding residues of (**b**) kojic acid, (**d**) arbutin, and (**f**) DTA with tyrosinase.

3. Discussion

Although previous research indicated that docosatrienoic acid (DTA) accumulate in human fibroblast phospholipids when cultured in a basal nutrient medium (MCDB 110) with reduced fetal bovine serum levels (0.4%), the role of this lipid in skin aging is not well understood. The findings of this study support the anti-melanogenic properties of DTA, showcasing its potential in modulating melanogenesis. Previous studies have highlighted the role of various fatty acids in modulating melanogenesis, often by targeting tyrosinase activity or transcription factors like MITF. For instance, alpha-linolenic acid and linoleic acid, structurally similar to DTA, have been shown to inhibit melanogenesis through both direct and indirect pathways. Our study further supports these findings, demonstrating that DTA also reduces melanin production, primarily through the inhibition of MITF translocation [21].

Melanin pigmentation plays a critical role in protecting the skin from ultraviolet (UV) radiation, as melanin absorbs and dissipates the energy from UV rays, thereby preventing DNA damage in skin cells [22,23]. However, the role of melanin extends beyond simple photoprotection. Melanin is also involved in modulating immune responses, neuroprotection, and regulating reactive oxygen species (ROS) [5,24,25]. These additional roles highlight the importance of maintaining balanced melanin production, as both excessive and insufficient melanin can have significant physiological consequences.

UV radiation, particularly UVB, is a well-established inducer of melanogenesis. UV exposure triggers a cascade of molecular events within melanocytes, leading to increased melanin production as a protective response. However, the effects of UV radiation are not confined to the skin alone [26]. UV exposure influences various biological systems, including the neuroendocrine and immune systems, through mechanisms collectively known as "photo-neuro-immuno-endocrinology" [8]. This complexity underscores the need for a comprehensive understanding of UV radiation's impact when considering therapeutic strategies aimed at modulating melanogenesis.

Melanogenesis, the process of melanin production in the skin, is a multifaceted and tightly regulated biological pathway involving a complex network of enzymes and regulatory proteins. Central to this process is the MITF, which acts as a master regulator by controlling the expression of key melanogenic enzymes such as tyrosinase, *TRP-1*, and *TRP-2* [7]. These enzymes are essential for the biosynthesis of melanin, the pigment responsible for skin color and protection against UV radiation. Given MITF's pivotal role, it represents a strategic target for developing anti-melanogenic therapies aimed at treating hyperpigmentation disorders. Our study has provided insights into the molecular mechanisms by which DTA exerts its effects. We found that DTA effectively inhibits the nuclear translocation of MITF, resulting in a marked decrease in the transcription of melanogenic enzymes. This suppression of MITF activity consequently leads to reduced melanin production, highlighting the potential of DTA as a novel therapeutic agent for skin pigmentation disorders.

However, we believe that DTA does not directly inhibit tyrosinase activity. This conclusion is supported by the observation that DTA exhibited only a very mild inhibitory effect on mushroom tyrosinase at a high concentration of 60 μM. In contrast, significant inhibitory effects on cellular tyrosinase activity and melanin content were observed at much lower concentrations, starting from 1 μM. Therefore, we propose that the inhibitory effects of DTA on cellular tyrosinase and melanogenesis are primarily due to its impact on the mRNA expression levels of tyrosinase, likely resulting from the inactivation of MITF. This distinction may be important as it highlights the indirect mechanism by which DTA modulates melanogenesis. The indirect mechanism of action of DTA might offer several advantages in therapeutic applications. Targeting the transcriptional regulation of melanogenesis could provide a longer-lasting effect as it intervenes earlier in the melanogenic pathway. This may reduce the frequency of application needed for therapeutic effectiveness, improving patient compliance and overall treatment outcomes. Moreover, by modulating MITF activity, DTA may also influence other MITF-regulated pathways involved in cell survival and differentiation, potentially offering additional benefits in skin health and regeneration. Further research is needed to fully understand the broader implications of MITF inhibition by DTA. Investigating the long-term effects of DTA on skin cells, including potential impacts on cell viability and the expression of other MITF target genes, will be essential for developing safe and effective skin care treatments. Additionally, exploring the effects of DTA in various skin types and conditions can help tailor therapies to individual needs, enhancing the efficacy and safety of treatments for hyperpigmentation disorders.

The structural resemblance between DTA and other well-documented anti-melanogenic lipids, such as palmitoleic acid, alpha-linolenic acid, and linoleic acid, was a pivotal component of our research. These lipids are known for their capacity to inhibit melanogenesis, and our findings indicate that DTA shares this functional characteristic. This resemblance suggests that DTA might operate through similar biochemical pathways, potentially offering comparable efficacy in reducing melanin production. Utilizing SwissSimilarity for structural and functional predictions highlights the importance of bioinformatics tools in identifying and validating potential bioactive compounds [17]. These tools enable researchers to predict the functional capabilities of new compounds based on structural similarities to known active molecules. In our study, SwissSimilarity provided critical insights that guided our experimental focus, helping to prioritize DTA as a candidate for further investigation. By leveraging these predictions, we were able to streamline the research process, ensuring a more targeted and efficient exploration of DTA's anti-melanogenic potential. The application of such bioinformatics tools is not only useful for predicting the functional properties of compounds but also for understanding their potential interactions within biological systems.

Although further studies are necessary, DTA may also hold considerable promise for the cosmetic industry, offering benefits that span beyond its anti-melanogenic properties. Fatty acids and their derivatives are fundamental components in cosmetic formulations due to their multifaceted roles in enhancing product stability, functionality, and aesthetic appeal. They are crucial not only for maintaining the skin's lipid barrier, thus preventing transepidermal water loss and ensuring optimal hydration—key considerations for anti-aging and sensitive skin products—but also for reinforcing the skin's protective shield against environmental stressors such as UV radiation and pollutants.

In cosmetic formulations, fatty acid derivatives such as esters play an indispensable role in creating emulsions, particularly in formulations like water-in-oil (W/O) and oil-in-water (O/W). These derivatives significantly enhance the sensory attributes and spreadability of products, thereby improving consumer experience and acceptance. Additionally, fatty acid-derived surfactants are crucial in micellar solubilization processes, which are pivotal for increasing the bioavailability and efficacy of hydrophobic active ingredients in aqueous-based formulations. This capability is particularly advantageous for incorporating potent anti-aging compounds like retinoids into skincare products.

Beyond their emulsifying and solubilizing properties, fatty acids serve as effective moisturizers and skin conditioners, contributing to the overall sensory profile and efficacy of cosmetic formulations [27]. They play a key role in maintaining skin suppleness, smoothness, and elasticity—attributes that are essential for anti-aging and moisturizing products. Moreover, fatty acids possess soothing and anti-inflammatory properties, making them suitable for formulations aimed at addressing sensitive or irritated skin conditions. Further investigation is warranted to explore the potential application of DTA in these cosmetic fields. Its structural similarity to other effective anti-melanogenic and skincare-active lipids suggests that DTA could offer similar or complementary benefits in cosmetic formulations. Research into its specific mechanisms of action, compatibility with other ingredients, and efficacy in diverse product formulations will be essential for fully realizing its potential in skincare and cosmetic applications.

4. Materials and Methods

4.1. Material

Docosatrienoic acid (DTA): DTA was obtained as part of a fatty acid library purchased from Enzo Life Sciences (Catalog No. BML-L1120-0001) The equipment was sourced from Lausen, Switzerland. This library includes a variety of fatty acids, which were screened for potential anti-melanogenic compounds. Enzo Life Sciences is known for providing high-quality biochemical products, and this library has been extensively used in lipid research studies.

Other Reagents and Materials: The mushroom tyrosinase, NaOH, DCFDA, esterase, Trolox, DHR123, penicillamine, and most other reagents used in this study were purchased from Sigma (St. Louis, MO, USA). Additionally, primers for tyrosinase, microphthalmia-associated transcription factor (MITF), tyrosinase-related protein 1 (*TRP*-1), and tyrosinase-related protein 2 (*TRP*-2) were mostly ordered from Bioneer (Daejeon, Republic of Korea). The anti-MITF antibody used for staining was obtained from Santa Cruz Biotechnology (Santa Cruz, CA, USA). The chemical structure images of lipids used in this study were sourced from PubChem.

4.2. Structural Analysis Using SwissSimilarity

We utilized the web-based tool SwissSimilarity to identify compounds structurally similar to DTA and predict its potential biological functions. DTA (docosatrienoic acid, PubChem CID 5312557) showed high similarity scores with several fatty acids, including palmitoleic acid (PubChem CID 445638), cis-vaccenic acid (PubChem CID 5282761), ethanolamine oleate (PubChem CID 16759), oleic acid (PubChem CID 445639), alpha-linolenic acid (PubChem CID 5280934), gondoic acid (PubChem CID 5282768), gamolenic acid (PubChem CID 5280933), dihomo-gamma-linolenic acid (PubChem CID 5280581), arachidonic acid (PubChem CID 444899), alpha-hydroxylinoleic acid (PubChem CID 21158511), and linoleic acid (PubChem CID 5280450). The chemical structure images for these similar lipids were obtained from PubChem. Based on these similarities, we hypothesized that DTA might inhibit melanogenesis. To test this hypothesis, we conducted in vitro and cell-free experiments, applying various concentrations of DTA to melanocyte cultures and related cell lines to assess its impact on melanin synthesis and the expression of melanogenesis-related genes.

4.3. Cell Line and Culture Condition

The cells used in this study were B16F10 mouse melanoma cells and HS68 human primary fibroblasts. B16F10 cells were cultured in Dulbecco's Modified Eagle's Medium (DMEM) supplemented with 10% fetal bovine serum and 1% penicillin/streptomycin, incubated at 37 °C in a 5% CO_2 atmosphere. HS68 cells were cultured in DMEM supplemented with 10% fetal bovine serum and 1% penicillin/streptomycin under the same conditions (37 °C in a 5% CO_2 atmosphere).

4.4. Cell Viability Assay

B16F10 cells were cultured in a 96-well plate at a seeding density of 5×10^3; cells/well for 48 h. Subsequently, they were treated with DTA at concentrations ranging from 1 to 100 μM and cultured for 24 h. All wells were incubated with 5 μL of MTS reagent from the Promega MTS assay kit (CellTiter96® AQueous One Solution, Promega Corporation, Madison, WI, USA) for 1 h, and absorbance was measured at 490 nm using a microplate reader (Molecular Devices, San Jose, CA, USA).

HS68 cells were cultured in a 96-well plate at a seeding density of 8×10^3; cells/well for 48 h. They were treated with DTA at the same concentrations (1 to 100 μM) and under the same conditions as the B16F10 cells.

4.5. Melanin Contents

B16F10 cells (5×10^3;) treated with DTA were incubated in 1 N NaOH solution at 60 °C for 1 h to induce lysis. The resulting lysates (100 μL each) were then transferred to a 96-well plate. Absorbance readings to measure melanin content were taken at 409 nm using a spectrophotometer. To quantify protein levels in the same samples, 5 μL of each lysate was used for the BCA assay, with absorbance measured at 560 nm. The melanin absorbance values at 409 nm were then normalized to the protein content determined by the BCA assay to ensure accurate comparisons across samples [28–30].

4.6. *Real-Time PCR*

After treating B16F10 cells with DTA, we investigated its effects on melanogenesis by analyzing the expression of *tyrosinase*, *TRP-1*, and *TRP-2* genes. Total RNA (1 μg) was extracted using the RiboEXTM extraction kit (GeneAll, Seoul, Republic of Korea), followed by cDNA synthesis using the Primer Script RT Reagent kit (SMART GENE, Daejeon, Republic of Korea). For real-time PCR analysis, 2 μL of cDNA was added to each well of a PCR plate, mixed with 18 μL of buffer containing specific primers for tyrosinase, *TRP-1*, and *TRP-2*. Subsequently, 50 μL of TOPrealTM SYBR Green qPCR PreMIX (Enzynomics, Daejeon, Republic of Korea) was added to each well. Real-time PCR reactions were conducted using the QuantStudioTM 1 Real-Time PCR System (Applied Biosystems, Foster City, CA, USA). Gene expression levels were normalized using β-actin as a housekeeping gene, and ΔΔCt values were calculated for analysis.

The primer sequences are as follows. Tyrosinase: F: 5′-TTCTGCCTTGGCACAGACTT-3′, R: 5′-CTGCCAGGAGGAGAAGAAGG-3′, TRP-1: F: 5′-GCTGCAGGAGCCTTCTTTCTC-3′, R: 5′-GTCATCAGTGCAGACATCGC-3′, TRP-2: F: 5′-CTCAGAGCTCGGGCTCAGTT-3′, R: 5′-CTGCCAGGAGGAGAAGAAGG-3′.

4.7. *Immunofluorescence Staining*

Immunofluorescence staining was performed according to previously established protocols. B16F10 cells were treated with 1 μM and 5 μM of DTA, and then 1 h later, they were treated with 500 nM α-MSH and stimulated for 6 days. Cells were washed twice with PBS and fixed with 4% paraformaldehyde for 15 min. After fixation, the membrane was washed again with PBS and treated with 0.5% Triton X-100 for 5 min to permeabilize the membrane. Next, cells were incubated with MITF 1 antibody (1:100, sc-515925, Santa Cruz Biotechnology, Santa Cruz, CA, USA) overnight in the dark. Cells were washed with PBS and incubated with FSD™ 488-conjugated secondary antibody (1:500, RSA1145, BioActs, Incheon, Republic of Korea) for 1 h. Cell nuclei were counterstained with DAPI (4′,6-diamidino-2-phenylindole dihydrochloride), cells were observed under a fluorescence microscope, and images were taken.

4.8. *Mushroom Tyrosinase Activity*

To measure tyrosinase activity, 10 μL of DTA at various concentrations was added to each well of a 96-well microplate, followed by mixing with 180 μL of phosphate buffer (pH 6.8) containing 1 mM L-Tyrosine. Then, 10 μL of mushroom tyrosinase (1000 units) was added, and the reaction was allowed to proceed in the dark at 37 °C for 30 min. Absorbance at 492 nm was measured using a microplate reader.

4.9. *CUPRAC Assay*

The CUPRAC solution was prepared by mixing $CuCl_2$ (10 mM), neocuproine (75 mM) diluted in MeOH, and distilled water in specific ratios. Each sample was added to a 96-well plate at a volume of 2 μL per well. Then, 198 μL of the prepared solution was added to each well. The plate was incubated in a dry oven at 37 °C for 10 min, protected from oxygen and light. After incubation, absorbance was recorded at 450 nm. Ascorbic acid served as the standard.

4.10. *$ONOO^-$ Assay*

Peroxynitrite ($ONOO^-$) was measured using dihydrorhodamine 123 (DHR 123). DHR 123 was dissolved in PBS to achieve a final concentration of 5 μM. 3-Morpholinosydnonimine

(SIN-1), an $ONOO^-$ donor, was added to the DHR 123 solution to a final concentration of 1 mM in a test tube. The mixture was incubated in the dark at 37 °C for 30 min. The fluorescence intensity was measured using a fluorescence spectrophotometer with an excitation wavelength of 500 nm and an emission wavelength of 536 nm. An increase in fluorescence intensity indicated the generation of $ONOO^-$.

4.11. Protein-Ligand Docking Simulation

Protein-ligand docking simulations were executed using AutoDock Vina 1.1.2. Predictions of binding affinity were based on the 3D structure of the tyrosinase protein from Agaricus bisporus (PDB ID: 2Y9X), accessed through the Protein Data Bank. For comparing binding affinity with tyrosinase, arbutin and kojic acid, recognized for their inhibitory effects on tyrosinase, were the primary ligands under investigation. Utilizing the binding site of tropolone as a reference for each protein structure, the tyrosinase binding sites for arbutin (CID: 440936) and kojic acid (CID: 3840) were delineated, with an additional exploration into the potential binding of DTA (HMDB ID: HMDB0002823) to the same site. Ligand structures for arbutin and kojic acid were obtained from PubChem via database searches, while the structure for DTA was obtained from the Human Metabolome Database (HMDB).

4.12. Statistical Analysis

Statistical analyses were performed using GraphPad Prism version 5.0 (GraphPad Software, San Diego, CA, USA). All experiments were conducted in triplicate, and data are presented as mean ± standard deviation (SD). Comparisons between multiple groups were made using one-way analysis of variance (ANOVA), followed by Tukey's post-hoc test for multiple comparisons. All statistical tests were two-tailed, and significance levels were set at $p < 0.05$, $p < 0.01$, and $p < 0.001$, as indicated in the figure legends.

5. Conclusions

In summary, this study demonstrates that while DTA does not directly inhibit tyrosinase activity, it significantly impacts melanogenesis by modulating MITF activity and reducing tyrosinase mRNA expression. This modulation leads to a decrease in melanin production, indicating that DTA operates through an indirect mechanism that targets the transcriptional regulation of melanogenesis. These findings highlight DTA's potential as a novel and targeted approach for skin depigmentation, offering an effective alternative for managing hyperpigmentation disorders.

Moreover, the ability of DTA to influence melanin production through the regulation of MITF and associated pathways suggests that it could provide more sustained and comprehensive effects compared to direct enzyme inhibitors. This indirect mechanism positions DTA as a promising candidate for both therapeutic and cosmetic applications aimed at improving skin aesthetics. These findings lay a strong foundation for further research to explore the practical implementation of DTA in skincare products, particularly for conditions involving excessive pigmentation.

Author Contributions: Writing—review and editing, K.M.M. and B.L.; funding acquisition, K.M.M. and B.L.; data curation, M.-K.L. and A.-r.K.; formal analysis, M.-K.L.; investigation, S.-Y.P. and J.S.; visualization, S.-Y.P.; resources, J.S.; validation, A.-r.K.; supervision, B.L. All authors have read and agreed to the published version of the manuscript.

Funding: This work was supported by the Pukyong National University Industry–University Cooperation Research Fund in 2023 (202312160001). This research was also supported by a National Research Foundation of Korea (NRF) grant funded by the Ministry of Education (NRF-2021R1A6A1A03039211 and NRF-2022R1C1C2005467).

Institutional Review Board Statement: Not applicable.

Informed Consent Statement: Not applicable.

Data Availability Statement: Data are contained within the article.

Conflicts of Interest: The authors declare no conflicts of interest.

References

1. Snyman, M.; Walsdorf, R.E.; Wix, S.N.; Gill, J.G. The metabolism of melanin synthesis—From melanocytes to melanoma. *Pigment. Cell Melanoma Res.* **2024**, *37*, 438–452. [CrossRef] [PubMed]
2. Qian, W.; Liu, W.; Zhu, D.; Cao, Y.; Tang, A.; Gong, G.; Su, H. Natural skin-whitening compounds for the treatment of melanogenesis (Review). *Exp. Ther. Med.* **2020**, *20*, 173–185. [CrossRef] [PubMed]
3. Dabas, G.; Vinay, K. Psychological disturbances in patients with pigmentary disorders: A cross-sectional study. *J. Eur. Acad. Dermatol. Venereol.* **2020**, *34*, 392–399. [CrossRef] [PubMed]
4. Vinardell, M.P.; Maddaleno, A.S.; Mitjans, M. Melanogenesis and Hypopigmentation: The Case of Vitiligo. *Indian J. Dermatol.* **2022**, *67*, 524–530. [CrossRef]
5. Slominski, R.M.; Sarna, T.; Płonka, P.M.; Raman, C.; Brożyna, A.A.; Slominski, A.T. Melanoma, melanin, and melanogenesis: The Yin and Yang relationship. *Front. Oncol.* **2022**, *12*, 842496. [CrossRef]
6. Lee, M.K.; Ryu, H.; Lee, J.Y.; Jeong, H.H.; Baek, J.; Van, J.Y.; Kim, M.J.; Jung, W.K. Potential Beneficial Effects of *Sargassum* spp. in Skin Aging. *Mar. Drugs* **2022**, *20*, 540. [CrossRef]
7. Pillaiyar, T.; Manickam, M.; Jung, S.-H. Recent development of signaling pathways inhibitors of melanogenesis. *Cell. Signal.* **2017**, *40*, 99–115. [CrossRef] [PubMed]
8. Slominski, R.M.; Chen, J.Y.; Raman, C.; Slominski, A.T. Photo-neuro-immuno-endocrinology: How the ultraviolet radiation regulates the body, brain, and immune system. *Proc. Natl. Acad. Sci. USA* **2024**, *121*, e2308374121. [CrossRef] [PubMed]
9. Kelm, G.R.; Wickett, R.R. Chapter 12—The Role of Fatty Acids in Cosmetic Technology. In *Fatty Acids*; Ahmad, M.U., Ed.; AOCS Press: Champaign, IL, USA, 2017; pp. 385–404.
10. Ando, H.; Ryu, A.; Hashimoto, A.; Oka, M.; Ichihashi, M. Linoleic acid and α-linolenic acid lightens ultraviolet-induced hyperpigmentation of the skin. *Arch. Dermatol. Res.* **1998**, *290*, 375–381. [CrossRef]
11. Yamada, H.; Hakozaki, M.; Uemura, A.; Yamashita, T. Effect of fatty acids on melanogenesis and tumor cell growth in melanoma cells. *J. Lipid Res.* **2019**, *60*, 1491–1502. [CrossRef]
12. Chocarro-Calvo, A.; Jociles-Ortega, M.; Garcia-Martinez, J.M.; Louphrasitthiphol, P.; Vivas-Garcia, Y.; Ramírez-Sánchez, A.; Chauhan, J.; Fiuza, M.C.; Duran, M.; García-Jiménez, C. Phenotype-specific melanoma uptake of fatty acid from human adipocytes activates AXL and CAV1-dependent beta-catenin nuclear accumulation. *bioRxiv* **2024**. [CrossRef]
13. Innocenzi, D.; Alo, P.; Balzani, A.; Sebastiani, V.; Silipo, V.; La Torre, G.; Ricciardi, G.; Bosman, C.; Calvieri, S. Fatty acid synthase expression in melanoma. *J. Cutan. Pathol.* **2003**, *30*, 23–28. [CrossRef]
14. Shabani, F.; Sariri, R. Increase of melanogenesis in the presence of fatty acids. *Pharmacologyonline* **2010**, *1*, 314–323.
15. Krutetskaia, Z.I.; Lebedev, O.E.; Roshchina, N.G.; Butov, S.N. The effect of docosatrienoic acid on the potassium channels of outward rectification in the membrane of rat peritoneal macrophages. *Fiziol. Zhurnal Im. I.M. Sechenova* **1995**, *81*, 111–119.
16. Chen, Y.; Qiu, X.; Yang, J. Comparing the in vitro antitumor, antioxidant and anti-inflammatory activities between two new very long chain polyunsaturated fatty acids, docosadienoic acid (DDA) and docosatrienoic acid (DTA), and docosahexaenoic acid (DHA). *Nutr. Cancer* **2021**, *73*, 1697–1707. [CrossRef]
17. Zoete, V.; Daina, A.; Bovigny, C.; Michielin, O. SwissSimilarity: A Web Tool for Low to Ultra High Throughput Ligand-Based Virtual Screening. *J. Chem. Inf. Model.* **2016**, *56*, 1399–1404. [CrossRef]
18. Karmiol, S.; Bettger, W.J. Accumulation of (n-9)-eicosatrienoic and docosatrienoic acids in human fibroblast phospholipids. *Lipids* **1988**, *23*, 891–898. [CrossRef] [PubMed]
19. Yoon, W.J.; Kim, M.J.; Moon, J.Y.; Kang, H.J.; Kim, G.O.; Lee, N.H.; Hyun, C.G. Effect of palmitoleic acid on melanogenic protein expression in murine b16 melanoma. *J. Oleo Sci.* **2010**, *59*, 315–319. [CrossRef]
20. Mustonen, A.M.; Nieminen, P. Dihomo-γ-Linolenic Acid (20:3n-6)-Metabolism, Derivatives, and Potential Significance in Chronic Inflammation. *Int. J. Mol. Sci.* **2023**, *24*, 2116. [CrossRef]
21. Ando, H.; Wen, Z.-M.; Kim, H.-Y.; Valencia, J.C.; Costin, G.-E.; Watabe, H.; Yasumoto, K.-i.; Niki, Y.; Kondoh, H.; Ichihashi, M. Intracellular composition of fatty acid affects the processing and function of tyrosinase through the ubiquitin–proteasome pathway. *Biochem. J.* **2006**, *394*, 43–50. [CrossRef]
22. Solano, F. Photoprotection and skin pigmentation: Melanin-related molecules and some other new agents obtained from natural sources. *Molecules* **2020**, *25*, 1537. [CrossRef] [PubMed]
23. Eller, M.S.; Ostrom, K.; Gilchrest, B.A. DNA damage enhances melanogenesis. *Proc. Natl. Acad. Sci. USA* **1996**, *93*, 1087–1092. [CrossRef] [PubMed]
24. Lee, M.; Kim, D.; Park, S.-H.; Jung, J.; Cho, W.; Yu, A.R.; Lee, J. Fish Collagen Peptide (Naticol®) Protects the Skin from Dryness, Wrinkle Formation, and Melanogenesis Both In Vitro and In Vivo. *Prev. Nutr. Food Sci.* **2022**, *27*, 423. [CrossRef]
25. Lee, H.-S.; Cho, H.-J.; Lee, K.-W.; Park, S.-S.; Seo, H.-C.; Suh, H.-J. Antioxidant activities and melanogenesis inhibitory effects of Terminalia chebula in B16/F10 melanoma cells. *Prev. Nutr. Food Sci.* **2010**, *15*, 213–220. [CrossRef]
26. Panich, U. Antioxidant defense and UV-induced melanogenesis: Implications for melanoma prevention. In *Current Management of Malignant Melanoma*; IntechOpen: Rijeka, Croatia, 2011; pp. 227–252.
27. Slipicevic, A.; Jørgensen, K.; Skrede, M.; Rosnes, A.K.R.; Trøen, G.; Davidson, B.; Flørenes, V.A. The fatty acid binding protein 7 (FABP7) is involved in proliferation and invasion of melanoma cells. *BMC Cancer* **2008**, *8*, 276. [CrossRef] [PubMed]

28. Lee, M.-K.; Ryu, H.; Jeong, H.H.; Lee, B. Brassinin abundant in Brassicaceae suppresses melanogenesis through dual mechanisms of tyrosinase inhibition. *Foods* **2022**, *12*, 121. [CrossRef]
29. Moon, K.M.; Yang, J.-H.; Lee, M.-K.; Kwon, E.-B.; Baek, J.; Hwang, T.; Kim, J.-I.; Lee, B. Maclurin exhibits antioxidant and anti-tyrosinase activities, suppressing melanogenesis. *Antioxidants* **2022**, *11*, 1164. [CrossRef]
30. Moon, K.M.; Kim, C.Y.; Ma, J.Y.; Lee, B. Xanthone-related compounds as an anti-browning and antioxidant food additive. *Food Chem.* **2019**, *274*, 345–350. [CrossRef]

pharmaceuticals

MDPI

Article

Enhanced Anti-Obesity Effects of Euphorbia Kansui Extract through Macrophage and Gut Microbiota Modulation: A Real-World Clinical and In Vivo Study

Ji-Won Noh, Jung-Hwa Yoo and Byung-Cheol Lee *

Department of Clinical Korean Medicine, College of Korean Medicine, Graduate School, Kyung Hee University, 26 Kyungheedae-ro, Dongdaemun-gu, Seoul 02447, Republic of Korea; oiwon1002@khu.ac.kr (J.-W.N.); yoojh872@gmail.com (J.-H.Y.)

* Correspondence: hydrolee@khu.ac.kr; Tel.: +82-2-958-9182

Abstract: Rising obesity and associated multi-systemic complications amplify the health burden. Euphorbia kansui (EK) extract is clinically recognized for managing obesity. In a human study, 240 obese individuals were categorized into two cohorts: those receiving solely herbal medicine (HM group) and those administered EK concomitantly with herbal medicine (EK group). An in vivo examination using C57BL/6-Lep^{ob}/Lep^{ob} mice elucidated mechanisms involving macrophages and gut microbiota with associated metabolic advantages. The clinical study revealed a significant 7.22% body weight reduction during 91.55 average treatment days and examined 16.71% weight loss at 300 days after treatment. In whole subjects, 60.4%, 21.3%, and 6.3% achieved weight reductions exceeding 5%, 10%, and 15%, respectively. Impressively, the EK group exhibited superior weight loss compared to the HM group (EK: −7.73% vs. HM: −6.27%, $p = 0.012$). The anti-obesity effect was positively associated with EK therapy frequency and herbal medicine duration. In the in vivo study, EK significantly improved insulin sensitivity and mitigated infiltration of adipose tissue macrophages (ATMs) by modulating the CD11c+ and CD206+ subtypes. EK also correlated with increased *Bacteroidetes* and *Firmicutes* populations and reduced *Proteobacteria* and *Verrucomicrobia*. Consequently, EK is an effective adjunctive anti-obesity therapy offering metabolic benefits by modulating ATMs and gut microbiota profiles.

Keywords: anti-obesity; herbal remedies; Euphorbia kansui; insulin resistance; gut microbiota; adipose tissue macrophage; weight management

1. Introduction

The global attention on obesity is driven by its detrimental effect on a range of health problems; however, there are few effective treatments to target both body weight reduction and improvement of insulin resistance, such as lifestyle, pharmaceutical, and surgical options, which are limited by hard maintenance or adverse effects involving psychological, gastrointestinal, or cardiovascular events [1,2].

The intricate interplay between the accumulation of body fat and its resultant impact on systemic metabolism and immune equilibrium underscores the overarching significance of this issue [3]. Obesity evolves into a chronic inflammatory state with low grade derived by adipose tissue macrophages (ATMs), primarily connecting obesity to the development of insulin resistance, which initiates from aberrant lipolysis and cytokine secretion in adipose tissue [4]. In obese individuals, the precursor monocytes infiltrate adipose tissue in greater numbers, and the ATMs are frequently polarized toward the M1 pro-inflammatory profile, releasing cytokines that impair insulin signaling [5,6]. Recently, the intestinal microbiome has been suggested as a therapeutic target for metabolic problems because the changes in microbial phyla have been reported to affect body composition [7]. High-fat diet feeding changes gut permeability and elevates lipopolysaccharide (LPS) levels, which is essential in triggering infiltration of ATMs. However, weight gain, as well as insulin intolerance, also arise upon modification of intestinal microbiota, irrespective of microbiota-induced LPS production [8].

Euphorbia kansui radix (EK), also known as Gan Sui, is a traditional Korean medicinal herb belonging to the Euphorbiaceae family and was first recorded "Shen nong ben cao jing" to attack the water by diarrhea [9]. The therapeutic properties of EK have been reported on cirrhotic ascites [10], pleural effusion [11], diuresis [12], and various cancers [13,14]. The immunomodulatory activities were especially reported, in which EK suppressed Th17 and Th1 differentiation related to excessive inflammation and autoimmune diseases [15]. Van et al. demonstrated that Euphorbia tirucalli, a plant in the Euphorbiaceae family, suppressed CD4+ and CD8+ T cells associated with interleukin-2 and interferon and also inhibited the migration of leukocytes [16]. With respect to metabolic diseases, previous studies revealed that other species in Euphorbiaceae had anti-diabetic [17] and anti-obesity properties [18]; however, there are few studies on EK, though EK therapy has been applied in obese patients in Republic of Korea [19]. Therefore, we collected the clinical data about EK therapy, confirmed the in vivo effects on body weight and insulin resistance, and investigated the mechanisms via monocytes, ATMs, and intestinal microbiota.

2. Results

2.1. Clinical Results from the Human Study

2.1.1. Baseline Characteristics

A total of 480 patients who first visited the Weight Management Center to lose weight took herbal medicine (HM) treatment based on the TKM theory. Among them, 240 patients were studied, while the other 240 patients were excluded from the analysis due to overweight, not obesity, or a lack of follow-up visits (Figure 1).

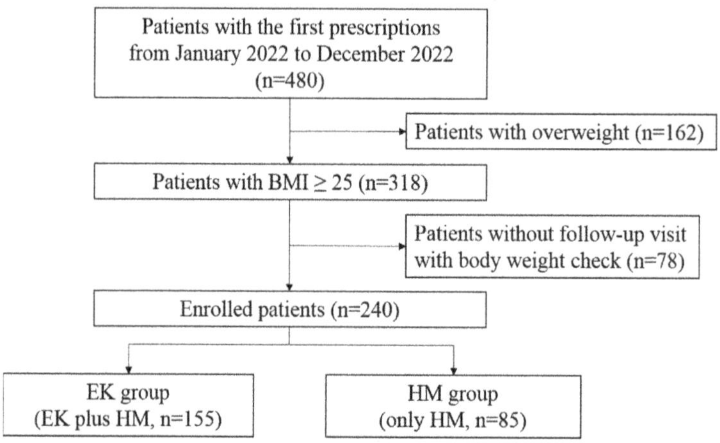

Figure 1. The flow chart of clinical study. BMI, body mass index; EK, Euphorbia kansui; HM, herbal medicine.

The number of patients who took EK therapy was 155. Demographic characteristics at baseline did not differ significantly between the EK group and the HM group, including age, height, smoking and drinking habits, and follow-up duration. However, we confirmed the significant tendency of patients with high body weight, BMI, and body fluid to perform EK therapy on the first visit (Table 1). The primary procedure of EK therapy entails inducing diarrhea and vomiting, typically lasting for 6 to 8 h. In the EK group, 58.95% of patients experienced only diarrhea without vomiting, and the number of diarrhea and vomiting was 5.51 ± 2.38 and 0.79 ± 1.24, respectively. The compliance rates of both groups were 68.3 ± 23.5 and 67.2 ± 24.5%, respectively.

Table 1. Baseline characteristics of enrolled patients.

Variables	Total	EK Group [1]	HM Group	p Value
N	240	155	85	
Age (years)	41.28 ± 12.17	41.75 ± 12.20	40.42 ± 12.14	0.442
Male:Female (%)	29.58:70.42	34.19:65.80	21.18:78.82	0.034
Height (cm)	164.6 ± 8.41	165.4 ± 8.78	163.3 ± 7.52	0.062
Body weight (kg)	81.25 ± 14.73	84.75 ± 15.38	74.88 ± 10.97	<0.001
BMI (kg/m^2)	29.84 ± 4.12	30.85 ± 4.34	28.01 ± 2.94	<0.001
Follow-up duration (days)	91.55 ± 66.77	93.30 ± 70.43	88.36 ± 59.78	0.903
Fat weight (kg)	32.27 ± 15.75	33.93 ± 17.89	28.31 ± 7.49	<0.001
Muscle weight (kg)	27.91 ± 6.41	28.81 ± 6.60	25.80 ± 5.42	<0.001
Body fluid (kg)	36.95 ± 7.76	38.09 ± 7.96	34.26 ± 6.58	<0.001
Smokers (%)	16.35	18.71	12.05	
Non-drinkers (%)	41.66	38.06	51.81	

[1] Patients in the EK group received EK and HM treatments. *p* values show the results from Mann–Whitney U test and student's *t*-test between EK and HM groups. BMI, body mass index.

2.1.2. Effects on Body Weight

Significant changes in the percentage of body weight reduction were observed from baseline to the final visit of each participant in the trial period (−7.22 ± 5.16%, $p < 0.001$). The impact on weight loss in the EK group was significantly greater than the corresponding effect in the HM group (−7.73 ± 4.98% vs. −6.27 ± 5.40%, $p = 0.012$) (Figure 2a). In total participants, the mean changes in BMI from baseline to each final visit was −2.14 ± 1.85 kg/m^2 (Figure 2c). The changes in both body weight and BMI demonstrated a statistically significant difference between the EK and HM groups ($p < 0.001$) (Figure 2b,c). In total participants, the average body weight reduction increased over the course of the treatment, and the estimated mean body weight change from baseline to 300 days was −17.6 ± 7.01% (Figure 2d). At 30, 60, and 90 days, the average body weight changes were significantly greater in the EK group compared to the HM group (Figure 2d). The percentages of participants in the EK group who achieved ≥5%, ≥10%, and ≥15% body weight loss were 66.4%, 21.9%, and 7.09%, and those in the HM group were 57.9%, 20.4%, and 6.02%, respectively (Figure 2e). The trial number of EK therapy affected the mean body weight reduction by HM treatment (Figure 2f).

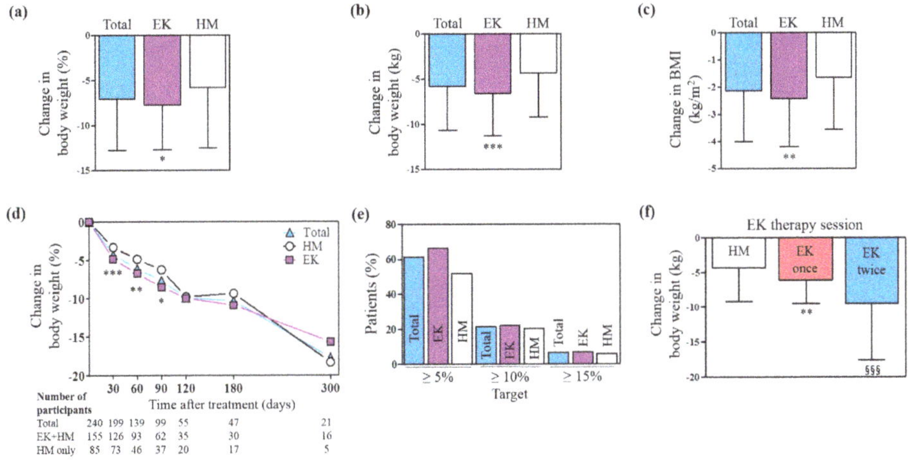

Figure 2. Anti-obesity outcomes of EK therapy and HM treatment. Change in body weight by (**a**) percentage and (**b**) kg, and (**c**) BMI from baseline to the final visit. (**d**) Mean changes from baseline in body weight. (**e**) Proportions of participants achieving body weight reductions of at least 5, 10, and 15%. (**f**) Mean body weight changes according to the trial number of EK therapy throughout the treatment period. * $p < 0.05$; ** $p < 0.01$; *** $p < 0.001$ versus HM group. §§§ $p < 0.001$ versus the EK once group. EK, Euphorbia kansui; HM, herbal medicine; BMI, body mass index.

2.1.3. Change in the Body Compositions

In the whole participants, fat weights were significantly changed at the final visit compared to the first visit (−3.35 ± 4.94 kg, $p < 0.001$), but muscle and body fluid were not significantly changed ($p > 0.05$). The changes in fat weight were not significantly different between the two groups ($p = 0.15$); however, the weights of body fluid and muscle decreased in the EK group and increased in the HM group with significant differences ($p < 0.01$) (Figure 3).

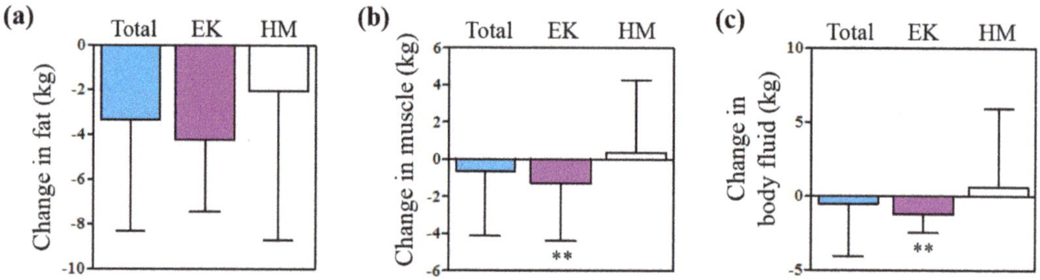

Figure 3. Change in (**a**) fat weight, (**b**) muscle weight, and (**c**) body fluid. Subgroup analysis divided by the number of EK therapy trials. ** $p < 0.01$ versus the HM group. EK, Euphorbia kansui; HM, herbal medicine.

2.1.4. Adverse Events after EK Therapy and during HM Treatment

There was no severe adverse event or unpredictable event after EK therapy, but two patients reported mild abdominal pain until the following day after EK therapy, and one patient reported mild dizziness on the day of EK therapy. There were two patients in the EK group who dropped out because of systolic blood pressure elevation above 200 mmHg and no favorable weight loss, respectively. Any serious adverse event was not reported throughout the duration of HM treatment. Among 200 patients observed at 30 days, 72.5% reported no side effects. The most frequently reported side effect experienced by patients during HM treatment was poor sleep quality; however, its severity was not sufficient to result in treatment discontinuation. Mild constipation, dry mouth, diarrhea, and nausea were the subsequent most commonly reported adverse events.

2.2. *Results from Animal Model*

2.2.1. Body Weight, Glucose Metabolism, and Lipid Profile

Both the ob/ob and EK groups demonstrated no significant difference in body and epi fat weights. At 4 and 8 weeks, the fasting blood glucose (FBG) of the EK group was significantly lower than that of the ob/ob group (Figure 4). In oral glucose tolerance tests (OGTT), the blood glucose levels at 30, 60, 90, and 120 min were significantly reduced in the EK group compared to the ob/ob group. The area under the curve (AUC) also showed a similar propensity. The EK group showed decreased fasting serum insulin (FSI) and homeostatic model assessment for insulin resistance (HOMA-IR) compared to the ob/ob group (FSI: 2.62 ± 0.58 ng/mL vs. 5.66 ± 1.36 ng/mL, $p = 0.07$; HOMA-IR: 48.30 ± 14.29 vs. 175.13 ± 42.40, $p < 0.05$). Among lipids, triglyceride (TG) and non-esterified fatty acid (NEFA) concentrations in the EK group were significantly decreased compared to the ob/ob group (Figure 4).

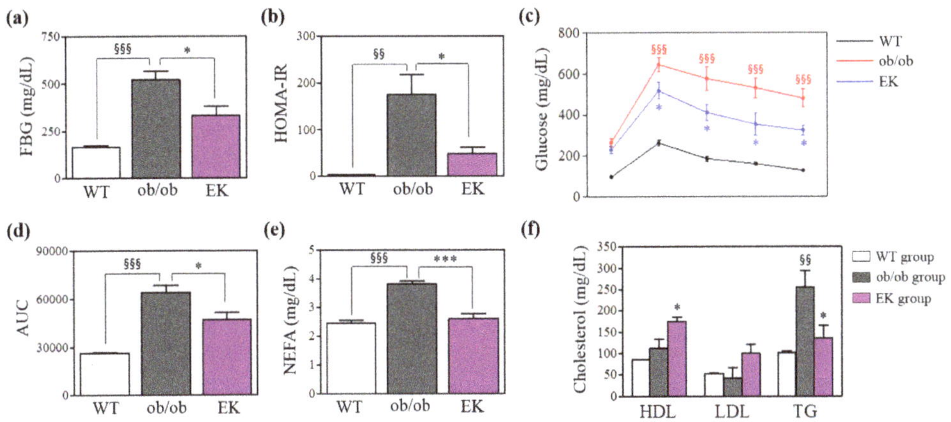

Figure 4. Metabolic benefits of Euphorbia kansui in the animal study. Comparison between three groups in (**a**) FBG, (**b**) HOMA-IR, (**c**) oral glucose tolerance test (OGTT) results, (**d**) AUC of OGTT, (**e**) NEFA, and (**f**) cholesterols. * $p < 0.05$; *** $p < 0.01$ versus the ob/ob group. §§ $p < 0.01$; §§§ $p < 0.001$ versus the WT group. FBG, fasting blood glucose; WT, wild-type; EK, Euphorbia kansui; HOMA-IR, homeostatic model assessment for insulin resistance; AUC, area under the curve; NEFA, non-esterified fatty acid; HDL, high-density lipoprotein; LDL, low-density lipoprotein; TG, triglyceride.

2.2.2. Safety Profile

To determine the toxic effect of EK on the liver and kidney function, serum levels of aspartate aminotransferase (AST), alanine aminotransferase (ALT), and creatinine were investigated. The creatinine and AST levels were not influenced by EK administration, and the difference in ALT levels between the EK and ob/ob groups was not significant.

2.2.3. Mechanism of EK Therapy in Macrophages and Monocytes

A significantly increased percentage of total and CD11c+ ATMs and a decrease in the percentage of CD206+ in the ob/ob group compared to the WT group was demonstrated. The EK group showed a significantly reduced percentage of total and CD11c+ ATMs and an enhanced percentage of CD206+ ATMs (Figure 5). The number of ATMs per epi fat weight was significantly decreased in the ob/ob group compared to the WT group but significantly increased in the EK group compared to the ob/ob group. In monocyte analysis, the ob/ob group had a lower percentage of $CD11b^+/Ly6c^{low}$ and a higher percentage of $CD11b^+/Ly6c^{high}$ than the WT group. However, the EK group demonstrated a significantly elevated percentage of $CD11b^+/Ly6c$ and a decreased percentage of $CD11b^+/Ly6c^{high}$ compared to the ob/ob group (Figure 6).

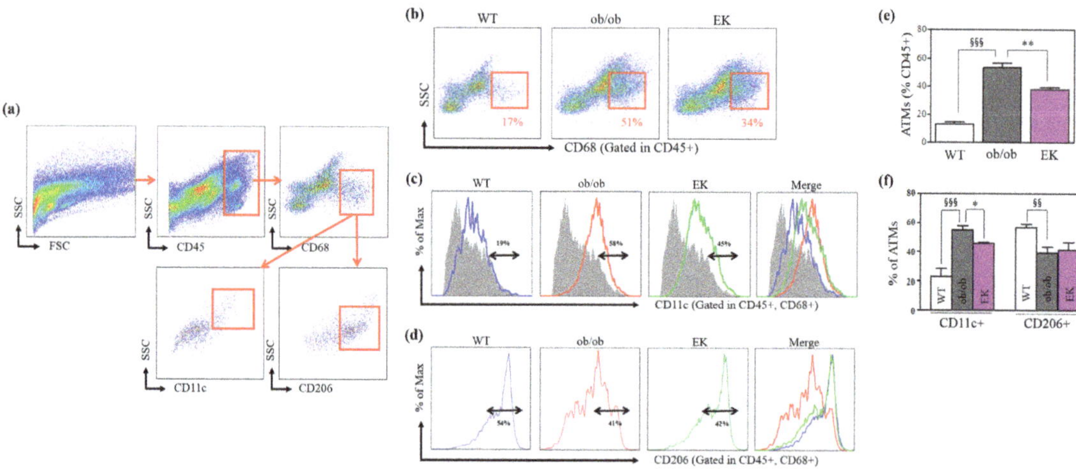

Figure 5. Anti-inflammatory changes in adipose tissue macrophages. (**a**) Flow cytometry results showing adipose tissue macrophage gating (CD45+ leukocytes, CD68 + macrophages, CD11C + macrophage and CD206 macrophages). (**b–f**) Percentages of adipose tissue macrophages in total, CD11c+, and CD206+ subtypes of WT (blue), ob/ob (red) and EK (green line). Gray shadow indicates fluorescence minus one control. * $p < 0.05$; ** $p < 0.01$ versus the ob/ob group. §§ $p < 0.01$; §§§ $p < 0.001$ versus WT group. WT, wild-type; EK, Euphorbia kansui; ATMs, adipose tissue macrophages.

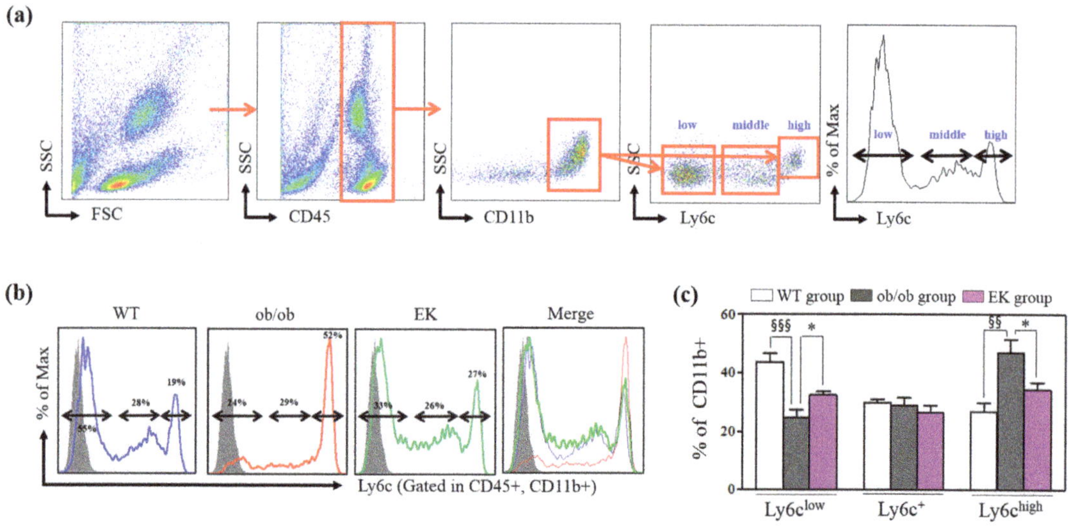

Figure 6. Anti-inflammatory changes in monocytes. (**a**) Flow cytometry showing monocyte gating (CD45+ leukocytes, CD11b + monocytes, and Ly6C low, middle and high subtypes monocytes). (**b**,**c**) Populations of $Ly6^{-}$, $Ly6c^{+}$, and $Ly6c^{++}$ monocytes of WT (blue), ob/ob (red) and EK (green line). Gray shadow indicates fluorescence minus one control. * $p < 0.05$ versus the ob/ob group. §§ $p < 0.01$; §§§ $p < 0.001$ versus WT group. WT, wild-type; EK, Euphorbia kansui.

2.2.4. Mechanism of EK Therapy in Gut Microbiota

In the phylum analysis, the two major phyla, both *Bacteroidetes* and *Firmicutes*, showed as significantly reduced in the ob/ob group compared to the WT group; however, the EK group demonstrated significant increments in both of them (*Bacteroidetes:* 73.13 ± 0.42% vs. 58.49 ± 2.39%; *Firmicutes:* 18.79 ± 1.64% vs. 13.93 ± 0.55%). *Verrucomicrobia* was the second most abundant in the ob/ob group; however, the proportion of *Verrucomicrobia* substantially decreased in the EK group (2.59 ± 2.16%). The other increasing fecal microbial species in the ob/ob group compared to the WT group were *Actinobacteria* and *Proteobacteria*, both of which were decreased in the EK group. *Deferribacteres* phylum was significantly increased in the EK group compared to the ob/ob group (6.24 ± 1.73% vs. 0.38 ± 0.18%). According to Simpson's method, the diversity indexes of all three groups were not significantly different from each other. However, the results of Principal Coordinate Analysis (PCoA) and Unweighted Pair Group Method with Arithmetic mean (UPGMA) suggested similar patterns of microbiota composition between the WT and EK groups, distinctly different from the ob/ob group (Figure 7).

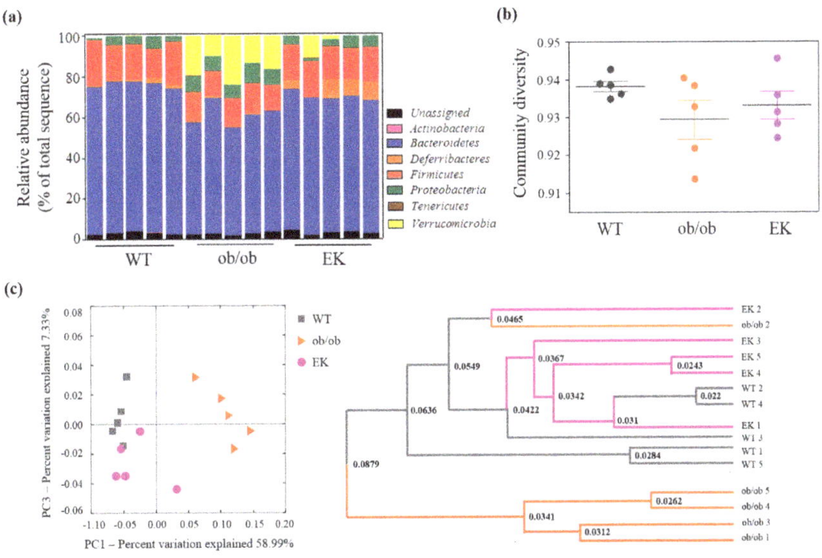

Figure 7. The changes in gut microbiota structure and diversity. (**a**) Percentage of each phylum in the gut microbiota. (**b**) Diversity of gut microbiota. (**c**) Principal coordinate analysis (PCoA) analysis of individuals and UPGMA clustering. WT, wild-type; EK, Euphorbia kansui.

3. Discussion

The current study was the first real-world clinical study with EK therapy and HM treatment for obesity in Republic of Korea, and it also investigated its mechanism. The patients who took only HM treatment significantly lost 6.27 ± 5.40% of body weight; however, the other patients who additionally took EK therapy once or twice significantly demonstrated additional weight loss of 1.45%. In demographic features, patients in the EK group showed a tendency to have higher BMI, fat, muscle, and body fluid. Moreover, the EK therapy during HM treatment significantly attributed to additional effects on the change in BMI, muscle, and body fluid. According to an in vivo mechanism study, EK therapy showed significant effects on adipose tissue inflammation at macrophage and monocyte levels and changed the gut microbiota towards the pattern of the lean, not that of the obese. Therefore, this article proposed EK therapy as an effective adjunctive treatment to be combined with HM treatment for obesity.

The EK therapy plus HM treatment showed 7.7% body weight and significant reductions in BMI, muscle, and body fluid compared to only HM treatment. In regard to body fat loss, the two groups were not statistically different. As the anti-obesity efficacy increased over the HM treatment time, the EK group showed significantly greater weight loss until 90 days; however, the mean change of body weight at 300 days was greater in the HM group. We confirmed that anti-obesity efficacy significantly increased according to the number of undergoing EK therapies ($p < 0.01$). Notably, the trial number of EK therapy was concentrated during the early treatment period. In the EK group, all subjects underwent EK therapy within 30 days from baseline, and the number of subjects undergoing EK therapy substantially diminished to 13, 10, 6, 5, 3, and 2 at 60, 90, 120, 180, and 300 days, respectively. In a previous prospective study with EK therapy [20], one trial of EK therapy contributed to a significant body weight loss of 1.27 kg. Our HM group was shown as similar to the results from the previous studies treated with various polyherbal decoctions, such as Bofutsushosan [21], Gambisan [22], Taeeumjowee-Tang [23], and Chegamuiyiin-Tang [24]. Gambisan showed 6.2% of body weight loss and 2.87% of body fat. The compliance rate of the Gambisan study was higher than 70%, and the weight loss effect of adjunctive EK therapy was potent, losing 7.73% of body weight and 2.47% of body fat [22].

Our study assessed the safety of EK therapy by self-reported adverse events during the treatment period and laboratory blood tests in mice. We observed no toxic effect on the liver and kidney in mice, and Lee et al. [20] confirmed no significant difference in AST, ALT, GGT, BUN, creatinine, and eGFR before and after EK therapy in humans. Also, the adverse events of EK therapy were similar to the results that Lee had reported, such as mild to moderate abdominal pain, which lasted 1–2 days. All our prescriptions for HM treatments included Ma-huang, and no severe adverse effect was reported in common with previous studies, including dry mouth, constipation, diarrhea, palpitation, and insomnia.

The importance of this study is assessing the anti-inflammation effect through various values at the cellular level. In obese patients, persistent, low-grade inflammation is triggered by ATM infiltration and its derived cytokines, which disrupts the insulin signaling cascade-like feedback loop [25]. We investigated the effects of EK on inflammation in this respect. EK therapy decreased the number of ATMs in the quantitative aspect and also significantly improved adipose tissue inflammation in the qualitative aspect. EK treatment significantly decreased CD11C+ ATMs, namely M1 ATMs, which stands for the pro-inflammatory activity of ATMs in adipose tissue, and the same results were shown in the analysis of blood Ly6c monocyte types. Lee also suggested EK-modulated ATMs and pro-inflammatory cytokines, including TNF-α and IL-6, in the same manner as our results.

Ly6c^{hi} monocytes representing pro-inflammatory traits are recruited to the inflammation site by chemo-attractants and differentiate into macrophages or dendritic cells depending on the local cytokines [26]. Ly6c^{low} monocytes are patrolling to differentiate into resident macrophages and promote wound healing [27]. In the obesity inflammation, Ly6c^{hi} and Ly6c^{low} monocytes may differentiate into M1 and M2 macrophages [5,28]. As per our expectation, Ly6c^{hi} in monocyte-related pro-inflammation was decreased, while Ly6c^{low}-type of monocyte-related anti-inflammation was increased by EK.

Alteration of gut microbiota and resultant modulation of intestinal permeability could be a key strategy to ameliorate obesity inflammation [7]. The most definite result in microbiota was the increase in *Verrucomicrobia* in the ob/ob group. *Verrucomicrobia* were counted at 16.85% in the ob/ob group; however, the WT group and EK group showed only 0.00% and 2.59%. The relationship between *Verrucomicrobia* and obesity was reported that high-fat feeding induced the increase in *Verrucomicrobia* and also the increasing ratio of *Verrucomicrobia* to *Bacteroidetes* [29]. Our study showed similar results to this previous study. The mean ratio of *Verrucomicrobia* to *Bacteroidetes* was significantly increased in the ob/ob group; however, the ratio was decreased in the EK group, demonstrating EK had effects on recovering harmful microbial transition.

In the Genus-level analysis, *Alistipes* belonging to *Bacteroidetes* were significantly decreased in the ob/ob group and recovered in the EK group, even higher than the WT group. *Alistipes* correlate negatively with leukocytes and present more abundantly in healthy subjects compared to non-alcoholic fatty liver disease patients mediated by inflammation [30,31]. Moreover, a human study confirmed that successful weight loss significantly enriched *Alistipes* [31]. Notably, the dominant phyla, *Firmicutes*, was decreased in the ob/ob group and increased in the EK group, contradicting other results. Turnbaugh et al. [32] found an increase in the abundance of *Firmicutes* associated with diet-induced obesity. These compositional changes were completely reversed after returning to a normal diet, which suggests that diet is the main contributing factor to obesity-associated changes in the gut microbiota [33]. In our study, the diets of all experimental groups were identical, and the results of genetically obese and obese individuals with high-fat dietary habits were thought to be different for microorganisms. Indeed, the critical biomarker of obesity is uncertain among *Firmicutes*, *Bacteroidetes*, *Firmicutes/Bacteroidetes* ratio, and other phyla and remains to be determined [34].

Deferribacteres showed a low proportion in both the WT group and the ob/ob group and obviously increased in the EK group. In a study of diet-induced weight modification, *Mucispirillum*, the only genus of *Deferribacteres*, was positively correlated with serum leptin levels [35] and also had several systems for scavenging reactive oxygen species induced by inflammation [36]. Interestingly, *Mucispirillum* was known not to be affected by the prebiotic treatment [37]. Therefore, EK could be a potent option to promote the growth of *Mucispirillum*, finally leading to weight reduction.

We had several limitations. In our pragmatic, real-world clinical study, a disparity in the number of follow-up bioelectrical impedance analyses (BIAs) resulted in limited sufficient analyses in body composition changes, such as fat, muscle, and body fluid, and attributed to the data imbalance between the EK and HM groups. Also, the fidelity of the intervention was restricted due to real-world conditions, lacking placebo or randomization. Second, the compliance of HM treatment and EK therapy was low compared to the other retrospective studies with HM treatment [22]. Additionally, the final body weight was not recorded at the end-of-treatment- but at the last-prescription-date during the study period. These approaches would have underestimated the potential weight loss effects associated with both HM treatment and EK therapy. Third, the numbers of each mouse groups were too small to make a generalization human, and additional studies are needed, with large numbers of animal and human studies. However, our study had enough patients to be the first real-world clinical study, although clinical trials with EK therapy were rare because of its toxicity. In the past, the anti-inflammatory benefits of EK were studied, focusing on various cancers and gastrointestinal tract-associated diseases. However, this study was also the first research of EK in obesity and glucometabolism to investigate potent anti-inflammatory mechanisms of macrophages and Ly6c monocytes, suggesting a positive role in host energy metabolism by the transition of microbiota. Finally, the biomarkers used in this study, such as AST, ALT, and creatinine, are typically only activated when the liver or kidneys have been damaged to some degree; therefore, ultrasensitive PCR methods are needed to detect inflammatory processes that may occur before organ damage. Future studies may also incorporate more sensitive markers than bilirubin, gamma-glutamyl transferase (GGT), liver biopsy, and creatinine to help detect liver and kidney dysfunction at an earlier stage.

In summary, EK therapy, when combined with HM treatment, significantly contributed to additional weight loss and improvements in various body metrics. Our findings from the in vivo mechanism study revealed that EK therapy influenced adipose tissue inflammation at the macrophage and monocyte levels. Specifically, EK therapy reduced the number of pro-inflammatory CD11c+ macrophages (M1 macrophages) and altered the balance between pro-inflammatory Ly6c^{hi} monocytes and anti-inflammatory Ly6c^{low} monocytes, suggesting a modulation of inflammatory responses associated with obesity. Furthermore, we noted significant changes in gut microbiota composition due to EK therapy. EK therapy shifted the microbiota towards a profile more typical of lean individuals, with reductions in the abundance of Verrucomicrobia, which is often elevated in obese conditions, and increased levels of beneficial genera such as Alistipes. These changes in gut microbiota are consistent with previous research linking microbiota modulation to improvements in obesity and metabolic health.

4. Materials and Methods

4.1. A Real-World Clinical Study

4.1.1. Study Design and Eligible Patients

This study was an open-label, pragmatic cohort study encompassing outpatients who visited the Weight Management Center at Kyunghee University Korean Medicine Hospital (Seoul, Republic of Korea) to treat obesity between 1 January 2022 and 31 December 2022. Eligible patients were included according to the following criteria:

(1) Men and women aged 15 years or older with BMI over 25.
(2) Those who decided to receive HM treatment among the patients who visited the hospital for weight loss,
(3) Each patient who visited the hospital at least twice within the entire treatment period to confirm the change in body weight.

The patients who denied taking HM for weight loss or could not be checked for the follow-up body weight were excluded. All eligible patients underwent HM treatment, of which the contents of the prescription were different for each patient. At the first visit, all patients measured their body weight and performed BIA using InBody720 (InBody Inc., Seoul, Republic of Korea) and were recommended not to take any other medicines or supplements for weight loss during the HM treatment period.

Patients were fully informed about the potential risks, including diarrhea, vomiting, and abdominal pain, associated with the susceptible EK treatment. We then assigned patients into either the EK treatment group or the HM group based on their choice: the EK group who underwent EK therapy at least once plus conventional HM and the HM group who were prescribed only conventional HM without EK therapy. We compared the changes in body weight and other body compositions before and after HM treatment between the EK group and HM group. For monitoring compliance, we checked how much of the prescribed medication was taken at each patient visit.

This real-world clinical study's protocol was approved by the Kyung Hee University Korean Medicine Hospital Institutional Review Board (KOMCIRB 2023-07-001), and written informed consent was obtained from all participants.

4.1.2. EK Therapy and HM Treatment

EK was provided by the Department of Pharmaceutical Preparation of the Kyunghee University Korean Medicine Hospital. An EK capsule contains 400 mg of EK powder. EK therapy is performed as a 1-day course at home. Patients were prescribed 8 to 12 EK capsules at a single time, taking 4–5 capsules every 2 min on an empty stomach. After 1–2 h, multiple episodes of diarrhea and vomiting would occur over a period of 6–8 h, along with abdominal pain or nausea. We notified in advance that (1) severe abdominal pain could be relaxed with a hot pack or antispasmodics and (2) dehydration might occur after more than 10 times of diarrhea, and a can of soft drink could be helpful. All participants were prescribed HM, which was *Gami-Samhwang-san* (by decocting Ephedra Herba 4 g, Armeniacae Semen 4 g, Acori Gramineri Rhizoma 4 g, Raphani Semen 4 g, Coicis Semen 4 g, Phellodendri Cortex 4 g, Atractylodes Chinensis Rhizome 4 g, Rhei Radix et Rhizoma 4 g in water), and TKM clinical doctors at the Weight Management Center in Kyunghee University Korean Medicine Hospital modulated the prescriptions according to health problems of each patient.

4.1.3. Lifestyle Modification

On the first visit, all patients were counseled on correcting their lifestyle based on a common diet and exercise regimen. Our center highlighted taking regular 2 or 3 meals in a day, avoiding fruits and confections, including sweet drinks and sauces, and walking for an hour, 1–2 times a week, until sweating.

4.2. Animal Study

4.2.1. Study Design and Animal and EK Preparations

The experimental animals were wild-type 19~21 g male C57BL/6 mice (WT group, n = 5) and obese 27~31 g male C57BL/6-Lepob/Lepob (ob/ob) mice (Central Lab Animals Inc., Seoul, Republic of Korea). The ob/ob mice were randomly assigned into two groups: the ob/ob group (n = 5) and the EK group (n = 5). Normal chow with 4.5% crude fat and water were supplied ad libitum. The EK group was treated with EK powder (200 mg/kg), orally administered twice a week for 8 weeks, while the WT and ob/ob groups took normal saline. EK was purchased from the Department of Pharmaceutical Preparation of Kyunghee University Korean Medicine Hospital (Seoul, Republic of Korea). All experiments were carried out in accordance with guidelines from the Korean National Institute of Health Animal Facility. The relative humidity in the room was maintained at 40~70%, and the light–dark cycle was set at 12 h. At the end of the study, the mice were euthanized by cervical dislocation.

4.2.2. Weight Measurements and Blood Analysis

Body weights were recorded at the beginning and end of the experiment using the CAS 2.5D scale (Seoul, Republic of Korea) in the morning. The weights of epididymal fat pads were measured at 8 weeks after scarification. To evaluate glucose metabolism, we examined FBG at 2, 4, and 8 weeks using ACCU-CHECK Performa (Australia) and performed OGTT at 6 weeks after glucose (2 g/kg body weight) feeding. Also, FSI was analyzed at 8 weeks using an ELISA reader by 450 nM, and HOMA-IR was calculated using FBG and FSI. We analyzed the lipid profiles, including total cholesterol (TC), high-density lipoprotein cholesterol (HDL-C), low-density lipoprotein cholesterol (LDL-C), TG, and NEFA, as well as the safety profile, including AST, ALT, and creatinine levels, using blood samples collected from the heart at 8 weeks.

4.2.3. Analysis of ATMs and Monocytes

Stromal vascular cells (SVCs) were segregated from the epi fat samples at the end of the study. The fat samples were soaked in the solution of phosphate-buffered saline (PBS) and 2% bovine serum albumin (BSA) and isolated by collagenase (Sigma, St. Louis, MO, USA) and DNase I (Roche, Brighton, MA, USA). The cell number of SVC was counted by a cellometer (Nexcelom Bioscience LLC., Lawrence, MA, USA). To prepare before fluorescence-activated cell sorting (FACS) analysis, FcBlock (BD Pharmingen, San Jose, CA, USA) was mixed at the ratio of 1:100, and the fluorophore-conjugated antibodies were added to react with the samples as follows: CD45-PerCP-Cy5.5 (Biolgend, San Diego, CA, USA), CD68-APC (Biolgend, USA), CD11c-phycoerythrin (Biolgend, USA), CD206-FITC (Biolgend, USA), CD11b-PE (Biolgend, USA), and Ly6c-APC. All samples were added into FACS tubes after washing with 2% FBS/PBS solution and analyzed by FACS Caliber (BD bioscience, San Jose, CA, USA). We calculated the percentage of macrophages with CD45+/CD68+, CD45+/CD68+/CD206+, CD45+/CD68+/CD11c+, and the percentage of monocytes with CD45+/CD11b+/Ly6c-, CD45+/CD11b+/Ly6c+, and CD45+/CD11b+/Ly6c++ using FlowJo (Tree star Inc., Ashland, OR, USA).

4.2.4. Analysis of the Composition of the Fecal Microbiota

At 8 weeks, the fecal samples were collected, and their DNA was extracted following amplification by polymerase chain reaction (PCR). The Basic Local Alignment Search Tool (*BLAST*) found regions of local similarity between sequences to analyze taxonomic composition for each sample from the Phylum to Species level. In diversity analysis, we used Simpson's diversity index to calculate alpha diversity. PCoA and UPGMA clustering trees were used to assess the variation.

4.3. Statistical Analysis

The continuous variables were reported in the clinical study using the mean and standard deviation (SD), presented as mean ± SD, and in the animal study using the mean and standard error of the mean (SEM), presented as mean ± SEM. We compared the continuous variables between the EK group and the other group using the Mann–Whitney U test only for baseline age and height using the student's *t*-test. Linear regression was performed to analyze the changes in weight loss between the EK and HM treatments using linear regression. In our model, we included age, gender, and treatment duration as covariates to control for these potential confounding factors.

We conducted an analysis of variance (ANOVA) and Tukey's post hoc to compare the weight loss outcomes across the number of EK therapy sessions in the clinical study and to analyze group differences in the animal study. The change in body weight before and after obesity treatment was analyzed by the Wilcoxon signed rank test. We also used a student's *t*-test to check if a final weight loss was different between different subgroups of gender and behavioral factors. All statistical analyses were performed using PRISM 7 (Graphpad software Inc., La Jolla, CA, USA). All p values were two-tailed, and significance was set at $p < 0.05$.

5. Conclusions

We can infer the effect of Euphorbia kansui treatment on the grounds of the results related to anti-inflammation and alteration of microbial community composition. These different types of microorganisms might be linked to changes in nutrient absorption and energy regulation. Additionally, we can also assert that leading changes in adipose tissue macrophage and blood Ly6c^{hi} monocytes level by Euphorbia kansui treatment can reduce systemic inflammation activity and finally impact the insulin signaling network.

Author Contributions: Conceptualization and methodology, J.-W.N. and B.-C.L.; investigation, data curation, and writing—original draft preparation, J.-W.N. and J.-H.Y.; writing—review and editing, J.-W.N. and B.-C.L.; funding acquisition and project administration, B.-C.L. All authors have read and agreed to the published version of the manuscript.

Funding: This research was supported by the Korea Health Technology R&D Project through the Korea Health Industry Development Institute (KHIDI), funded by the Ministry of Health and Welfare, Republic of Korea (grant number: HFD20C0022).

Institutional Review Board Statement: The human study's protocol was approved by the Kyung Hee University Korean Medicine Hospital Institutional Review Board (KOMCIRB 2023-07-001) and conducted in accordance with the guidelines of the Declaration of Helsinki. The animal study was approved by the Animal Care Committee at Kyunghee University (KHMC-IACUC 2016-032), and the ARRIVE guidelines were checked.

Informed Consent Statement: Written informed consent was obtained from all participants.

Data Availability Statement: Data is contained within the article.

Conflicts of Interest: The authors declare no conflicts of interest.

References

1. Wyatt, H.R. Update on treatment strategies for obesity. *J. Clin. Endocrinol. Metab.* **2013**, *98*, 1299–1306. [CrossRef] [PubMed]
2. Tham, K.W.; Abdul Ghani, R.; Cua, S.C.; Deerochanawong, C.; Fojas, M.; Hocking, S.; Lee, J.; Nam, T.Q.; Pathan, F.; Saboo, B.; et al. Obesity in South and Southeast Asia—A new consensus on care and management. *Obes. Rev.* **2023**, *24*, e13520. [CrossRef]
3. Furukawa, S.; Fujita, T.; Shimabukuro, M.; Iwaki, M.; Yamada, Y.; Nakajima, Y.; Nakayama, O.; Makishima, M.; Matsuda, M.; Shimomura, I. Increased oxidative stress in obesity and its impact on metabolic syndrome. *J. Clin. Investig.* **2004**, *114*, 1752–1761. [CrossRef]
4. Jin, X.; Qiu, T.; Li, L.; Yu, R.; Chen, X.; Li, C.; Proud, C.G.; Jiang, T. Pathophysiology of obesity and its associated diseases. *Acta Pharm. Sin. B* **2023**, *13*, 2403–2424. [CrossRef] [PubMed]
5. Russo, L.; Lumeng, C.N. Properties and functions of adipose tissue macrophages in obesity. *Immunology* **2018**, *155*, 407–417. [CrossRef]

6. Li, Y.H.; Zhang, Y.; Pan, G.; Xiang, L.X.; Luo, D.C.; Shao, J.Z. Occurrences and Functions of Ly6C(hi) and Ly6C(lo) Macrophages in Health and Disease. *Front. Immunol.* **2022**, *13*, 901672. [CrossRef]
7. Cox, A.J.; West, N.P.; Cripps, A.W. Obesity, inflammation, and the gut microbiota. *Lancet Diabetes Endocrinol.* **2015**, *3*, 207–215. [CrossRef] [PubMed]
8. Aron-Wisnewsky, J.; Warmbrunn, M.V.; Nieuwdorp, M.; Clement, K. Metabolism and Metabolic Disorders and the Microbiome: The Intestinal Microbiota Associated with Obesity, Lipid Metabolism, and Metabolic Health-Pathophysiology and Therapeutic Strategies. *Gastroenterology* **2021**, *160*, 573–599. [CrossRef]
9. Hou, J.J.; Wu, W.Y.; Liang, J.; Yang, Z.; Long, H.L.; Cai, L.Y.; Fang, L.; Wang, D.D.; Yao, S.; Liu, X.; et al. A single, multi-faceted, enhanced strategy to quantify the chromatographically diverse constituents in the roots of *Euphorbia kansui*. *J. Pharm. Biomed. Anal.* **2014**, *88*, 321–330. [CrossRef]
10. Tong, G.D.; Zhou, D.Q.; He, J.S.; Zhang, L.; Chen, Z.F.; Xiao, C.L.; Peng, L.S. Clinical research on navel application of Shehuang Paste combined with Chinese herbal colon dialysis in treatment of refractory cirrhotic ascites complicated with azotemia. *World J. Gastroenterol.* **2006**, *12*, 7798–7804. [CrossRef]
11. Shen, J.; Wang, J.; Shang, E.X.; Tang, Y.P.; Kai, J.; Cao, Y.J.; Zhou, G.S.; Tao, W.W.; Kang, A.; Su, S.L.; et al. The dosage-toxicity-efficacy relationship of kansui and licorice in malignant pleural effusion rats based on factor analysis. *J. Ethnopharmacol.* **2016**, *186*, 251–256. [CrossRef]
12. Li, H.; Lei, F.; Wang, Y.; Xiao, X.; Hu, J.; Cheng, X.; Xing, D.; Hua, L.; Lin, R.; Du, L. Effect of Euphorbia kansui on urination and kidney AQP2, IL-1beta and TNF-alpha mRNA expression of mice injected with normal saline. *China J. Chin. Mater. Med.* **2012**, *37*, 606–610.
13. Feng, X.; Li, J.; Li, H.; Chen, X.; Liu, D.; Li, R. Bioactive C21 Steroidal Glycosides from Euphorbia kansui Promoted HepG2 Cell Apoptosis via the Degradation of ATP1A1 and Inhibited Macrophage Polarization under Co-Cultivation. *Molecules* **2023**, *28*, 2830. [CrossRef] [PubMed]
14. Hou, J.J.; Shen, Y.; Yang, Z.; Fang, L.; Cai, L.Y.; Yao, S.; Long, H.L.; Wu, W.Y.; Guo, D.A. Anti-proliferation activity of terpenoids isolated from Euphorbia kansui in human cancer cells and their structure-activity relationship. *Chin. J. Nat. Med.* **2017**, *15*, 766–774. [CrossRef] [PubMed]
15. Kim, S.J.; Jang, Y.W.; Hyung, K.E.; Lee, D.K.; Hyun, K.H.; Park, S.Y.; Park, E.S.; Hwang, K.W. Therapeutic Effects of Methanol Extract from Euphorbia kansui Radix on Imiquimod-Induced Psoriasis. *J. Immunol. Res.* **2017**, *2017*, 7052560. [CrossRef]
16. Van Sickle, M.D.; Duncan, M.; Kingsley, P.J.; Mouihate, A.; Urbani, P.; Mackie, K.; Stella, N.; Makriyannis, A.; Piomelli, D.; Davison, J.S.; et al. Identification and functional characterization of brainstem cannabinoid CB_2 receptors. *Science* **2005**, *310*, 329–332. [CrossRef] [PubMed]
17. Guo, J.; Zhou, L.Y.; He, H.P.; Leng, Y.; Yang, Z.; Hao, X.J. Inhibition of 11b-HSD1 by tetracyclic triterpenoids from *Euphorbia kansui*. *Molecules* **2012**, *17*, 11826–11838. [CrossRef]
18. Kim, J.W.; Kim, E.Y. The effect of Hyungbangdojucksan-Gami and Kamsuchunilhwan on the obesity in the rats. *J. Sasang Const. Med.* **2000**, *12*, 184–194. [CrossRef]
19. Kim, D.H.; Noh, J.W.; Jeong, S.M.; Ahn, S.Y.; Ahn, Y.M.; Lee, B.C.; Yoo, J.H. A Retrospective Chart Review of the Clinical Use of Euphorbia kansui Radix, Melonis Calyx. *J. Intern. Korean Med.* **2019**, *40*, 1015–1025. [CrossRef]
20. Lee, S.W.; Na, H.Y.; Seol, M.H.; Kim, M.; Lee, B.C. Euphorbia kansui Attenuates Insulin Resistance in Obese Human Subjects and High-Fat Diet-Induced Obese Mice. *Evid. Based Complement. Alternat. Med.* **2017**, *2017*, 9058956. [CrossRef]
21. Uneda, K.; Kawai, Y.; Yamada, T.; Kaneko, A.; Saito, R.; Chen, L.; Ishigami, T.; Namiki, T.; Mitsuma, T. Japanese traditional Kampo medicine bofutsushosan improves body mass index in participants with obesity: A systematic review and meta-analysis. *PLoS ONE* **2022**, *17*, e0266917. [CrossRef] [PubMed]
22. Jo, D.H.; Lee, S.; Lee, J.D. Effects of Gambisan in overweight adults and adults with obesity: A retrospective chart review. *Medicine* **2019**, *98*, e18060. [CrossRef]
23. Lee, A.-R.; Lee, D.-Y.; Kim, M.-J.; Lee, H.-S.; Choi, K.-H.; Kim, S.-Y.; Lim, Y.-W.; Park, Y.-B. Gamitaeeumjowee-Tang for weight loss in diabetic patients: A retrospective chart review. *J. Korean Med.* **2021**, *42*, 46–58. [CrossRef]
24. Jung, S.-H.; Lee, J.-S.; Kim, S.-S.; Shin, H.-D. The Effect of Very Low Calorie Diet and Chegamuiyiin-tang on Bone Mineral Density. *J. Korean Med. Obes. Res.* **2005**, *5*, 87–95.
25. McArdle, M.A.; Finucane, O.M.; Connaughton, R.M.; McMorrow, A.M.; Roche, H.M. Mechanisms of obesity-induced inflammation and insulin resistance: Insights into the emerging role of nutritional strategies. *Front. Endocrinol.* **2013**, *4*, 52. [CrossRef] [PubMed]
26. Kratofil, R.M.; Kubes, P.; Deniset, J.F. Monocyte Conversion During Inflammation and Injury. *Arterioscler. Thromb. Vasc. Biol.* **2017**, *37*, 35–42. [CrossRef]
27. Auffray, C.; Fogg, D.; Garfa, M.; Elain, G.; Join-Lambert, O.; Kayal, S.; Sarnacki, S.; Cumano, A.; Lauvau, G.; Geissmann, F. Monitoring of blood vessels and tissues by a population of monocytes with patrolling behavior. *Science* **2007**, *317*, 666–670. [CrossRef]
28. Shi, C.; Pamer, E.G. Monocyte recruitment during infection and inflammation. *Nat. Rev. Immunol.* **2011**, *11*, 762–774. [CrossRef]
29. Li, X.; Guo, J.; Ji, K.; Zhang, P. Bamboo shoot fiber prevents obesity in mice by modulating the gut microbiota. *Sci. Rep.* **2016**, *6*, 32953. [CrossRef]

30. Jiang, W.; Wu, N.; Wang, X.; Chi, Y.; Zhang, Y.; Qiu, X.; Hu, Y.; Li, J.; Liu, Y. Dysbiosis gut microbiota associated with inflammation and impaired mucosal immune function in intestine of humans with non-alcoholic fatty liver disease. *Sci. Rep.* **2015**, *5*, 8096. [CrossRef]
31. Louis, S.; Tappu, R.M.; Damms-Machado, A.; Huson, D.H.; Bischoff, S.C. Characterization of the Gut Microbial Community of Obese Patients Following a Weight-Loss Intervention Using Whole Metagenome Shotgun Sequencing. *PLoS ONE* **2016**, *11*, e0149564. [CrossRef] [PubMed]
32. Turnbaugh, P.J.; Ley, R.E.; Mahowald, M.A.; Magrini, V.; Mardis, E.R.; Gordon, J.I. An obesity-associated gut microbiome with increased capacity for energy harvest. *Nature* **2006**, *444*, 1027–1031. [CrossRef] [PubMed]
33. Boulange, C.L.; Neves, A.L.; Chilloux, J.; Nicholson, J.K.; Dumas, M.E. Impact of the gut microbiota on inflammation, obesity, and metabolic disease. *Genome Med.* **2016**, *8*, 42. [CrossRef] [PubMed]
34. Murphy, E.F.; Cotter, P.D.; Healy, S.; Marques, T.M.; O'Sullivan, O.; Fouhy, F.; Clarke, S.F.; O'Toole, P.W.; Quigley, E.M.; Stanton, C.; et al. Composition and energy harvesting capacity of the gut microbiota: Relationship to diet, obesity and time in mouse models. *Gut* **2010**, *59*, 1635–1642. [CrossRef]
35. Ravussin, Y.; Koren, O.; Spor, A.; LeDuc, C.; Gutman, R.; Stombaugh, J.; Knight, R.; Ley, R.E.; Leibel, R.L. Responses of gut microbiota to diet composition and weight loss in lean and obese mice. *Obesity* **2012**, *20*, 738–747. [CrossRef]
36. Loy, A.; Pfann, C.; Steinberger, M.; Hanson, B.; Herp, S.; Brugiroux, S.; Gomes Neto, J.C.; Boekschoten, M.V.; Schwab, C.; Urich, T.; et al. Lifestyle and Horizontal Gene Transfer-Mediated Evolution of *Mucispirillum schaedleri*, a Core Member of the Murine Gut Microbiota. *mSystems* **2017**, *2*, e00171-16. [CrossRef]
37. Everard, A.; Lazarevic, V.; Gaia, N.; Johansson, M.; Stahlman, M.; Backhed, F.; Delzenne, N.M.; Schrenzel, J.; Francois, P.; Cani, P.D. Microbiome of prebiotic-treated mice reveals novel targets involved in host response during obesity. *ISME J.* **2014**, *8*, 2116–2130. [CrossRef]

pharmaceuticals

MDPI

Article

Lipid-Lowering and Anti-Inflammatory Effects of *Campomanesia adamantium* Leaves in Adipocytes and *Caenorhabditis elegans*

Paola dos Santos da Rocha †, Sarah Lam Orué †, Isamara Carvalho Ferreira, Priscilla Pereira de Toledo Espindola, Maria Victória Benites Rodrigues, José Tarcísio Giffoni de Carvalho, Debora da Silva Baldivia, Daniel Ferreira Leite, Helder Freitas dos Santos, Alex Santos Oliveira, Jaqueline Ferreira Campos, Edson Lucas dos Santos and Kely de Picoli Souza *

Research Group on Biotechnology and Bioprospecting Applied to Metabolism (GEBBAM), Federal University of Grande Dourados, Rodovia Dourados-Itahum, Km 12, Dourados 79804-970, MS, Brazil; paolasantosrocha@ufgd.edu.br (P.d.S.d.R.); sarah.orue005@academico.ufgd.edu.br (S.L.O.); isamara.ferreira137@academico.ufgd.edu.br (I.C.F.); priscatoledo@hotmail.com (P.P.d.T.E.); maria.rodrigues072@academico.ufgd.edu.br (M.V.B.R.); tarcisiogiffoni@outlook.com.br (J.T.G.d.C.); deborasbaldivia@ufgd.edu.br (D.d.S.B.); danielleitesci@gmail.com (D.F.L.); helderfsantos@ufgd.edu.br (H.F.d.S.); alexsantosoliveira@gmail.com (A.S.O.); jaquelinefcampos@ufgd.edu.br (J.F.C.); edsonsantosphd@gmail.com (E.L.d.S.)

* Correspondence: kelypicoli@gmail.com or kelypicoli@ufgd.edu.br

† These authors contributed equally to this work.

Abstract: Obesity is a pandemic disease characterized by lipid accumulation, increased proinflammatory cytokines, and reactive oxygen species. It is associated with the development of comorbidities that lead to death. Additionally, drug treatments developed to control obesity are insufficient and have a variety of adverse effects. Thus, the search for new anti-obesity therapies is necessary. *Campomanesia adamantium* is a species from the Brazilian Cerrado that has the potential to treat obesity, as described by the antihyperlipidemic activity of its roots. Therefore, this study aimed to investigate the activity of the aqueous extract of *C. adamantium* leaves (AECa) on the control of reactive species in vitro, on lipid accumulation in adipocytes and *Caenorhabditis elegans*, and on the production of proinflammatory cytokines in adipocytes. The antioxidant capacity of AECa was observed by its action in scavenging DPPH$^{\bullet}$ free radical, iron-reducing power, and inhibition of β-carotene bleaching. AECa reduced lipid accumulation in preadipocytes and in *C. elegans*. Moreover, AECa reduced the production of the proinflammatory cytokines MCP-1, TNF-α, and IL-6 in adipocytes. In summary, the antioxidant activity and the ability of AECa to reduce the accumulation of lipids and proinflammatory cytokines indicate, for the first time, the anti-obesity potential of *C. adamantium* leaves.

Keywords: guavira; oxidative stress; inflammation; obesity

1. Introduction

Obesity is a pandemic chronic inflammatory disease, mainly due to unhealthy eating and a sedentary lifestyle. It is currently the leading nutritional disorder in developed countries [1]. Obesity is characterized by the expansion of white adipose tissue, resulting from the processes of adipogenesis and lipogenesis, which are characteristics of adipocyte hyperplasia and hypertrophy, respectively [2]. Adipogenesis is upregulated in the mesenchymal stem cells of adipose tissue by fatty acid-activated transcription factors, which include PPAR-γ [3]. Furthermore, the activation of PPAR-γ in adipocytes also promotes the sensitivity of these cells to insulin, promoting the absorption of glucose and the accumulation of lipids through a process known as lipogenesis [4]. For lipid accumulation during lipogenesis, transcriptional factors, including SREBP-1c, are activated [5].

In addition, adipocyte hypertrophy contributes to the production of proinflammatory cytokines such as interleukin 6 (IL-6) and tumor necrosis factor-alpha (TNF-α) and increases the secretion of chemokines such as monocyte chemoattractant protein 1 (MCP-1) [6]. Hypertrophy upregulates a cycle of continuous cellular recruitment of inflammation that leads to the increased production of reactive oxygen species [7]. If not neutralized, these reactive oxygen species generate an oxidative stress condition. The inflammatory and oxidative stress conditions in adipocytes that characterize obesity are associated with the development of comorbidities such as type 2 diabetes, cardiovascular disease, and cancer, which are among the leading causes of death in the world today [8].

Drug treatments developed to control obesity are insufficient and have several adverse effects [9]. Therapeutic alternatives are, therefore, being sought to obtain products that modulate adipogenesis, lipogenesis, and the production of proinflammatory cytokines and possess antioxidant activities.

Among the therapeutic alternatives, medicinal plants have gained prominence for their biological activities, with fewer adverse effects and low costs to public health [10]. *Campomanesia adamantium* O. Berg, popularly known as guavira, is a medicinal plant from the Myrtaceae family, native to the Brazilian Cerrado [11]. *C. adamantium* is traditionally used to treat diarrhea, urinary tract infections, and stomach disorders [11]. Its biological properties include anti-inflammatory, pro-longevity, and cyclooxygenase-inhibiting activities [12–14].

In a previous study, we verified the antioxidant and antihyperlipidemic effects of *Campomanesia adamantium* O. Berg roots [15]. Furthermore, another study found that the aqueous extract of *C. adamantium* leaves has quinic acid and phenolic compounds, such as flavonoids, with myricetin and quercetin as its main constituents [16]. Therefore, in this study, we investigated the effect of *C. adamantium* leaves on controlling reactive oxygen species, lipid accumulation, and the production of proinflammatory cytokines.

2. Results

2.1. Antioxidant Activity of AECa

AECa showed antioxidant activity observed by the DPPH•, FRAP, and β-carotene bleaching methods (Table 1). The concentration of AECa capable of inhibiting 50% (IC_{50}) of DPPH• radicals was approximately 1.6 times higher than that of the Controls, ascorbic acid, and BHA. The FRAP test's average effective concentration (EC_{50}) of AECa was approximately 1.4 times higher than ascorbic acid. In the β-carotene bleaching test, AECa had an IC_{50} approximately 15 times higher than BHA, and a value the IC_{50} of ascorbic acid was not detected (Table 1).

Table 1. Antioxidant activity of aqueous extract of *Campomanesia adamantium* leaves (AECa).

Sample	DPPH•	FRAP	β-Carotene Bleaching
	IC_{50} (μg/mL)	EC_{50} (μg/mL)	IC_{50} (μg/mL)
AECa	10.41 ± 1.06	56.54 ± 3.00	229.87 ± 5.92
AA	6.09 ± 2.28	40.16 ± 4.96	ND
BHA	6.45 ± 2.28	-	15.14 ± 2.07

AA: ascorbic acid; BHA: butyl-4-hydroxyanisole; IC_{50}: half-maximal inhibitory concentration; EC_{50}: median effective concentration; -: not performed; ND: not detected. Results are expressed as means ± SEM.

2.2. Effect of AECa on Preadipocytes

AECa did not reduce the viability of preadipocytes regardless of the concentration at 24 h. At 48 h, the concentrations of AECa maintained viability above 90% (Figure 1).

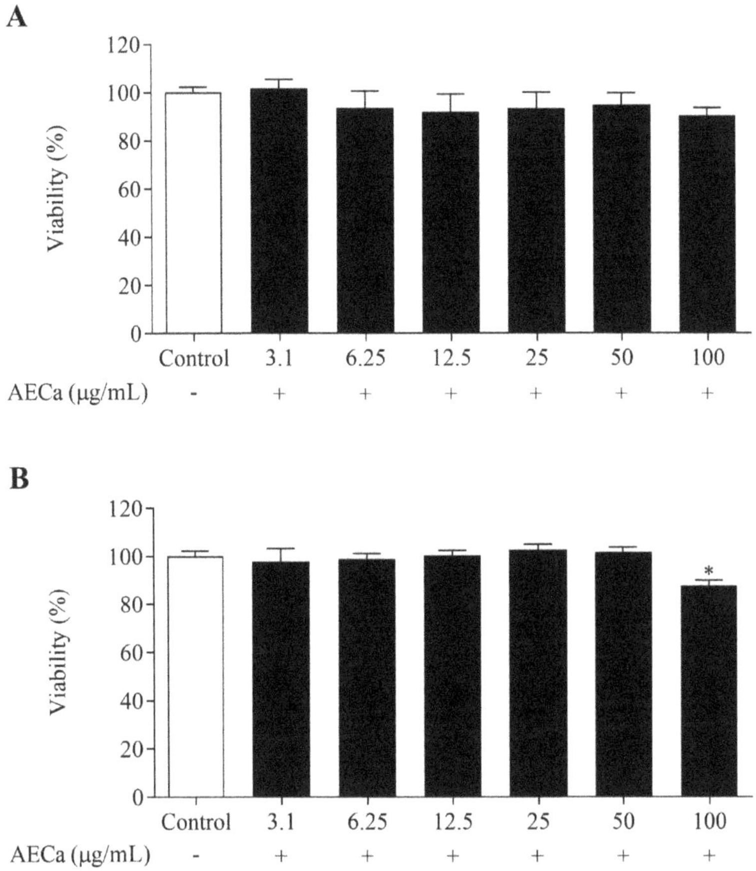

Figure 1. Cellular viability of preadipocytes incubated with different concentrations (3.1, 6.25, 12.5, 25, 50, and 100 μg/mL) of aqueous extract of *C. adamantium* leaves (AECa): (**A**) 24 h and (**B**) 48 h. Results are expressed as means ± SEM. * $p < 0.05$ versus Control.

2.3. Effect of AECa on Lipid Accumulation in Cells

The induction of differentiation using adipogenic medium in preadipocytes increased lipid content by 35% compared to the lipid content of undifferentiated cells (Control). AECa prevented lipid accumulation in a concentration-independent manner by approximately 31% compared to the cells differentiated using adipogenic medium (Figure 2A,B).

In differentiated adipocytes, AECa reduced lipid accumulation by approximately 30%, 25%, and 19% at 12.5, 25, and 50 μg/mL concentrations, respectively, compared to the Control (Figure 2C).

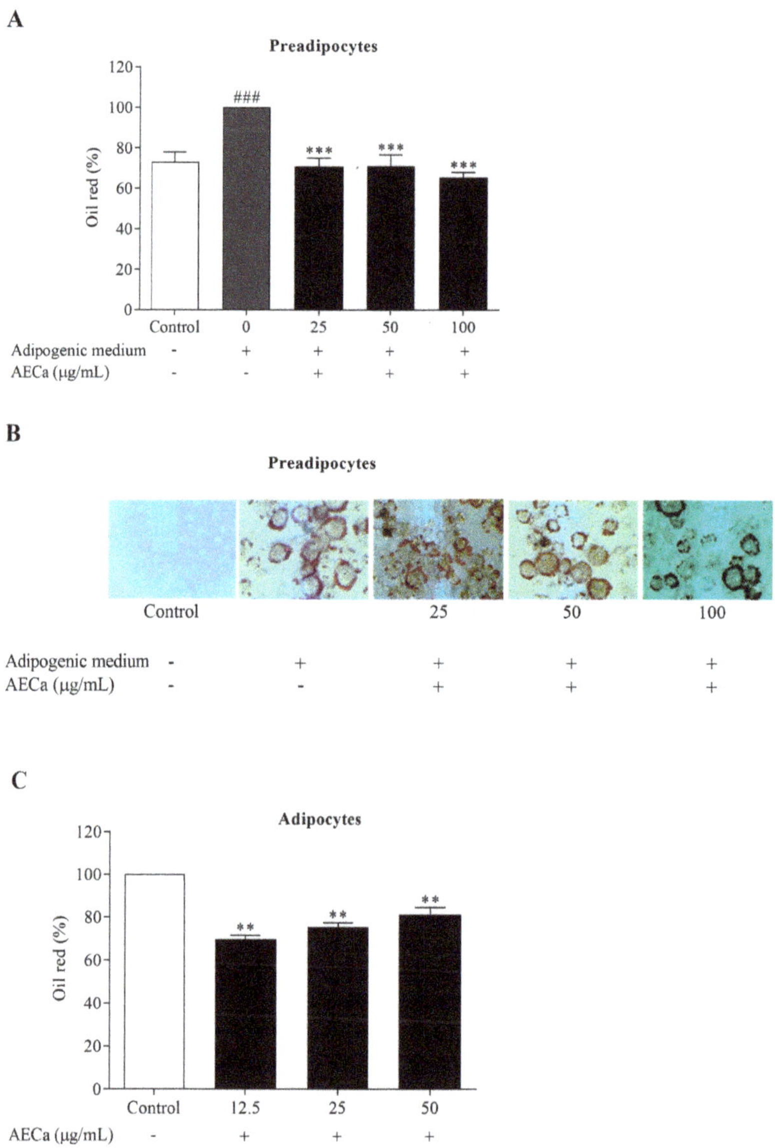

Figure 2. Lipid content observed by the percentage of Oil red in preadipocytes and differentiated adipocytes treated with different concentrations (0, 25, 50, and 100 µg/mL) of aqueous extract of *C. adamantium* leaves (AECa): (**A**) percentage of Oil red in preadipocytes treated with AECa followed by an 8-day induction of differentiation; (**B**) photomicrographs of preadipocytes treated with AECa followed by an 8-day induction of differentiation at 400× magnification; (**C**) percentage of Oil red in adipocytes by an 8-day differentiation induction followed by 48 h AECa treatment. Results are expressed as means ± SEM. ### $p < 0.001$ versus Control; ** $p < 0.01$, *** $p < 0.01$ versus adipogenic medium (0 µg/mL).

2.4. *Effect of AECa on Cytokine Production*

The induction of differentiation by the adipogenic medium in preadipocytes increased the production of the proinflammatory cytokines MCP-1, TNF-α, and IL-6 compared to undifferentiated cells (Control). AECa reduced MCP-1 production by 13, 27, and 43% at 25, 50, and 100 µg/mL concentrations, respectively. AECa reduced TNF-α production by approximately 25%. AECa reduced IL-6 production by 37 and 50% at concentrations of 50 and 100 µg/mL. AECa did not alter the production of the anti-inflammatory cytokine IL-10 (Figure 3).

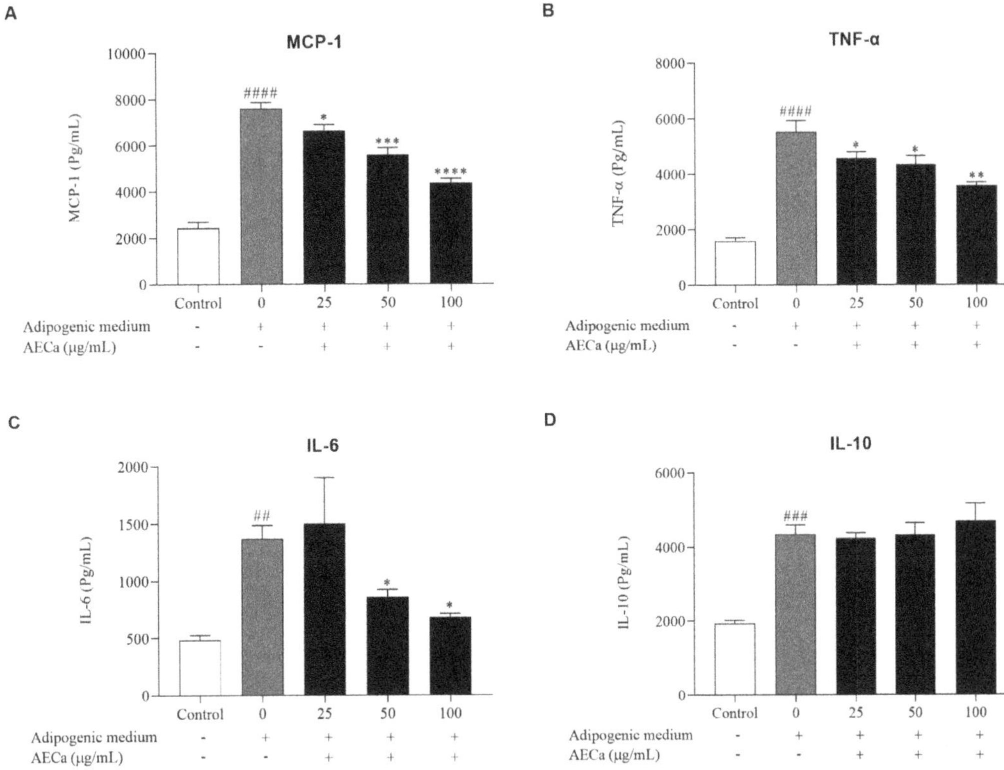

Figure 3. Cytokine production in preadipocytes and hypertrophied adipocytes treated with different concentrations (0, 25, 50, and 100 µg/mL) of aqueous extract of *C. adamantium* leaves (AECa): (**A**) MCP-1; (**B**) TNF-α; (**C**) IL-6; and (**D**) IL-10. Results are expressed as means ± SEM. ## $p < 0.01$, ### $p < 0.001$, and #### $p < 0.0001$ versus Control; * $p < 0.05$, ** $p < 0.01$, *** $p < 0.001$, and **** $p < 0.0001$ versus adipogenic medium.

2.5. *Effect of AECa on Caenorhabditis elegans Nematodes*

AECa did not alter the viability of the nematode *C. elegans*, except at a concentration of 1000 µg/mL over 24 h, where viability remained above 85%. At 48 h, the highest concentrations of AECa (750 and 1000 µg/mL) kept the viability of the nematodes above 75% (Figure 4A).

AECa reduced the lipid content in *C. elegans* by approximately 20% and 24% at concentrations of 250 and 500 µg/mL, respectively, compared to the Control (Figure 4B,C).

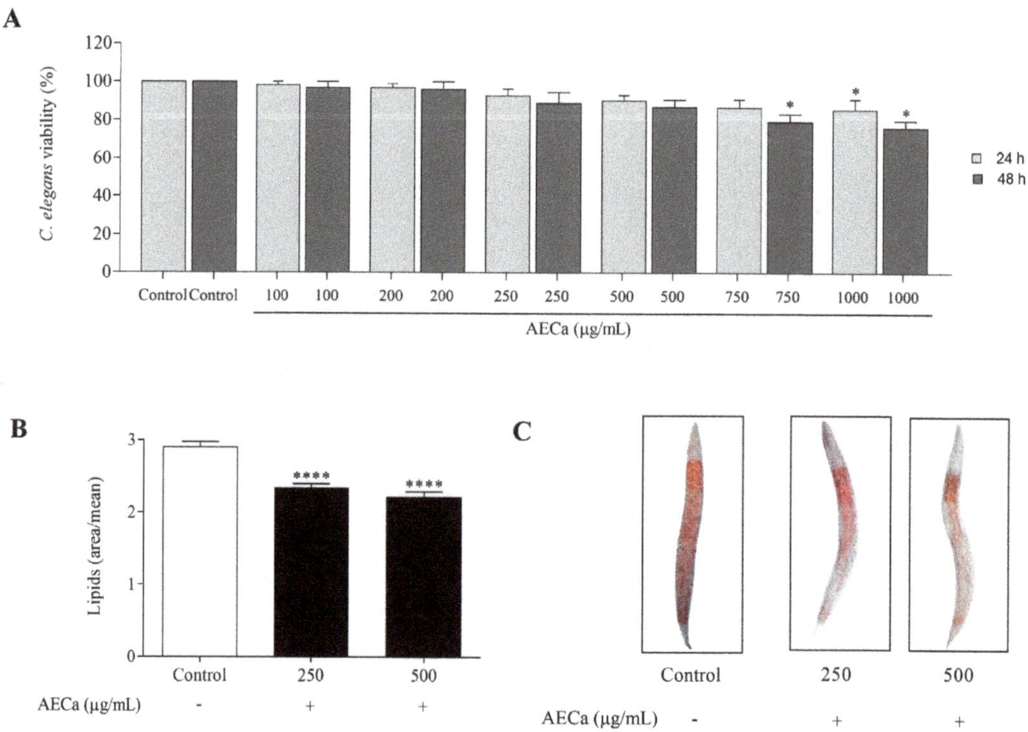

Figure 4. Viability and lipid content of *C. elegans* treated with different concentrations (100, 200, 250, 500, 750, and 1000 μg/mL) of aqueous extract of *C. adamantium* leaves (AECa): (**A**) 24 h and 48 h; (**B**) lipids (area/average); (**C**) photomicrographs of *C. elegans* at 100× magnification. Results are expressed as means ± SEM. * $p < 0.05$ and **** $p < 0.0001$ versus Control.

3. Discussion

This study reports, for the first time, the ability of the aqueous extract of *C. adamantium* leaves to reduce lipid content in preadipocytes, and in the in vivo model *C. elegans*, the production of proinflammatory cytokines in these cells, besides its antioxidant activity in vitro. In a previous study, we found that the main phytochemical constituents of AECa are quinic acid and phenolic compounds such as myricetin and quercetin [16]. Phenolic compounds are widely described for their antioxidant potential, as they have a chemical structure consisting of an aromatic ring and free hydroxyls that confer on them the ability to donate hydrogen and electrons [17,18]. AECa showed antioxidant activity in the DPPH$^•$, FRAP, and β-carotene bleaching assays, probably mediated by donating electrons from its phenolic compounds to stabilize radical molecules, reduce stable molecules, and prevent oxidative processes in lipids, respectively.

In addition, some phenolic compounds have been described as having anti-obesity potential, either through their ability to reduce adipogenesis and lipogenesis or to activate lipolysis [19–21]. In this study, we found that AECa reduced lipid accumulation when preadipocytes were treated with the extract simultaneously with the induction of differentiation with adipogenic medium. This reduction occurred in a concentration-independent manner of the AECa, which is probably related to the maximum sustained activity of the active compound in the extract, as observed for other plant extracts [22]. Probably, the AECa lowers adipogenesis (reduced differentiation) or reduces lipogenesis in differentiated cells, as some compounds present in AECa, such as quercetin and myricetin, have already been described as negative regulators of adipogenic and lipogenic genes and transcription factors such as PPAR-γ and SREBP-1c [23,24]. In this way, we can suggest that the effect of AECa is related to the group of compounds present in the extract that probably promote a reduction in the differentiation and lipogenesis of preadipocytes and adipocytes, respectively.

Additionally, AECa was able to promote lipolysis in differentiated and hypertrophied cells. Among the compounds in the extract, quercetin and myricetin may be associated with the lipolytic potential observed, as they have already been described in other studies for their lipolytic activity in adipocytes [23,25,26]. In a study by Yun-Soo et al. [25], quercetin promoted lipolysis by increasing the expression of hormone-sensitive lipase (HSL). In another study, Brasaemle et al. [26] found that myricetin downregulated the expression of perilipin A, the most abundant protein associated with lipid droplets in adipocytes that control basal and stimulated lipolysis [27].

The progression of obesity and its comorbidities is directly related to the increased production of proinflammatory cytokines and reduced production of anti-inflammatory cytokines [28]. In obesity, hypertrophied adipose tissue is accompanied by inadequate vascularization, making the cells dysfunctional and hypoxic and consequently increasing the production of proinflammatory cytokines, promoting immune cell recruitment [29]. Proinflammatory cytokines produced by immune cells and secreted by the adipose tissue, such as TNF-α, IL-4, and IL-6, stimulate obesity-associated diseases, including insulin resistance, dyslipidemia, and cardiovascular diseases. These comorbidities are related to the increased production of reactive oxygen species, which characterizes obesity-related oxidative stress [30–33]. Therefore, the in vitro antioxidant activity observed in this study may contribute to reducing the damage caused by obesity, as already observed in other studies [34].

AECa reduced the production of proinflammatory cytokines in the hypertrophied adipocytes in this study, which was probably mediated by the phenolic compounds and quinic acid present in AECa. In other studies, compounds present in AECa, such as phenolic compounds and quinic acid, have been shown to modulate cytokines such as TNF-α, IL-6, and MCP-1 [35–37]. Quinic acid, quercetin, and myricetin reduce TNF-α and IL-6 production levels by blocking the nuclear translocation of nuclear factor-κB [35,36]. Additionally, quercetin reduces the levels of MCP-1 in vitro and in vivo [37].

In the same way that AECa reduced lipid content in cells, it also reduced lipid accumulation in *C. elegans*, a complete organism. This free-living nematode is widely used as a model organism for evaluating the effect of different substances due to genes homologous to humans [38] and has been suggested as a model for obesity and drug studies [39]. *C. elegans* does not have adipocytes, so the lipid droplets are stored mainly in intestinal cells, called enterocytes. The lipid droplets of *C. elegans* mainly store triglycerides and cholesterol esters [40]. Lipid storage in *C. elegans* occurs through the activation of pathways orthologous to human pathways related to lipid metabolism, such as SBP-1, and those orthologous to SREBP [41].

In our study, *C. elegans* nematodes were treated with AECa from the first larval stage after the eggs had hatched. Therefore, the reduction in lipid content observed in the nematode intestinal cells is probably related to the suppression of the SBP-1 pathway by the compounds present in the extract. As previously mentioned, compounds present in AECa, such as myricetin, have been reported to modulate SREBP-1c negatively [42]. Moreover, another study observed that quercetin and myricetin reduced the lipid content in *C. elegans* [42].

Additionally, lipolysis in *C. elegans* can be mediated by hormone-sensitive lipase (HSL) [41]. As we saw earlier, among the compounds present in the extract, quercetin may be associated with the lipolytic potential observed by increasing the expression of HSL [23,25], thereby contributing to the reduction in the lipid content in *C. elegans* once the nematodes were treated until the L4 stage.

In conclusion, our results indicate that the aqueous extract of *C. adamantium* leaves has anti-obesity potential, with the ability to reduce adipogenesis and lipogenesis, activate lipolysis, and reduce the inflammatory processes and oxidative stress associated with the development and progression of obesity and its comorbidities.

4. Materials and Methods

4.1. Plant Material and Extract Preparation

C. adamantium O. Berg leaves were collected after authorization from SISBIO (Biodiversity Authorization and Information System, number 54470) in Dourados, Mato Grosso do Sul, Brazil (coordinates: 22°02′47.9″ S and 055°08′14.3″ W). An exsiccate was deposited in the Herbarium of the Federal University of Grande Dourados, Mato Grosso do Sul, Brazil (DDMS registration number 4108). The leaves were sanitized, dried in an air circulation oven at 45 °C, and pulverized in a knife mill. The aqueous extract of *C. adamantium* leaves (AECa) was prepared as described by Espindola et al. [15].

4.2. Evaluation of the Antioxidant Activity of AECa

4.2.1. DPPH• Free Radical Scavenging Assay

The antioxidant capacity of AECa was evaluated using the 2,2-Diphenyl-1-picrylhydrazyl (DPPH•) free radical capture method described by Bobo-García et al. [43]. Briefly, 20 µL of AECa (10–1000 µg/mL) was mixed with 180 µL of DPPH• 150 µmol/L solution and incubated for 40 min at room temperature in the dark. The absorbance was measured at 515 nm. The Control consisted of 20 µL of distilled water and 180 µL of DPPH• solution. Ascorbic acid and 2,3-tert-butyl-4-hydroxyanisole (BHA) (10–1000 µg/mL) were used as the standards. Three independent experiments were carried out in triplicate. The DPPH• inhibition percentage was obtained using the following equation:

$$\text{DPPH}^{\bullet}\text{ inhibition } (\%) = (1 - \text{Abs}_{\text{extract}}/\text{Abs}_{\text{control}}) \times 100. \quad (1)$$

The free radical 50% inhibition values (IC_{50}) were calculated.

4.2.2. Ferric Reducing Antioxidant Power (FRAP) Assay

The antioxidant capacity was assessed by its potential to reduce iron, as described by Ustundag et al. [44]. Briefly, 20 µL of AECa (20–200 µg/mL) was mixed with 280 µL of FRAP reagent. The mixture was incubated at 37 °C for 30 min. The absorbance was measured at 593 nm. The Control consisted of 20 µL of distilled water mixed with 280 µL of the FRAP reagent. BHA (20–200 µg/mL) was used as a standard. Three independent experiments were carried out in triplicate. The mean effective concentration (EC_{50}) values of the extract were calculated.

4.2.3. β-Carotene Bleaching Inhibitory Activity Assay

The antioxidant capacity was evaluated by inhibiting the bleaching of β-carotene, resulting from the oxidation induced by linoleic acid degradation products, as described by Koleva et al. [45] and Rocha et al. [46]. Briefly, 30 µL of AECa (100–1000 µg/mL) was mixed with 250 µL of β-carotene emulsion. The mixture was stirred and the absorbance was measured at 492 nm immediately after adding the emulsion (Abs1). The mixture was kept at 50 °C under stirring for 120 min. The absorbance was measured at 492 nm (Abs2). The Control consisted of 30 µL of distilled water and 250 µL of the emulsion. BHA was used as a standard (1–100 µg/mL). Three independent experiments were carried out in triplicate. The percentage of inhibition of β-carotene bleaching in the samples was obtained using the following equation:

$$\text{Inhibition of } \beta\text{-carotene bleaching } (\%) = [1 - (\text{Abs2}_{\text{extract}} - \text{Abs1}_{\text{extract}})/(\text{Abs2}_{\text{control}} - \text{Abs1}_{\text{control}})] \times 100. \quad (2)$$

IC_{50} values were calculated.

4.3. Evaluation of the Effect of AECa on Preadipocytes and Adipocytes

4.3.1. Cell Culture

Preadipocytes (3T3-F442A cells) were grown to 90% confluence in high-glucose Dulbecco's Modified Medium (DMEM) containing 3.7 g/L of sodium bicarbonate and 5.77 g/L of HEPES, supplemented with 10% Fetal Bovine Serum (FBS) and 1% penicillin/streptomycin (10,000 U mL^{-1}), all from Gibco/Invitrogen, Minneapolis, MN, USA. The cells were kept at 37 °C in a humidified atmosphere of 5% CO_2.

4.3.2. Cell Viability Assay Using MTT

Preadipocytes were plated in 96-well microplates (6×10^3 cells/well) and incubated for 24 h. After this period, different concentrations of AECa (3.12–100 µg/mL) were added to the cell culture medium, and the cells were incubated for 24 h and 48 h. Subsequently, the cells were incubated for 4 h with 1 mg/mL of 3-(4,5-dimethylthiazol-2-yl)-2,5-diphenyltetrazolium bromide (MTT). The reduction in MTT in the mitochondria resulted in the formation of violet-colored formazan crystals, which were dissolved in DMSO (100 µL/well), and the absorbance was measured at 630 nm in a microplate reader. Three independent experiments were performed in triplicate.

4.3.3. Lipid Accumulation in Cells

The effect of AECa on preadipocytes was evaluated according to the methods described by Elfakhani et al. [47] with modifications. For this purpose, preadipocytes were plated in 6-well plates (1×10^4 cells/well). When 70% confluence was reached (day 0), the adipogenic medium was added for differentiation: cell culture medium, insulin 5 µg/mL, and rosiglitazone 3 mM.

To assess the antiadipogenic effect of AECa, the cells induced to differentiate with the adipogenic medium were simultaneously given different concentrations of AECa (25–100 µg/mL) on day 0 and incubated for 48 h. The adipogenic medium without AECa was replaced every 48 h until day 8. In the end, the cells were fixed with 10% formaldehyde for 1 h and stained with a 0.3% Oil red solution for 30 min. The cells were photographed in representative fields with a camera attached to an inverted microscope at 400× magnification for analysis. The stained lipid content was removed with 100% isopropanol, and the absorbance was measured at 492 nm.

To assess the lipolytic effect of AECa, hypertrophied cells were treated with different concentrations of AECa (25–100 µg/mL) on day 8 after differentiation. After 48 h of treatment, the cells were fixed with 10% formaldehyde for 1 h and stained with a 0.3% Oil red solution for 30 min. The stained lipid content was removed with 100% isopropanol, and the absorbance was measured at 492 nm.

The cells in the Control group were incubated with the cell culture medium without the adipogenic medium while untreated cells induced to differentiation were incubated with the adipogenic medium. Two independent experiments were performed in duplicate.

4.3.4. Cytokine Quantification

To evaluate the effect of AECa on cytokine production (MCP-1, TNF-α, IL-6, and IL-10), the cells were treated with different concentrations of AECa (25–100 µg/mL) on day 0. On day 8, the adipocyte supernatant was collected and subjected to the Cytometric Bead Array (CBA) method (BD Biosciences). The evaluation was carried out by Flow Cytometry (BD LSRFortessa, BD biosciences) according to the manufacturer's instructions, and analysis was performed using the (BD biosciences). Two independent experiments were performed in duplicate.

4.4. Evaluation of the Effect of AECa on Caenorhabditis elegans

4.4.1. *C. elegans* Culture

The in vivo tests were carried out using the wild strain N2 of the nematode *C. elegans*, obtained from the Caenorhabditis Genetics Center (CGC), Minneapolis, MN, USA. The nematodes were incubated at 20 °C in Petri dishes containing nematode growth medium (NGM) and fed with *Escherichia coli* OP50 bacteria, inactivated with 10 mM kanamycin antibiotic. The nematodes were synchronized for the tests with an alkaline medium containing 2% sodium hypochlorite and 5 M sodium hydroxide. Eggs resistant to alkaline lysis were transferred to Petri dishes containing NGM and *E. coli*.

4.4.2. Sub-Chronic Toxicity

The effect of AECa on the viability of *C. elegans* was evaluated according to the method described by Leite et al. [48]. Briefly, the nematodes were synchronized at the L4 stage of development (10 nematodes N2/well) and transferred to 96-well microplates containing 100 µL of M9 buffer and 100 µL of AECa at different concentrations (3.1–100 µg/mL). The nematodes were incubated at 20 °C for 24 h and 48 h. The nematodes in the Control group were incubated with M9 buffer (200 µL). In the end, nematode viability was assessed by touch sensitivity using a platinum wire. Three independent experiments were carried out in triplicate.

4.4.3. Lipid Accumulation in *C. elegans*

For the quantification of lipids in *C. elegans*, the method described by Escorcia et al. [49] was used. For this purpose, synchronized *C. elegans* nematodes (L1 stage) were transferred to Petri dishes containing NGM and 300 µL of different concentrations of AECa (250–500 µg/mL) diluted in *E. coli* OP50. Upon reaching the L4 stage of development (approximately 48 h after synchronization), the nematodes were stained with 0.3% Oil red for 2 h. In the end, a slide was prepared with a volume of 5 µL, covered with a coverslip, and photographed under a microscope at 100× magnification. The images were analyzed using the ImageJ (version 1.52a) program. Three independent experiments were performed in duplicate.

4.5. Statistical Analysis

The data obtained were expressed as means ± standard error of the mean (SEM). Analysis of variance (ANOVA) with a Newman–Keuls post-test in GraphPad Prism 9 software (San Diego, CA, USA) was used to analyze and compare the experimental groups. The results were considered significant when $p < 0.05$.

Author Contributions: Conceptualization, P.d.S.d.R., S.L.O., I.C.F., M.V.B.R., J.F.C., E.L.d.S., and K.d.P.S.; methodology, P.d.S.d.R., S.L.O., I.C.F., P.P.d.T.E., M.V.B.R., J.T.G.d.C., D.d.S.B., D.F.L., H.F.d.S., and A.S.O.; software, P.d.S.d.R., S.L.O., I.C.F., P.P.d.T.E., M.V.B.R., J.F.C., E.L.d.S., and K.d.P.S.; validation, P.d.S.d.R., S.L.O., J.T.G.d.C., D.d.S.B., J.F.C., E.L.d.S., and K.d.P.S.; formal analysis, P.d.S.d.R., S.L.O., J.T.G.d.C., J.F.C., E.L.d.S., and K.d.P.S.; investigation, P.d.S.d.R., S.L.O., I.C.F., M.V.B.R., J.T.G.d.C., D.d.S.B., D.F.L., H.F.d.S., A.S.O., J.F.C., E.L.d.S., and K.d.P.S.; resources, J.F.C., E.L.d.S., and K.d.P.S.; data curation, P.d.S.d.R., S.L.O., J.T.G.d.C., J.F.C., E.L.d.S., and K.d.P.S.; writing—original draft preparation, P.d.S.d.R., S.L.O., I.C.F., M.V.B.R., D.d.S.B., D.F.L., H.F.d.S., A.S.O., J.F.C., E.L.d.S., and K.d.P.S.; writing—review and editing, P.d.S.d.R., S.L.O., I.C.F., M.V.B.R., J.T.G.d.C., D.d.S.B., D.F.L., H.F.d.S., A.S.O., J.F.C., E.L.d.S., and K.d.P.S.; visualization, P.d.S.d.R., S.L.O., J.T.G.d.C., D.d.S.B., J.F.C., E.L.d.S., and K.d.P.S.; supervision, J.F.C., E.L.d.S., and K.d.P.S.; project administration, J.F.C., E.L.d.S., and K.d.P.S.; funding acquisition, J.F.C., E.L.d.S., and K.d.P.S. All authors have read and agreed to the published version of the manuscript.

Funding: This research was funded by Fundação de Apoio ao Desenvolvimento do Ensino, Ciência e Tecnologia do Estado de Mato Grosso do Sul (FUNDECT), Pró-Reitoria de Ensino de Pós-Graduação e Pesquisa da Universidade Federal da Grande Dourados (PROPP-UFGD); Coordenação de Aperfeiçoamento de Pessoal de Nível Superior (CAPES), Conselho Nacional de Desenvolvimento Científico e Tecnológic (CNPq); and Financiadora de Estudos e Projetos (Finep). The APC was funded by FUNDECT grant number TO 230/2022.

Institutional Review Board Statement: Not applicable.

Informed Consent Statement: Not applicable.

Data Availability Statement: The data presented in this study are available upon request from the corresponding author.

Acknowledgments: This work was supported by Pró-Reitoria de Ensino de Pós-Graduação e Pesquisa da Universidade Federal da Grande Dourados (PROPP-UFGD); Fundação de Apoio ao Desenvolvimento do Ensino, Ciência e Tecnologia do Estado de Mato Grosso do Sul (FUNDECT); Coordenação de Aperfeiçoamento de Pessoal de Nível Superior (CAPES), Conselho Nacional de Desenvolvimento Científico e Tecnológic (CNPq); and Financiadora de Estudos e Projetos (Finep).

Conflicts of Interest: The authors declare no conflicts of interest.

References

1. Jakab, J.; Miškić, B.; Mikšić, Š.; Juranić, B.; Ćosić, V.; Schwarz, D.; Včev, A. Adipogenesis as a Potential Anti-Obesity Target: A Review of Pharmacological Treatment and Natural Products. *Diabetes Metab. Syndr. Obes. Targets Ther.* **2021**, *14*, 67–83. [CrossRef] [PubMed]
2. Jo, J.; Gavrilova, O.; Pack, S.; Jou, W.; Mullen, S.; Sumner, A.E.; Cushman, S.W.; Periwal, V. Hypertrophy and/or Hyperplasia: Dynamics of Adipose Tissue Growth. *PLoS Comput. Biol.* **2009**, *5*, e1000324. [CrossRef] [PubMed]
3. Kershaw, E.E.; Schupp, M.; Guan, H.-P.; Gardner, N.P.; Lazar, M.A.; Flier, J.S. PPARγ Regulates Adipose Triglyceride Lipase in Adipocytes in Vitro and in Vivo. *Am. J. Physiol. Metab.* **2007**, *293*, E1736–E1745. [CrossRef] [PubMed]
4. Janani, C.; Ranjitha Kumari, B.D. PPAR Gamma Gene—A Review. *Diabetes Metab. Syndr. Clin. Res. Rev.* **2015**, *9*, 46–50. [CrossRef] [PubMed]
5. Shimano, H. SREBPs: Physiology and Pathophysiology of the SREBP Family. *FEBS J.* **2009**, *276*, 616–621. [CrossRef] [PubMed]
6. Monserrat-Mesquida, M.; Quetglas-Llabrés, M.; Capó, X.; Bouzas, C.; Mateos, D.; Pons, A.; Tur, J.A.; Sureda, A. Metabolic Syndrome Is Associated with Oxidative Stress and Proinflammatory State. *Antioxidants* **2020**, *9*, 236. [CrossRef] [PubMed]
7. Monteiro, R.; Azevedo, I. Chronic Inflammation in Obesity and the Metabolic Syndrome. *Mediat. Inflamm.* **2010**, *2010*, 289645. [CrossRef] [PubMed]
8. Salmon, A. Beyond Diabetes: Does Obesity-Induced Oxidative Stress Drive the Aging Process? *Antioxidants* **2016**, *5*, 24. [CrossRef]
9. Heymsfield, S.B.; Wadden, T.A. Mechanisms, Pathophysiology, and Management of Obesity. *N. Engl. J. Med.* **2017**, *376*, 254–266. [CrossRef]
10. Saad, B.; Zaid, H.; Shanak, S.; Kadan, S. Introduction to Medicinal Plant Safety and Efficacy. In *Anti-Diabetes and Anti-Obesity Medicinal Plants and Phytochemicals*; Springer International Publishing: Cham, Switzerland, 2017; pp. 21–55. [CrossRef]
11. Cardoso, C.A.L. *Plantas Do Gênero Campomanesia: Potenciais Medicinal e Nutracêutico*; Carvalho, E.S.d., Ed.; UEMS: Dourados, Brazil, 2021.
12. Lescano, C.H.; Freitas de Lima, F.; Mendes-Silvério, C.B.; Justo, A.F.O.; da Silva Baldivia, D.; Vieira, C.P.; Sanjinez-Argandoña, E.J.; Cardoso, C.A.L.; Mónica, F.Z.; Pires de Oliveira, I. Effect of Polyphenols from *Campomanesia adamantium* on Platelet Aggregation and Inhibition of Cyclooxygenases: Molecular Docking and in Vitro Analysis. *Front. Pharmacol.* **2018**, *9*, 617. [CrossRef]
13. Ferreira, L.C.; Grabe-Guimarães, A.; de Paula, C.A.; Michel, M.C.P.; Guimarães, R.G.; Rezende, S.A.; de Souza Filho, J.D.; Saúde-Guimarães, D.A. Anti-Inflammatory and Antinociceptive Activities of *Campomanesia adamantium*. *J. Ethnopharmacol.* **2013**, *145*, 100–108. [CrossRef]
14. de Araújo, L.C.A.; Leite, N.R.; Rocha, P.d.S.d.; Baldivia, D.d.S.; Agarrayua, D.A.; Ávila, D.S.; da Silva, D.B.; Carollo, C.A.; Campos, J.F.; Souza, K.d.P.; et al. *Campomanesia adamantium* O Berg. Fruit, Native to Brazil, Can Protect against Oxidative Stress and Promote Longevity. *PLoS ONE* **2023**, *18*, e0294316. [CrossRef] [PubMed]
15. Espindola, P.P.d.T.; Rocha, P.d.S.d.; Carollo, C.A.; Schmitz, W.O.; Pereira, Z.V.; Vieira, M.D.C.; dos Santos, E.L.; Souza, K.d.P. Antioxidant and Antihyperlipidemic Effects of *Campomanesia adamantium* O. Berg Root. *Oxid. Med. Cell. Longev.* **2016**, *2016*, 7910340. [CrossRef] [PubMed]
16. Campos, J.F.; Espindola, P.P.d.T.; Torquato, H.F.V.; Vital, W.D.; Justo, G.Z.; Silva, D.B.; Carollo, C.A.; Souza, K.d.P.; Paredes-Gamero, E.J.; dos Santos, E.L. Leaf and Root Extracts from *Campomanesia adamantium* (Myrtaceae) Promote Apoptotic Death of Leukemic Cells via Activation of Intracellular Calcium and Caspase-3. *Front. Pharmacol.* **2017**, *8*, 466. [CrossRef]
17. Platzer, M.; Kiese, S.; Tybussek, T.; Herfellner, T.; Schneider, F.; Schweiggert-Weisz, U.; Eisner, P. Radical Scavenging Mechanisms of Phenolic Compounds: A Quantitative Structure-Property Relationship (QSPR) Study. *Front. Nutr.* **2022**, *9*, 882458. [CrossRef]
18. Anttonen, M.J.; Karjalainen, R.O. High-Performance Liquid Chromatography Analysis of Black Currant (*Ribes nigrum* L.) Fruit Phenolics Grown Either Conventionally or Organically. *J. Agric. Food Chem.* **2006**, *54*, 7530–7538. [CrossRef] [PubMed]
19. Gómez-Zorita, S.; Lasa, A.; Abendaño, N.; Fernández-Quintela, A.; Mosqueda-Solís, A.; Garcia-Sobreviela, M.P.; Arbonés-Mainar, J.M.; Portillo, M.P. Phenolic Compounds Apigenin, Hesperidin and Kaempferol Reduce in Vitro Lipid Accumulation in Human Adipocytes. *J. Transl. Med.* **2017**, *15*, 237. [CrossRef]
20. Aranaz, P.; Navarro-Herrera, D.; Zabala, M.; Romo-Hualde, A.; López-Yoldi, M.; Vizmanos, J.L.; Milagro, F.I.; González-Navarro, C.J. Phenolic Compounds Reduce the Fat Content in *Caenorhabditis elegans* by Affecting Lipogenesis, Lipolysis, and Different Stress Responses. *Pharmaceuticals* **2020**, *13*, 355. [CrossRef]

21. dos Santos da Rocha, P.; Orué, S.L.; Leite, D.F.; de Toledo Espindola, P.P.; Cassemiro, N.S.; da Silva, D.B.; Carollo, C.A.; Nunes-Souza, V.; Rabelo, L.A.; Campos, J.F.; et al. Beneficial Effects of *Bauhinia rufa* Leaves on Oxidative Stress, Prevention, and Treatment of Obesity in High-Fat Diet-Fed C57BL/6 Mice. *Oxid. Med. Cell. Longev.* **2022**, *2022*, 8790810. [CrossRef]
22. Oh, M.-J.; Lee, H.-B.; Yoo, G.; Park, M.; Lee, C.-H.; Choi, I.; Park, H.-Y. Anti-Obesity Effects of Red Pepper (*Capsicum annuum* L.) Leaf Extract on 3T3-L1 Preadipocytes and High Fat Diet-Fed Mice. *Food Funct.* **2023**, *14*, 292–304. [CrossRef]
23. Wang, Q.; Wang, S.; Yang, X.; You, P.; Zhang, W. Myricetin Suppresses Differentiation of 3 T3-L1 Preadipocytes and Enhances Lipolysis in Adipocytes. *Nutr. Res.* **2015**, *35*, 317–327. [CrossRef]
24. Lee, C.W.; Seo, J.Y.; Lee, J.; Choi, J.W.; Cho, S.; Bae, J.Y.; Sohng, J.K.; Kim, S.O.; Kim, J.; Park, Y.I. 3-O-Glucosylation of Quercetin Enhances Inhibitory Effects on the Adipocyte Differentiation and Lipogenesis. *Biomed. Pharmacother.* **2017**, *95*, 589–598. [CrossRef]
25. Yun-Soo, S.; Ok-Hwa, K.; Sung-Bae, K.; Su-Hyun, M.; Da-Hye, K.; Da-Wun, Y.; Jang-Gi, c.; Young-Mi, L.; Dae-Kil, K.; Ho-Seog, L.; et al. Quercetin Prevents Adipogenesis by Regulation of Transcriptional Factors and Lipases in OP9 Cells. *Int. J. Mol. Med.* **2015**, *35*, 1779–1785. [CrossRef]
26. Brasaemle, D.L.; Subramanian, V.; Garcia, A.; Marcinkiewicz, A.; Rothenberg, A. Perilipin A and the Control of Triacylglycerol Metabolism. *Mol. Cell. Biochem.* **2009**, *326*, 15–21. [CrossRef]
27. Sztalryd, C.; Brasaemle, D.L. The Perilipin Family of Lipid Droplet Proteins: Gatekeepers of Intracellular Lipolysis. *Biochim. Biophys. Acta Mol. Cell Biol. Lipids* **2017**, *1862*, 1221–1232. [CrossRef] [PubMed]
28. Fernández-Sánchez, A.; Madrigal-Santillán, E.; Bautista, M.; Esquivel-Soto, J.; Morales-González, Á.; Esquivel-Chirino, C.; Durante-Montiel, I.; Sánchez-Rivera, G.; Valadez-Vega, C.; Morales-González, J.A. Inflammation, Oxidative Stress, and Obesity. *Int. J. Mol. Sci.* **2011**, *12*, 3117–3132. [CrossRef] [PubMed]
29. Wang, R.; Sun, Q.; Wu, X.; Zhang, Y.; Xing, X.; Lin, K.; Feng, Y.; Wang, M.; Wang, Y.; Wang, R. Hypoxia as a Double-Edged Sword to Combat Obesity and Comorbidities. *Cells* **2022**, *11*, 3735. [CrossRef] [PubMed]
30. Hall, J.E.; Mouton, A.J.; da Silva, A.A.; Omoto, A.C.M.; Wang, Z.; Li, X.; do Carmo, J.M. Obesity, Kidney Dysfunction, and Inflammation: Interactions in Hypertension. *Cardiovasc. Res.* **2021**, *117*, 1859–1876. [CrossRef]
31. Van Raemdonck, K.; Umar, S.; Szekanecz, Z.; Zomorrodi, R.K.; Shahrara, S. Impact of Obesity on Autoimmune Arthritis and Its Cardiovascular Complications. *Autoimmun. Rev.* **2018**, *17*, 821–835. [CrossRef]
32. Matsuda, M.; Shimomura, I. Roles of Oxidative Stress, Adiponectin, and Nuclear Hormone Receptors in Obesity-Associated Insulin Resistance and Cardiovascular Risk. *Horm. Mol. Biol. Clin. Investig.* **2014**, *19*, 75–88. [CrossRef]
33. Khan, S.S.; Ning, H.; Wilkins, J.T.; Allen, N.; Carnethon, M.; Berry, J.D.; Sweis, R.N.; Lloyd-Jones, D.M. Association of Body Mass Index With Lifetime Risk of Cardiovascular Disease and Compression of Morbidity. *JAMA Cardiol.* **2018**, *3*, 280–287. [CrossRef] [PubMed]
34. Khutami, C.; Sumiwi, S.A.; Khairul Ikram, N.K.; Muchtaridi, M. The Effects of Antioxidants from Natural Products on Obesity, Dyslipidemia, Diabetes and Their Molecular Signaling Mechanism. *Int. J. Mol. Sci.* **2022**, *23*, 2056. [CrossRef]
35. Nam, S.-Y.; Han, N.-R.; Rah, S.-Y.; Seo, Y.; Kim, H.-M.; Jeong, H.-J. Anti-Inflammatory Effects of *Artemisia scoparia* and Its Active Constituent, 3,5-Dicaffeoyl-Epi-Quinic Acid against Activated Mast Cells. *Immunopharmacol. Immunotoxicol.* **2018**, *40*, 52–58. [CrossRef]
36. Zhong, R.; Miao, L.; Zhang, H.; Tan, L.; Zhao, Y.; Tu, Y.; Angel Prieto, M.; Simal-Gandara, J.; Chen, L.; He, C.; et al. Anti-Inflammatory Activity of Flavonols via Inhibiting MAPK and NF-KB Signaling Pathways in RAW264.7 Macrophages. *Curr. Res. Food Sci.* **2022**, *5*, 1176–1184. [CrossRef]
37. Le, N.H.; Kim, C.-S.; Park, T.; Park, J.H.Y.; Sung, M.-K.; Lee, D.G.; Hong, S.-M.; Choe, S.-Y.; Goto, T.; Kawada, T.; et al. Quercetin Protects against Obesity-Induced Skeletal Muscle Inflammation and Atrophy. *Mediat. Inflamm.* **2014**, *2014*, 834294. [CrossRef]
38. Shen, P.; Yue, Y.; Zheng, J.; Park, Y. *Caenorhabditis elegans*: A Convenient In Vivo Model for Assessing the Impact of Food Bioactive Compounds on Obesity, Aging, and Alzheimer's Disease. *Annu. Rev. Food Sci. Technol.* **2018**, *9*, 1–22. [CrossRef] [PubMed]
39. Yue, Y.; Li, S.; Shen, P.; Park, Y. *Caenorhabditis elegans* as a Model for Obesity Research. *Curr. Res. Food Sci.* **2021**, *4*, 692–697. [CrossRef] [PubMed]
40. Dyczkowska, A.; Chabowska-Kita, A. *Caenorhabditis elegans* as a Model Organism in Obesity Research. *BioTechnologia* **2021**, *102*, 337–362. [CrossRef]
41. An, L.; Fu, X.; Chen, J.; Ma, J. Application of *Caenorhabditis elegans* in Lipid Metabolism Research. *Int. J. Mol. Sci.* **2023**, *24*, 1173. [CrossRef]
42. Lin, Y.; Yang, N.; Bao, B.; Wang, L.; Chen, J.; Liu, J. Luteolin Reduces Fat Storage in *Caenorhabditis elegans* by Promoting the Central Serotonin Pathway. *Food Funct.* **2020**, *11*, 730–740. [CrossRef]
43. Bobo-García, G.; Davidov-Pardo, G.; Arroqui, C.; Vírseda, P.; Marín-Arroyo, M.R.; Navarro, M. Intra-Laboratory Validation of Microplate Methods for Total Phenolic Content and Antioxidant Activity on Polyphenolic Extracts, and Comparison with Conventional Spectrophotometric Methods. *J. Sci. Food Agric.* **2015**, *95*, 204–209. [CrossRef] [PubMed]
44. Ustundag, Y.; Huysal, K.; Kahvecioglu, S.; Demirci, H.; Yavuz, S.; Sambel, M.; Unal, D. Establishing Reference Values and Evaluation of an In-House Ferric Reducing Antioxidant Power (FRAP) Colorimetric Assay in Microplates. *Eur. Res. J.* **2016**, *2*, 126–131. [CrossRef]
45. Koleva, I.I.; van Beek, T.A.; Linssen, J.P.H.; de Groot, A.; Evstatieva, L.N. Screening of Plant Extracts for Antioxidant Activity: A Comparative Study on Three Testing Methods. *Phytochem. Anal.* **2002**, *13*, 8–17. [CrossRef] [PubMed]

46. Rocha, P.d.S.d.; de Araújo Boleti, A.P.; do Carmo Vieira, M.; Carollo, C.A.; da Silva, D.B.; Estevinho, L.M.; dos Santos, E.L.; de Picoli Souza, K. Microbiological Quality, Chemical Profile as Well as Antioxidant and Antidiabetic Activities of *Schinus terebinthifolius* Raddi. *Comp. Biochem. Physiol. Part C Toxicol. Pharmacol.* **2019**, *220*, 36–46. [CrossRef] [PubMed]
47. Elfakhani, M.; Torabi, S.; Hussein, D.; Mills, N.; Verbeck, G.F.; Mo, H. Mevalonate Deprivation Mediates the Impact of Lovastatin on the Differentiation of Murine 3T3-F442A Preadipocytes. *Exp. Biol. Med.* **2014**, *239*, 293–301. [CrossRef] [PubMed]
48. Leite, N.R.; de Araújo, L.C.A.; Rocha, P.d.S.d.; Agarrayua, D.A.; Ávila, D.S.; Carollo, C.A.; Silva, D.B.; Estevinho, L.M.; Souza, K.d.P.; dos Santos, E.L. Baru Pulp (*Dipteryx alata* Vogel): Fruit from the Brazilian Savanna Protects against Oxidative Stress and Increases the Life Expectancy of *Caenorhabditis elegans* via SOD-3 and DAF-16. *Biomolecules* **2020**, *10*, 1106. [CrossRef]
49. Escorcia, W.; Ruter, D.L.; Nhan, J.; Curran, S.P. Quantification of Lipid Abundance and Evaluation of Lipid Distribution in *Caenorhabditis elegans* by Nile Red and Oil Red O Staining. *J. Vis. Exp.* **2018**, *2018*, e57352. [CrossRef]

pharmaceuticals MDPI

Article

Neuroprotective Effects of *Glycyrrhiza glabra* Total Extract and Isolated Compounds

Ali O. E. Eltahir [1,†], Sylvester I. Omoruyi [2], Tanya N. Augustine [2], Robert C. Luckay [3] and Ahmed A. Hussein [1,*]

1 Chemistry Department, Cape Peninsula University of Technology, Symphony Rd. Bellville, Cape Town 7535, South Africa; aliomers250@gmail.com
2 School of Anatomical Sciences, Faculty of Health Sciences, University of the Witwatersrand, Parktown, Johannesburg 2193, South Africa; sylvester.omoruyi@wits.ac.za (S.I.O.); tanya.augustine@wits.ac.za (T.N.A.)
3 Department of Chemistry and Polymer Science, Stellenbosch University, Matieland, Stellenbosch 7602, South Africa; rcluckay@sun.ac.za
* Correspondence: mohammedam@cput.ac.za; Tel.: +27-21-959-6193; Fax: +27-21-959-3055
† Current address: Department of Chemistry, Faculty of Education, Omdurman Islamic University, Omdurman 14415, Sudan.

Abstract: *Glycyrrhiza glabra* L. is a plant commonly utilized in herbal medicine and stands out as one of the more extensively researched medicinal plants globally. It has been documented with respect to several pharmacological activities, notably, neuroprotective effects, among others. However, the neuroprotective activity of pure phenolic compounds has not been reported yet. The chromatographic of a methanolic extract yielded twenty-two compounds, viz.: naringenin 4′-*O*-glucoside (**1**), 3′,4′,7-trihydroxyflavanone (butin) (**2**), liquiritin (**3**), liquiritin apioside (**4**), abyssinone (**5**), glabrol (**6**), isoliquiritin (**7**), neoisoliquiritin (**8**), isoliquiritin apioside (**9**), licuraside (**10**). 3′[*O*], 4′-(2,2-dimethylpyrano)-3,7-dihydroxyflavanone (**11**), glabrocoumarin (**12**), glabrene (**13**), isomedicarpin (**14**), 7-hydroxy-4′-methoxyflavone (formononetin) (**15**), ononin (**16**), glycyroside (**17**), (3*S*)-7,4′-dihydroxy-2′-methoxyisoflavan (**18**), glabridin (**19**), neoliquiritin (**20**), 3,11-dioxooleana-1,12-dien-29-oic acid (**21**), and 3-oxo-18β-glycyrrhetinic acid (**22**). The results of the neuroprotection evaluation showed that *G. glabra* total extract (TE) and compounds **1**, **7**, **11**, **16**, and **20** protected SH-SY5Y cells by inhibiting the depletion of ATP and elevated caspase 3/7 activities induced by MPP+. Indeed, this study reports for the first time the structure and activity of compound **11** and the neuroprotective activity of some phenolic constituents from *G. glabra*.

Keywords: *Glycyrrhiza glabra*; licorice; phenolic compounds; neuroprotection

1. Introduction

Neurodegenerative diseases are a group of diseases characterized by the loss of neurons in the brain [1]. Notable amongst them are Parkinson's disease and Alzheimer's disease. Specifically, Parkinson's disease (PD) involves the loss of dopaminergic neurons in the substantia nigra pars compacta of the midbrain [2]. Classical symptoms of PD include tremors, bradykinesia, akinesia, and postural imbalance [3]. At the molecular level, the progressive loss of dopaminergic neurons is triggered by a cascade of events, including the alteration of the mitochondrial electron transport chain following the accumulation of reactive oxygen species and the loss of adenosine triphosphate (ATP) in the cells [4]. This cascade of events will eventually lead to the death of neurons [5]. Although the actual cause of PD is yet to be fully understood, the onset is believed to result from an interplay between the environment and genetic factors [2]. For instance, exposure to certain neurotoxins such as 1-methyl-4-phenyl-1,2,3,6-tetrahydropyridine (MPTP), a heroin analogue, has been implicated in the onset of the disease [6]. Age is also a major contributing factor, as PD mainly affects people aged 60 and above [7]. To date, treatment of PD remains daunting, as existing treatments only treat symptoms, and levodopa in particular, a dopamine replacement agent which is the current standard care, can nevertheless also lead to Parkinsonism symptoms after prolonged usage [8]. In this regard, medicinal and natural products have continued to serve as a resource base for exploiting biochemical entities that could offer neuroprotective activities [9–11].

Licorice is a name given to different species of the *Glycyrrhiza* (Licorice) genus. Notable amongst them is *G. glabra*, one of the most valuable medicinal plants. It consists of about 30 taxa, of which only 15 taxa have been studied so far [12], mainly including the species *G. glabra* L., *G. uralensis* Fisch., *G. inflata* Bat., *G. echinata* L., *G. lepidota*., *G. pallidflora* Maxim., and *G. macedonica*, [13–15]. The plants, renowned for their medicinal properties, are widely used in herbal medicine and are among the most extensively studied medicinal plants globally. They have a notable pharmaceutical history in regions such as China, India, Iran, Spain, Italy, Russia, and North Africa, and remain crucial in the exploration of new pharmaceuticals. Several modern medical research studies have concentrated on their chemical constituents and biological effects, aiming to understand the underlying mechanisms. Numerous pharmacological studies, including clinical investigations, have explored the effects of licorice root extract or its isolated compounds on the nervous system. These plants exhibit various pharmacological activities, including neuroprotective, anti-inflammatory, antimicrobial, anticancer, gastroprotective, hepatoprotective, and cardioprotective effects. Additionally, they have been found to be effective treatments for influenza, cough, lung diseases, pneumonia, bronchitis, skin diseases, and hormone replacement therapy [16–23]. Recently, the plant was used for the treatment of immunostimulating effects in the contexts of coronavirus disease 2019 (COVID-19) and severe acute respiratory syndrome coronavirus 2 (SARS-CoV-2) virus [24,25]. *G. glabra* and *G. uralensis* are the most studied species of this genus. Furthermore, the literature has reported up to 400 compounds from the *Glycyrrhiza* genus, which have been categorized into various classes such as phenolics (flavanones, flavones, flavanonols, chalcones and dihydrochalcones, isoflavones, and coumestans/phenyldihydrocoumarins, and their methoxylated, prenylated, and glycosolated derivatives) and triterpenoids, including their glycosides [26].

Although licorice species have been extensively studied for their biological activities, including their neuroprotective activities, the present study investigates the neuroprotective activities of the TE of *G. glabra* and its isolated compounds in an in vitro model of PD in the neuroblastoma cell line, SH-SY5Y, using the neurotoxin 1-methyl-4-phenylpyridinium (MPP^+). Indeed, several studies have demonstrated that MPP+, which is a byproduct of MPTP, a toxin known to induce parkinsonism, induces neurotoxicity in the SH-SY5Y cells [27,28]. We also report for the first time the activities of novel compounds isolated and identified from licorice species and show for the first time the neuroprotective activities of these compounds in a PD model.

2. Results

2.1. Chemical Characterization of the Isolated Compounds

Chromatographic purification of the total extract using different techniques, including semi-prep HPLC, resulted in the isolation of twenty-two (22) pure compounds, which were identified as naringenin 4′-*O*-glucoside (**1**) [29,30], 3′, 4′, 7-trihydroxyflavanone (butin) (**2**) [31,32], liquiritin (**3**) [33,34], liquiritin apioside (**4**) [33], abyssinone (**5**) [35], glabrol (**6**) [33,36,37], isoliquiritin (**7**) [38,39], neoisoliquiritin (**8**) [38,39], isoliquiritin apioside (**9**) [40–42], licuraside (**10**) [40–43], 3′[*O*],4′-(2,2-dimethylpyrano)-3,7-dihydroxyflavanone (**11**), glabrocoumarin (**12**) [44], glabrene (**13**) [37,45], isomedicarpin (**14**) [33,46], 7-hydroxy-4′-methoxyflavone (formononetin) (**15**) [33], ononin (**16**) [30,33], glycyroside (**17**) [30,33], (3*S*)-7,4′-dihydroxy-2′-methoxyisoflavan (**18**) [47], glabridin (**19**) [33,34,37], neoliquiritin (**20**) [48], 3,11-dioxooleana-1,12-die-29-oic acid (**21**) [49], and 3-oxo-18β-glycyrrhetinic acid (22) [50]. The isolated compounds were identified based on detailed spectroscopic analyses and comparison with those reported in the literature (Figure 1).

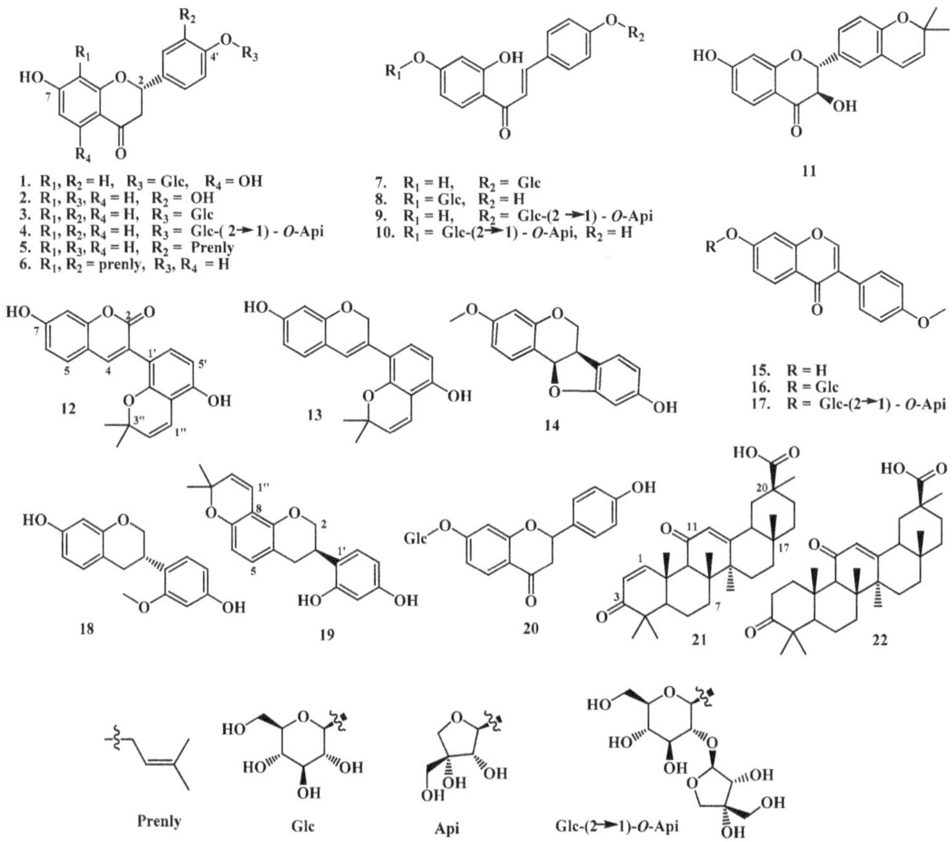

Figure 1. Chemical structures of the compounds isolated from *G. glabra*.

Compound **11** was isolated as a whitish-yellow powder, and its molecular formula was determined to be $C_{20}H_{18}O_5$ by its HRESIMS (High Resolution Electrospray Ionization Mass Spectrometry). The UV spectrum of **11** had absorption maxima at 313 and 276 nm, whereas the IR spectrum showed absorption bands at 3374, 1673, 1608, 1502, and 1463 cm^{-1} for OH, CO, and aromatic groups.

The ^1H NMR spectrum of **11** showed signals assignable to six aromatic protons belonging to two 1,3,4-trisubstituted aromatic rings [δ_H 7.72 (*d*, *J* = 8.5 Hz), 6.51 (*dd*, *J* = 8.5, 2.0 Hz), and 6.30 (*d*, *J* = 2.0 Hz); δ_H 7.25 (*d*, *J* = 7.9 Hz), and 6.76 (*br d*, *J* = 7.9 Hz), 7.23 (*br s*)]; two oxygenated methines [δ_H 4.92 and 4.50 (*d* each, *J* = 11.8 Hz)], and a 2,2-dimethyl pyrane ring [δ_H 6.43 and 5.58 (*d* each, *J* = 9.7 Hz), and two methyls at 1.37 (6H, s)]. The ^{13}C NMR and DEPT-135 showed 20 carbons which could be classified as CO (192.7); 14 olefinic signals, 12 of them aromatics (see Table 1); three oxy carbons (83.7, 76.3 and 72.9); and two methyls (27.7, 2C's). The above data showed similarity with (2*R*,3*R*)-3,4′,7-trihydroxy-3′-prenylflavanone isolated from the same source by Kuroda et. al. (2010) [51]; the only differences are lying on the chemical shifts of the prenyl signals. This similarity indicates that **11** could be a 3-hydroxyflavanol derivative attached to a pyrane ring. Heteronuclear Multiple Bond Correlation (HMBC) correlations between H-5 and C-4, C-7, C-9; H-8/C-7, C-9, C-10; H-6′/C-2, C-4′; H-2′/C-2, C-4′, H-1″/C-4′, C-2′, C-3″ indicate connectivity of the molecule and the linkage of the pyrane ring at C3′, C4′ of ring B (Figure 2).

Table 1. NMR data of compound **11** (DMSO-d_6) and 3,4′,7-trihydroxy-3′-prenylflavanone (acetone-d_6).

Position	Compound 11		3,4′,7-Trihydroxy-3′-prenylflavanone [51]	
	δ_C	δ_H, *multi, J* (Hz)	δ_C	δ_H, *multi, J* (Hz)
2	83.7	4.92 (*d*, 11.8)	84.6	5.03 (*d*, 11.9)
3	72.9	4.50 (*d*, 11.8)	73.4	4.59 (*d*, 11.9)
4	192.7	-	192.7	-
5	128.6	7.72 (*d*, 8.6)	129.3	7.74 (*d*, 8.6)
6	111.5	6.51 (*dd*, 8.6, 2.0)	111.2	6.64 (*dd*, 8.6, 2.2)
7	162.7	-	165.4	-
8	102.5	6.30 (*d*, 2.0)	103.1	6.41 (*d*, 2.2)
9	163.2	-	164.1	-
10	111.9	-	112.5	-
1′	129.6	-	128.9	-
2′	126.2	7.23 (*br s*)	130.0	7.35 (*d*, 2.0)
3′	120.7 s	-	128.1	-
4′	152.6	-	155.8	-
5′	115.5	6.76 (*d*, 7.9)	115.0	6.90 (d, 8.2)
6′	129.1 d	7.25 (*br d*, 7.9)	127.1	7.27 (*dd*, 8.2, 2.2)
1″	121.6	6.43 (*d*, 9.7)	28.7	3.38 (2H, *d*, 7.3)
2″	131.3	5.58 (*d*, 9.7)	123.1	5.39 (*m*)
3″	76.3	-	132.0	-
4″	27.7	1.37 (*s*)	25.4	1.72 (*br s*)
5″	27.7	1.37 (*s*)	17.4	1.74 (*br s*)

multi: multiplicity, *J* values in Hz, *s*: singlet, *br s*: broad singlet, *br d*: broad doublet, *d*: doublet, *dd*: doublet of doublet, *m*: multiple.

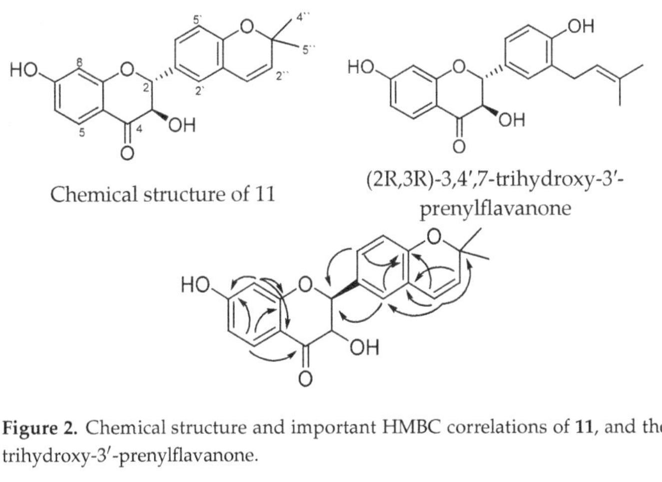

Figure 2. Chemical structure and important HMBC correlations of **11**, and the structure of 3,4′,7-trihydroxy-3′-prenylflavanone.

The known compounds were identified based on the extensive NMR data, including 2D (HSQC, COSY, and HMBC). The ^{1}H NMR spectrum of **1** displayed a typical flavanone skeleton, as well as a 2-3 dihydro ring C pattern [δ_H 5.50 (*d*, *J* = 12.7, 2.2 Hz, H-2; δ_C 78.4), δ_H 2.69 (*dd*, *J* = 17.1, 2.2 Hz, H-3β), and δ_H 3.24 (H-3α, overlapped; δ_C 42.4)]. The peaks at δ_H 7.43 (*d*, *J* = 8.6 Hz, H-2′, 6′) and δ_H 7.07 (*d*, *J* = 8.6 Hz, H-3′, 5′) indicated a 1,4-disubstituted ring B. The two protons at δ_H 5.85 and 5.83 (*br s*, δ_C 95.8 and 96.7) suggested free 6,8-positions of ring A. Additionally, the proton at δ_H 4.89 (*d*, *J* = 7.2 Hz, δ_C 100.7) was identified as an anomeric proton of a glucose unit. The ^{13}C NMR and DEPT-135 spectra revealed 19 signals corresponding to 21 carbons, including a signal at δ_C 196.1 (CO, C-4), supporting the presence of a flavanone skeleton. The attachment of the glucose unit to C-4′ is confirmed by the HMBC correlation of the anomeric proton with C-4′. The NMR data (Table S1) are identical to those of naringenin-4′-*O*-glucoside, previously isolated from the same source and *Salvia patens* [29,30].

Compounds **2**–**6** and **20** share a similar flavanone skeleton pattern with compound **1**. Compound **2** has characteristics similar to **1**, with the main differences being the absence of a glucose unit and the splitting of ring B into a typical 1,3,4-trisubstituted benzene ring, identified as 3′,4′,7-trihydroxyflavanone. The compound has been isolated previously from *Vernonia anthelmintica* and *Cotinus coggygria* [31,32]. Compounds **3** and **4** are also flavanones and are connected to a sugar at position C-4′. Compound **3** contains a glucose unit, which is supported by the presence of HMBC correlation between the anomeric proton (δ_H 4.89/δ_C 100.3) and C-4′, while compound **4** exhibits an additional signal of apiose at δ_H 5.36/δ_C 108.7. Both compounds were isolated from the same source [33,34].

Compounds **5** and **6** both exhibit additional signals from prenyl groups. In compound **5**, the prenyl signals are observed at the following chemical shifts (δ_H/δ_C): 3.22 (6.5, 2H-1″)/27.9; 5.28 (*br d*, 6.5, H-2″)/123.1; 1.68 (s, Me-4″)/26.0, and 1.67 (s, Me-5″)/18.1, in addition to a signal observed at δ_C 131.7 (C-3″). The prenyl group is attached to C-3′, as confirmed by HMBC correlation. Compound **6**, on the other hand, features two prenyl groups, at positions C-3′ and -8. (see Table S1 for more details). Both compounds **5** [35] and **6** [33,36,37] were derived from the same source. Compound **20** shares a similar profile with compound **3**, the only distinction being the attachment of the glucose unit at C-7 instead of C-3′ (as in compound **3**) [48].

Compounds **7**–**10** exhibit the same NMR pattern and are closely related to previous compounds, particularly compounds **2**, **3**, and **20**. However, in these compounds, ring C is replaced by a 1,4-enone system, as indicated by the signals corresponding to the carbonyl (CO), C_α and C_β. The change of glucose link between C-4 and C-4′ is evident and supported by HMBC correlations between the anomeric protons and the corresponding carbons [42,43]. For compounds **9** and **10**, the situation is analogous, with the glucose moiety being replaced by a glucose–apiose moiety. This replacement is supported by the similar NMR patterns and HMBC correlations, providing clear evidence of the structural changes [40–42].

Compound **12** exhibited a 1,2-benzopyrone nucleus (coumarin) with an OH group at C-7. The signal at δ_H 7.82/δ_C 142.5 indicates H-4, while the *o*-coupled protons at δ_H 7.52 (δ_C 129.6) and δ_H 6.79 (δ_C 113.1) correspond to H-5 and H-6. The *o*-coupled protons at δ_H 6.32 (δ_C 107.3) and δ_H 6.94 (δ_C 130.6) indicate H-5′ and H-6′, belonging to a 1,2,3,4-tetrasubstituted ring B. Additionally, the signals at δ_H 6.57 (d, J = 10 Hz, H-1″, δ_C 116.8), δ_H 5.53 (*d*, J = 10 Hz, H-2″, δ_C 128.3), and the two methyl groups at δ_H 1.37 (6H, s, δ_C 27.2 $\times$ 2C) indicate a pyrane ring attached to C-3 and C-2 of ring B. The data (see Table S1) are consistent with glabrocoumarins, and confirmed by 2D spectra. The compound has been previously isolated from the same source [44].

Compound **13** displayed signals similar to **12**, with the only difference being the absence of the carbonyl group at C-2 and the formation of another 2*H*-pyran ring. The data (see Table S1) are consistent with glabrene, also previously isolated from the same source [37,45].

Compound **14** displayed signals corresponding to a 1,2,4-trisubstituted benzene ring (see Table S1), as well as a 3,4-dihydro-2*H*-pyran ring [δ_H 3.56, 4.16 (CH_2-2)/δ_C 68.5; δ_H 3.52 (H-3)/δ_C 39.3; δ_H 5.47 (H-4)/δ_C 78.0]. Additionally, it showed an OMe group, at δ_H 3.65/δ_C 55.2, connected to C-7. These findings are consistent with isomedicarpin, which was isolated from the same source [33,46].

Compounds **15**–**17** share the same isoflavonoid skeleton, as indicated by the H-2 signals (δ_H ~ 8.40). Ring A is connected to different side chains at C-7, while ring B is 1,4-disubstituted with a methoxy group at C-4′ (see Table S1 for more details). Compound **15** has a hydroxyl group at C-7, compound **16** has a glucose moiety, and compound **17** has a glucose–apiose moiety, as evidenced by the anomeric H/C signals of the sugars. These three compounds were previously isolated from the same source [30,33].

Compound **18** displayed two 1,2,4-trisubstituted benzene rings (rings A and B) and a tetrahydropyrane ring (ring C), as evidenced by the presence of signals for two methylenes (δ_H 4.14, 4.61; δ_C 69.2 and δ_H 2.71, 2.87; δ_C 29.7) and a methine (δ_H 3.32; δ_C 31.0). Ring

A showed signals for two *o*-coupled protons (δ_H 6.85, d, *J* = 8.4 Hz, H-5 and δ_H 6.29, br *d*, *J* = 8.4 Hz, H-6) and a singlet at δ_H 6.19 (*br s*, H-8). Ring B exhibited signals for two *o*-coupled protons (δ_H 6.34, *br d*, *J* = 8.6 Hz, H-5′ and δ_H 6.97, *d*, *J* = 8.6 Hz, H-6′) and a singlet at δ_H 6.43 (*br s*, H-3′). The ^{13}C NMR and DEPT-135 spectra showed 16 well-resolved signals, corresponding to 16 carbons, including two methylenes, one sp^3 methine, six sp^2 methines, six sp^2 quaternary carbons, and a methoxy group. The NMR data matched those of 7,4′-dihydroxy-2′-methoxyisoflavan isolated from propolis [47]. Compound **19** is similar to compound **18**, with the only difference being the absence of the methoxy group at C-2′ and the appearance of a pyrane ring at C-8 and C-7 of ring A. The NMR data for compound **19** matched those of glabridin, which was isolated from the same source (see Table S1 for more details) [33,34,37].

Compounds **21** and **22** are oleanane-type triterpenes. Compound **22** exhibited seven methyl singlet signals at δ_H/δ_C: 1.12/26.3 (C-23), 1.09/21.4 (C-24), 1.29/15.6 (C-25), 1.19/18.5 (C-26), 1.40/23.3 (C-27), 0.87/28.5 (C-28), and 1.25/28.4 (C-29), along with a singlet at 5.47 (H-12). The ^{13}C NMR spectrum showed 29 well-resolved signals corresponding to 30 carbons, including two carbonyl carbons, at 217.0 and 199.7 ppm, the latter conjugated with a double bond at 169.8/128.4 ppm. Additionally, the spectrum included three methines, nine methylenes, and five quaternary carbons. The presence of the carbonyl carbon of the carboxylic group at 181.1 ppm and the conjugated double bond are characteristic fragments of glycyrrhetinic acid isolated from the same source. Based on the NMR data, the compound was identified as 3-oxo-glycyrrhetinic acid [50], with data matching reported values. It is important to note that, based on 2D NMR correlations, some chemical shifts were reassigned and corrected from reference [50], particularly for C-6, C-7, C-8, and C-14, and methyl groups at C-28 and C-29.

The NMR data for compound **21** are identical to those of compound **22**, with the exception of the presence of a double bond in ring A. This double bond is supported by signals at δ_H/δ_C 7.72/161.6 (both doublets, *J* = 10.4 Hz), and the high chemical shift of C-3 (204.6 ppm), as compared to compound **22**. Through the analysis of various 2D NMR experiments, a complete assignment of the carbons and protons was achieved (see Table S1). Compound **21** was identified as 3,11-dioxooleana-1,12-die-29-oic acid, which has been reported previously as a synthetic derivative [49]. Notably, this is the first comprehensive report of the NMR data for compound **21**.

The purity of the isolated compounds was confirmed by NMR, TLC, and HPLC (purity $\geq$ 95% for all compounds). Compound **11** is reported for the first time in this study, while **21** was reported previously as a synthetic product [49].

2.2. Biological Study

2.2.1. Dose–Response of Licorice TE and Compounds

To investigate the neuroprotective potentials of the TE and compounds, their effects on the cell viability of the SH-SY5Y were first determined. The total extract and 22 compounds were screened for their cytotoxicity using concentrations of 12.5, 25, and 50 μg/mL for the extract, and 2.5, 5, and 10 μg/mL for the compounds. The results show that the TE and compounds had minimal effects on the cell viability of the SH-SY5Y cells, especially at 2.5 μg/mL; however, with increased concentration, some compounds induced toxicity (Figure 3). In addition, the cells treated with compound 20 showed increased cell viability for all concentrations. In contrast, the cells treated with compound 6 showed significant reductions in cell viability at all concentrations tested. Following these results, the TE and five compounds, **1**, **7**, **11**, **16** and **20**, were selected to be investigated for their neuroprotective potentials, as they were not cytotoxic, and they improved cell viability the most compared to other compounds. In particular, compound **20** significantly increased cell viability at all concentrations tested.

2.2.2. Effects of Licorice TE and Compounds on MPP+-Induced Toxicity on SH-SY5Y Cells

To investigate the neuroprotective activities of the TE and compounds, their effects on cell viability in the presence of the MPP^+ neurotoxin were determined using the MTT cell viability assay. The results show that pretreatment with the TE and compounds resulted in significant improvements in cell viability of MPP+-treated cells, compared to cells treated with MPP alone (Figure 4). While MPP+ reduced cell viability to about 40% when compared to the control cells, pretreatment with the TE increased cell viability to 63, 69, and 73% for 12.5, 25, and 50 µg/mL, respectively (Figure 4A). Although all tested concentrations showed improvement in cell viability, the increase was more in 2.5 µg/mL concentrations for most of the compounds, and in 50 µg/mL for the TE. Considering this, the concentrations of 50 and 2.5 µg/mL were chosen for the TE and compounds, respectively, for further studies. Together, these results show that licorice TE and compounds confer neuroprotection on the SH-SY5Y cells.

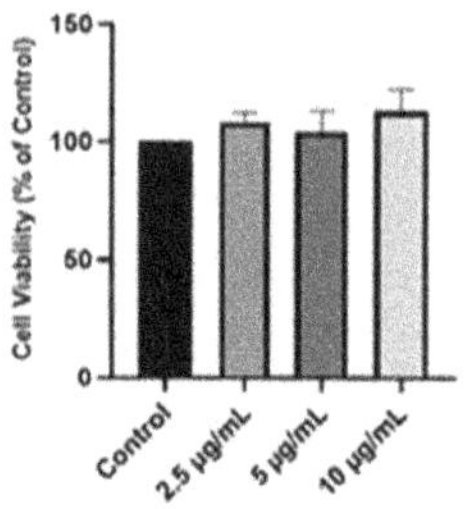

Naringenin 4′-O-glucoside (1)

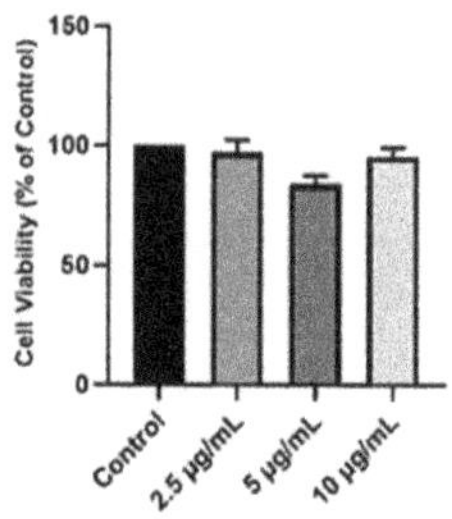

3′,4′,7-Trihydroxyflavanone (2)

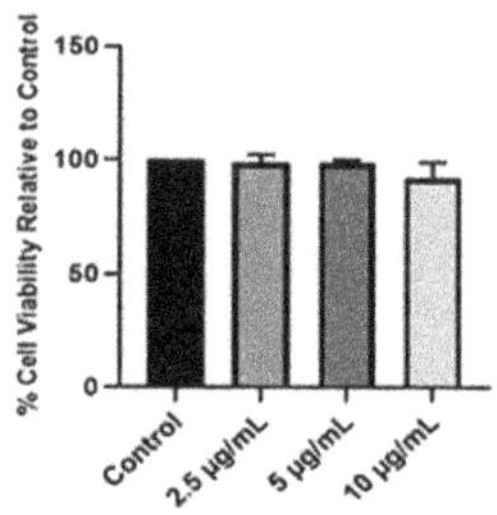

Liquiritin (3)

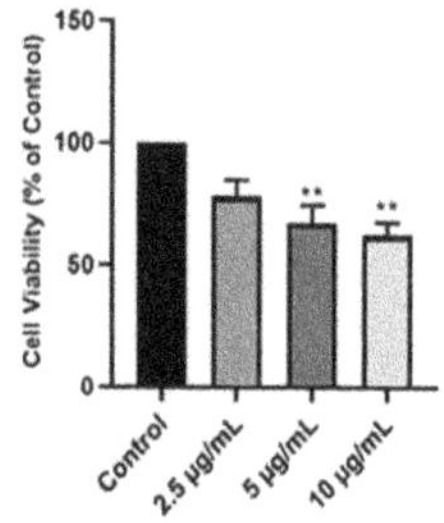

Liquiritin apioside (4)

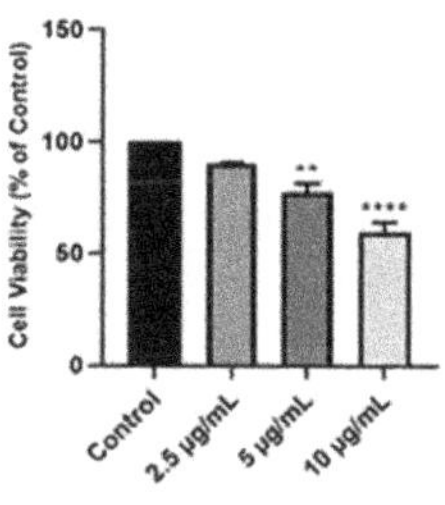

Abyssinone (5)

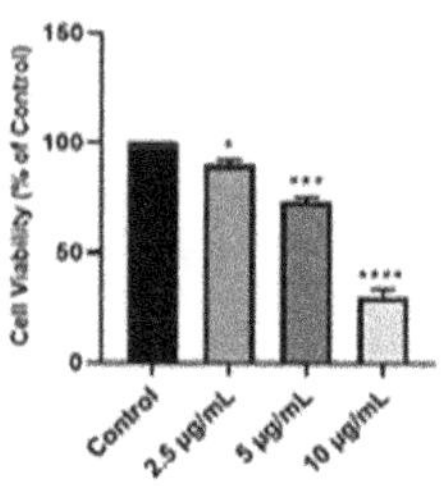

Glabrol (6)

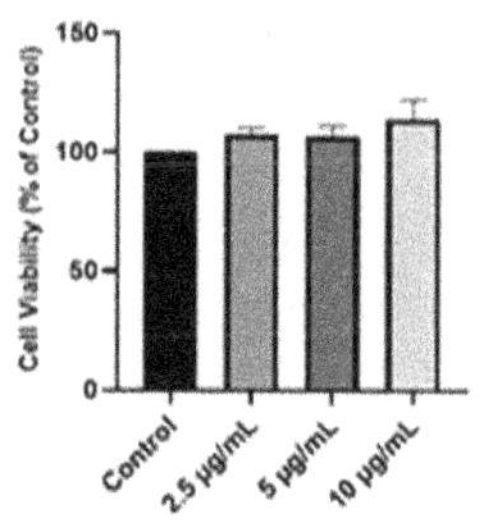

Isoliquiritin (7)

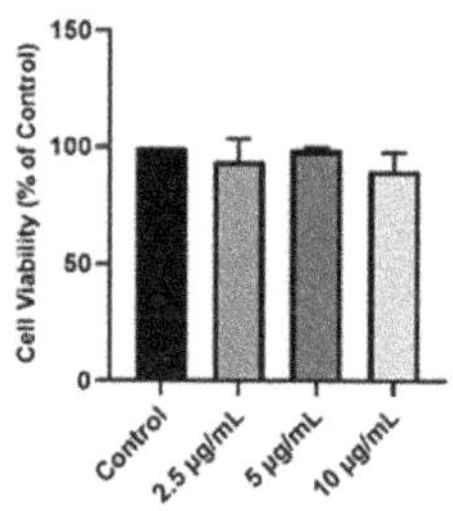

Neoisoliquiritin (8)

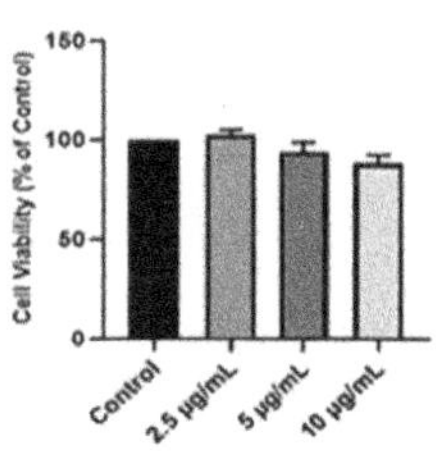

Isoliquiritin apioside (9)

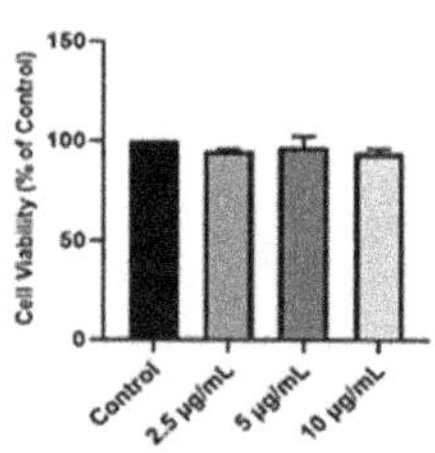

Licuraside (10)

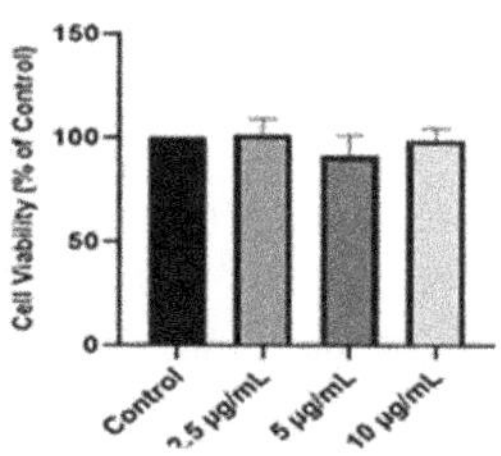

3′[O],4′-(2,2-Dimethylpyrano)-3,7-dihydroxyflavanone (11)

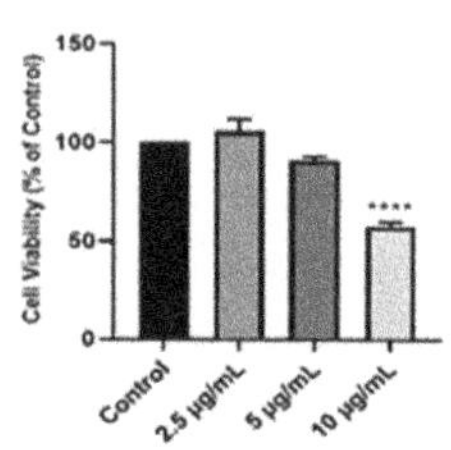

Glabrocoumarin (12)

Figure 3. *Cont.*

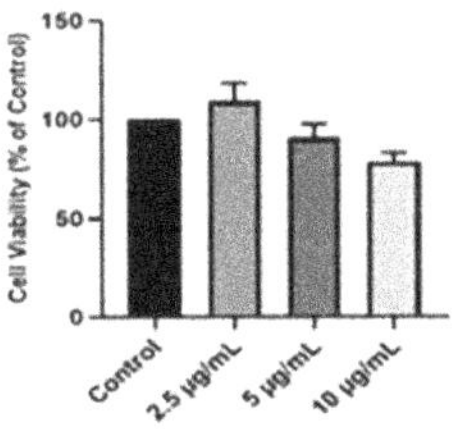

Glabrene (**13**)

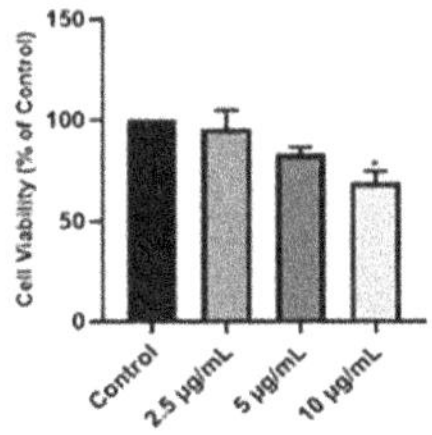

Isomedicarpin (**14**)

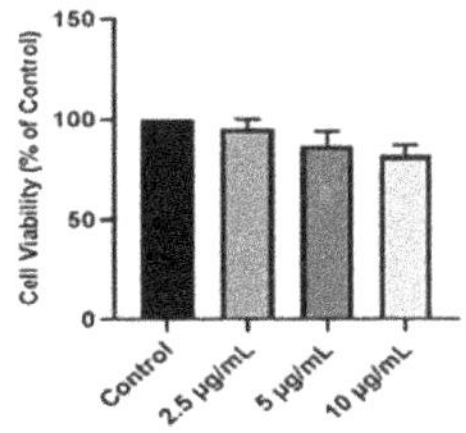

Formononetin (**15**)

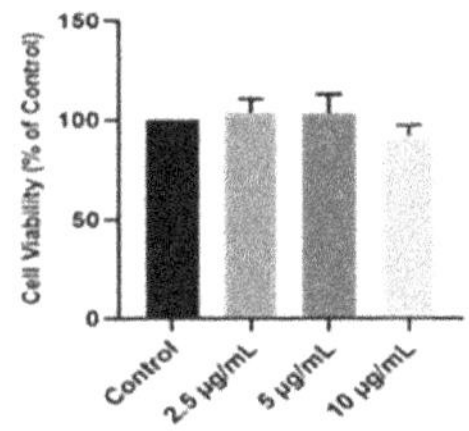

Ononin (**16**)

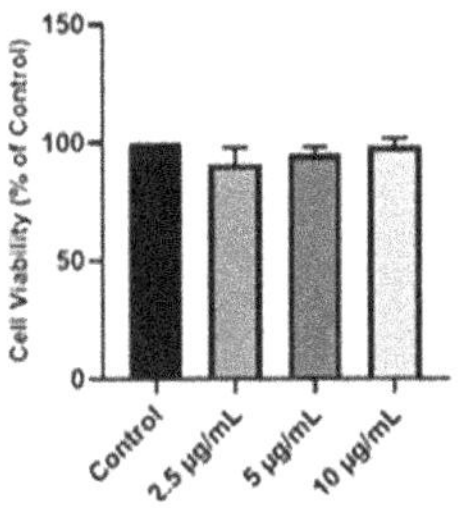

Glycyroside (**17**)

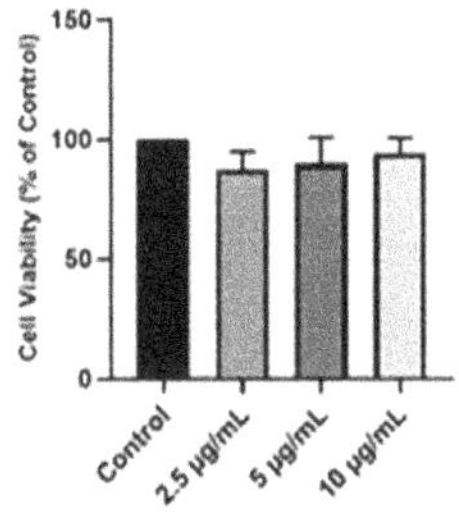

(3*S*)-7,4′-Dihydroxy-2′-methoxyisoflavan (**18**)

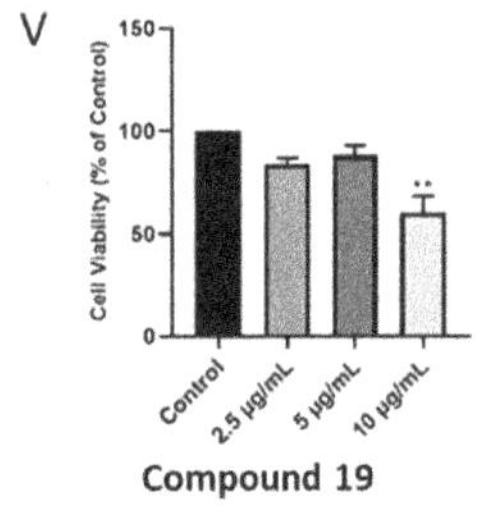

Glabridin (**19**)

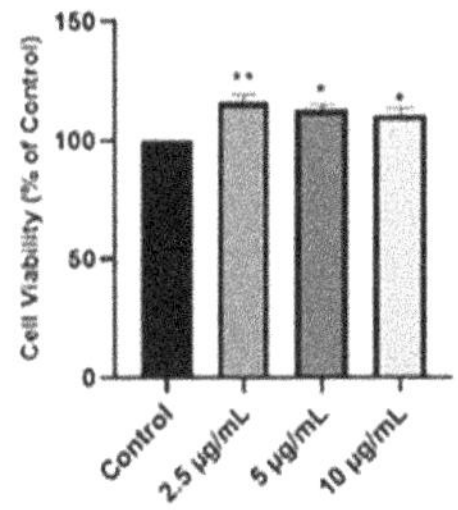

Neoliquiritin (**20**)

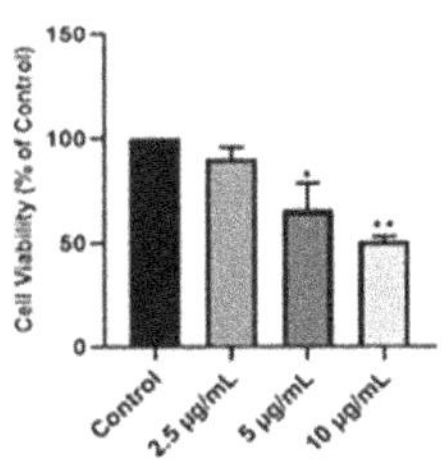

3, 11-Dioxooleana-1,12-dien-29-oic acid (**21**)

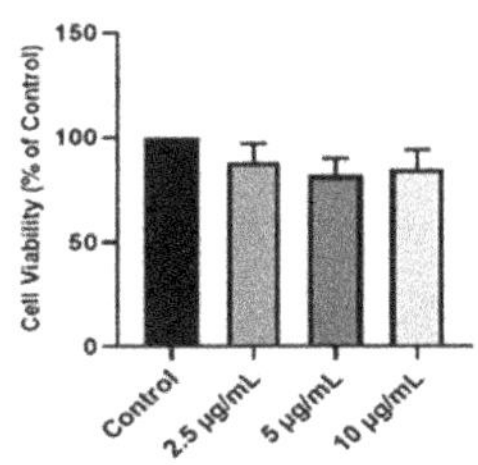

3-oxo-18β-Glycyrrhetinic acid (**22**)

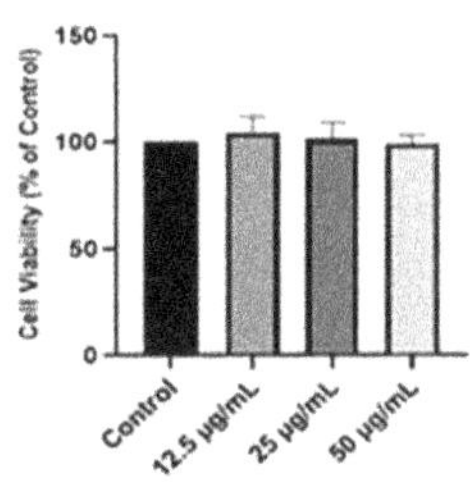

Total extract (TE)

Figure 3. Dose–response of licorice TE and compounds. MTT cytotoxicity assay on SH-SY5Y cells treated with increasing concentrations (12.5, 25, and 50 µg/mL) of licorice TE and compounds (2.5, 5, and 10 µg/mL) for 24 h. After assays, cell viability was expressed as a percentage of control, and each bar represents the mean + SEM of at least three replicate experiments obtained from quadruple wells. Treated cells were compared to control cells; significance levels are indicated. The significance of the difference when control cells were compared to treated cells is indicated by * $p < 0.05$, ** $p < 0.01$, *** $p < 0.001$, and **** $p < 0.0001$.

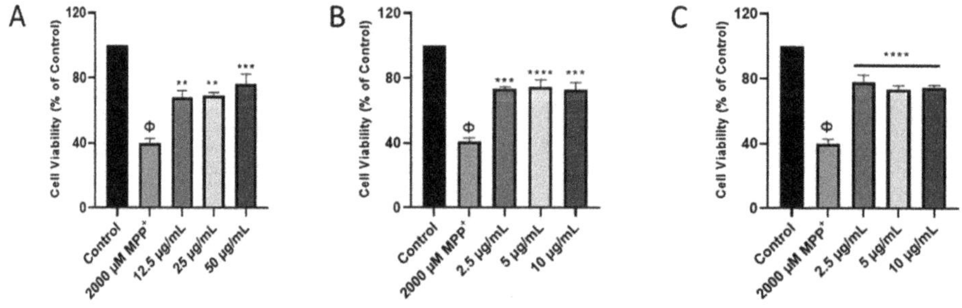

Total extract (TE) Treatment + MPP+

Neoliquiritin (**20**) Treatment + MPP+

Isoliquiritin (**7**) Treatment + MPP+

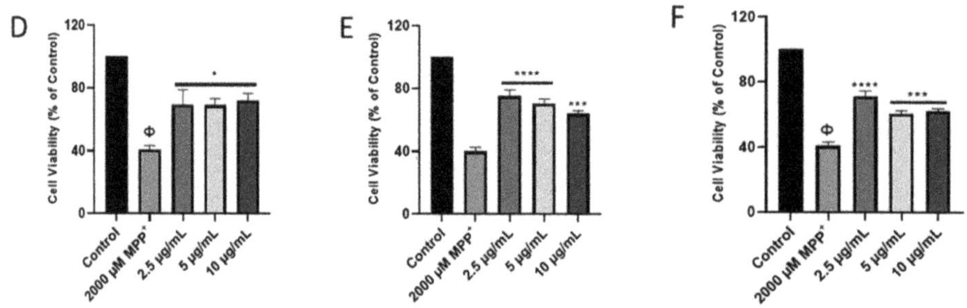

Naringenin 4′- *O*-glucoside (**1**) Treatment + MPP+

Ononin (**16**) Treatment + MPP+

3′[*O*],4′-(2,2-dimethylpyrano)-3,7-dihydroxyflavanone (**11**) Treatment MPP+

Figure 4. Licorice TE and compounds show protection in SH-SY5Y cells. Cells were pre-treated with TE (**A**) and compounds (**B–F**) before exposure to MPP^+ for 24 h. Each bar represents mean percentage cell viability relative to control, and significance of difference is indicated with * $p < 0.05$, ** $p < 0.01$, *** $p < 0.001$, and **** $p < 0.0001$ when TE/compounds are compared to MPP+, and Φ when MPP^+ -treated cells are compared to control.

2.2.3. Effect of TE and Compounds on ATP Production in the Cells

As a mechanism of neuronal toxicity, MPP+ induces ATP degeneration in neuronal cells by the inhibition of mitochondrial complex I [52]. To understand the mechanism of action of the licorice TE and compounds **1**, **7**, **11**, **16**, and **20**, we next investigated their effects on the levels of ATP in the cells following treatment with the MPP+ neurotoxin. Cells were plated in white-walled 96-well plates and treated with 50 µg/mL of the TE and 2.5 µg/mL of the compounds, as these concentrations showed better neuroprotective activity; ATP production was then measured using the MitotoxGlo Promega ATP kit. Figure 5 shows that MPP^+ treatment reduced ATP production in the cells to about 49%. However, pretreatment with the licorice TE and compounds improved ATP production in the cells undergoing MPP^+ treatment, while this was only significant for the cells pretreated with compounds **20**, **7** and **16**, with ATP levels of about 66, 65, and 75%, respectively. These results suggest that improving cellular ATP production is part of the mechanism of neuroprotection conferred by the extract and compounds.

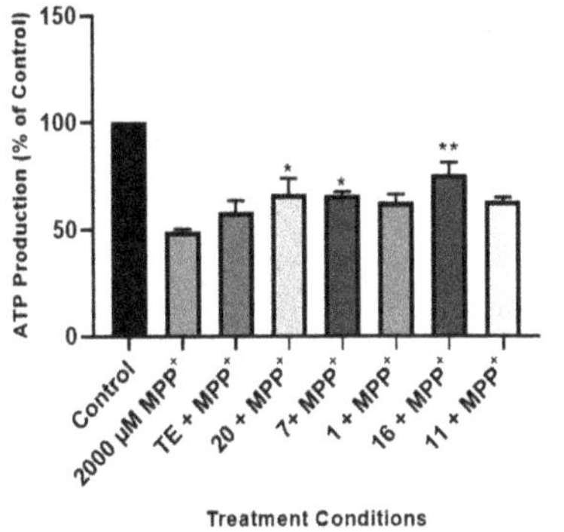

Figure 5. Effect of licorice TE and compounds on MPP+-induced depletion of ATP. Cells were pre-treated with 50 µg/mL of licorice TE and 2.5 µg/mL of compounds before exposure to 2000 µM of MPP+ for 24 h, and ATP levels were assessed. Each bar represents the mean percentage of ATP production relative to control, and the significance of the difference is indicated as * $p < 0.05$ and ** $p < 0.01$ when extract/compounds are compared to MPP+ and when MPP+-treated cells are compared to control.

2.2.4. Effect of TE and Compounds on Caspase 3/7 Activities in the Cells

To further ascertain the mechanism involved in the neuroprotective aspects of licorice TE and compounds in SH-SY5Y cells, the levels of apoptosis were assessed using caspase 3/7 as a marker. Caspases belong to the family of cysteine proteases, which drive apoptosis in cells and carry out their function by cleavage of substrates; thus, they are used as markers of apoptosis [24,53]. To investigate apoptosis, cells were pretreated with 50 µg/mL of the TE and 2.5 µg/mL of the compounds before exposure to MPP+, and caspase 3/7 activities were measured. Figure 6 shows that TE and compounds mitigate MPP+-increased levels of caspase 3/7 activity in the SH-SY5Y cells. Specifically, MPP+ increased levels of caspase 3/7 to about 3-fold of control and pre-treatment with TE reduced this activity to about 1.8-fold of control. Furthermore, all compounds also protected SH-Y5Y cells from MPP+-induced increase in caspase 3/7 activities. Altogether, these results indicate that inhibition of apoptosis is involved in the neuroprotective aspects of licorice TE and compounds.

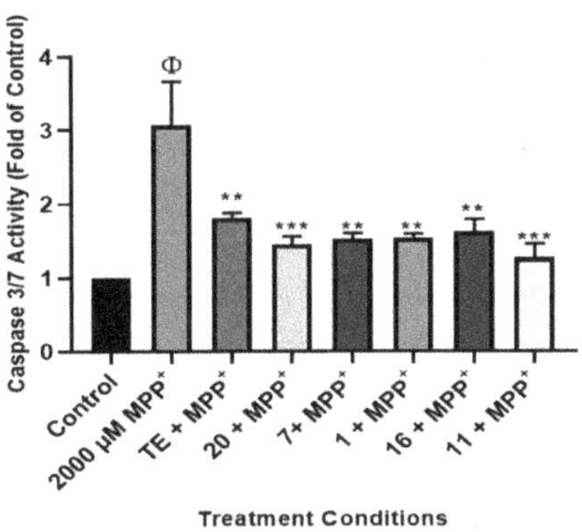

Figure 6. Licorice TE and compounds attenuate MPP+-induced increase in caspase 3/7 activities. Cells were pre-treated with 50 µg/mL of licorice TE and 2.5 µg/mL of compounds before exposure to 2000 µM of MPP+ for 24 h, and caspase 3/7 activities were determined. Each bar represents the level of caspase 3/7 expressed as a multiple of the control, and significance of difference is indicated by ** $p < 0.01$ and *** $p < 0.001$ when TE/compounds were compared to MPP+, and Φ when MPP+-treated cells were compared to control.

3. Discussion

The burden of PD continues to pose a challenge to the ageing population globally [54]. While the exact cause of the disease has yet to be fully elucidated, it has been proposed that PD is caused by a plethora of environmental events and genetic factors [55]. In clinical settings, PD is incurable, as it involves different clinical manifestations, including bradykinesia, resting tremor, and rigidity, along with postural instability; hence, medications are given to relieve symptoms [56]. One notable example of such medication is levodopa, but its prolonged use is associated with neuronal cell toxicity and other serious side effects, such as dyskinesias and psychosis [54]. Delaying the onset of PD is thought to effectively slow down the progression of the disease, so exploiting new approaches to achieve this remains critical.

In the present study, the neuroprotective effects of licorice TE and compounds were evaluated in an MPP^+ model of PD. Twenty-two compounds were isolated from the plant, with compound **11** being a new compound. The compounds were screened for their cytotoxicity, and some of them were observed to be cytotoxic to the SH-SY5Y cells. These compounds include glabrol (**6**), abyssinone (**5**) [35], liquiritin apioside (**4**), glabrocoumarin (**12**), isomedicarpin (**14**), and 3,11-dioxooleana-1,12-die-29-oic acid (**21**). In support of these findings, liquiritin apioside has been reported to induce toxicity on human cancer cell lines (HSC-2, HSC-3, HSC-4, and HL-60) which are derived from oral squamous cancers of the tongue [57], while glabrol showed cytotoxicity against C6 rat glioma cells [58]. In addition, 18β-glycyrrhetinic acid and formononetin have been reported to have cytotoxic potential against various cancer cell lines [59–64]. Despite the cytotoxicity observed for the compounds mentioned above, other compounds from the *Glycyrrhiza* genus have been demonstrated to have neuroprotective effects [20–23]. To this end, our findings show that the compounds naringenin 4′-*O*-glucoside (**1**), neoliquiritin (**20**), glabrol (**6**), isoliquiritin (**7**), and 3′[*O*],4′-(2,2-dimethylpyrano)-3,7-dihydroxyflavanone (**11**), alongside the TE, when investigated for their neuroprotective potentials, conferred neuroprotection on the cells. Supporting our findings, studies have demonstrated that neoliquiritin (**20**) protected rat cardiac myocytes from doxorubicin-induced reduction in cell proliferation [65], while naringenin, which is the parent compound from which neoliquiritin (**20**) and naringenin 4′-*O*-glucoside (**1**) were derived, is widely known to have cytoprotective potentials, including protecting neurons from toxin-mediated cell death in Alzheimer's disease and PD [66–68]. Isoliquiritin, on the other hand, has also shown to have neuroprotective potentials, as it inhibits monoamine oxidase and ameliorates depression [69,70], while 7-hydroxy-4′-methoxyflavone (formononetin) (**15**) was able to alleviate neuroinflammation in lipopolysaccharide-stimulated microglial cells by inhibiting TLR4/MyD88/MAPK signaling and activating the Nrf2/NQO-1 pathway [71].

As a mechanism of action, MPP+ is known to alter cellular energy levels in neuronal cells following the induction of oxidative stress [72]. Oxidative stress leads to impairment of the mitochondrial electron transport chain and, consequently, a decline in ATP production, as well as increased mitochondrial dysfunction [73,74]. Alteration of cellular ATP negatively impacts the ability of cells to carry out their normal metabolic functions, and in relation to humans, this could lead to cognitive decline, as neurotransmission will be affected [75]. Importantly, studies have shown that the ability to ameliorate oxidative stress and improve cellular energy and metabolism counteracts the effects of neurotoxins and, at the same time, improves neurotransmission and neuron function [75,76]. In line with this postulate, we show that the tested compounds and TE improved cellular ATP levels following exposure to MPP+. In support of these findings, it has been suggested that isoliquiritin provides protective action against corticosterone-induced cell damage by reducing oxidative stress and regulating mitochondrial dysfunction by preventing dissipation of mitochondrial membrane potential [77].

Consequently, neuronal cells proceed to programmed cell death following a decline in ATP, and this contributes to the reduction of dopaminergic neuronal cells in the substantia nigra pars compacta of the midbrain [72,78]. Thus, slowing or preventing neurons with respect to cell death via several mechanisms holds a future in the management of neurodegenerative diseases like PD. In the present study, our findings show that *G. glabra* TE and compounds **20**, **7**, **1**, **16**, and **11** inhibited elevated caspase 3/7 activities induced by MPP+. While this was the case for our study, previous studies have demonstrated that prunin (**20**) exerts its cytoprotective potential by inhibiting apoptosis triggered by cellular toxins in cardiac cells [65], In addition, naringenin showed hepatoprotective and neuroprotective properties against lead-induced oxidative stress, inflammation, and apoptosis in rats [68]. Moreover, isoliquiritin was also demonstrated to attenuate apoptosis by the inhibition of the overload of intracellular calcium Ca^{2+} ions; down-regulation of Bax, caspase 3, and cytochrome protein expression; and up-regulation of Bcl protein expression [77]. Thus, the findings are sufficient to state that prevention of cellular apoptosis is a critical component of the neuroprotective mechanism of *G. glabra* and compounds.

4. Materials and Methods

4.1. Chemicals, Materials, and Reagents

Root powder of *G. glabra* was purchased from the local market in Khartoum, Sudan in May 2020; the specimen (H614) was identified by Prof Hatil Elkamali (Department of Botany, Omdurman Islamic University, Omdurman, Sudan). Organic solvents, including methanol, acetonitrile (HPLC grade, Merck, Cape Town, South Africa), hexane, dichloromethane, ethanol, and ethyl acetate (analytical grade (AR), obtained from a local merchant (Kimix, Cape Town, South Africa)) were acquired. Silica gel 60 (0.063–0.200 mm), Sephadex (LH-20), and Aluminum TLC plate, silica gel PF254 were supplied by Merck (Cape Town, South Africa). The 1D NMR (^{1}H, ^{13}C and DEPT-135) and 2D spectra were measured using a Bruker spectrometer (Rheinstetten, Germany) operating at 400 MHz (for ^{1}H) and 100 MHz (for ^{13}C).

4.2. Method

Extraction and Purification of Compounds

The root powder (0.5 Kg) was extracted with methanol at 60 °C (3 L × 2 h × 2 time). After concentration, it yielded ~104.3 g. A quantity of 50.0 g of the total extract (TE) was applied to the silica gel column and eluted using a gradient of hexane and ethyl acetate with increasing polarity. Collected fractions were pooled together according to their profiles on the TLC to afford 24 major fractions coded as I to XXIV. The fractions were re-chromatographed to yield twenty-three major compounds as follows: Fraction XXIII (3.50 g) underwent chromatography on silica gel using a hexane: EtOAc gradient (80:20 to 0:100). Subsequently, sub-fraction 10 was subjected to purification on Sephadex with an isocratic 80% aqueous ethanol, followed by semi-preparative HPLC (Shimadzu, Kyoto, Japan) utilizing a MeOH and de-ionized water (DIW) gradient (40:60 to 60:80 in 30 min, then to 80:90 in 10 min, and finally to 100% MeOH in 10 min). This process yielded compounds **1** (4.8 mg), **3** (100.8 mg), **7** (45.6 mg), **8** (80.3 mg), and **16** (5.2 mg).

The main fraction, XXIV (4.30 g), was chromatographed on silica gel, and subsequent subfractions 2 and 3 were individually subjected to chromatography on Sephadex and semi-prep HPLC, as described earlier. This resulted in the isolation of compounds **4** (50.3 mg), **9** (39.8 mg), **10** (20 mg), **17** (15.6 mg), and **20** (5.3 mg).

Fraction XV (2.40 g) underwent chromatography on silica gel. Subfraction 16 was subsequently chromatographed on Sephadex and subjected to semi-prep HPLC as outlined before, resulting in the isolation of compound **2** (10.5 mg).

Fraction X (1.40 g) was chromatographed on silica gel using a hexane:EtOAc gradient (80:20 to 0:100), and sub-fraction 7 underwent purification on Sephadex and semi-prep HPLC with a MeOH and DIW mixture (1:1, isocratic) to yield compound **14** (5.8 mg).

Fraction IX (7.30 g) was chromatographed on silica gel using a hexane:EtOAc gradient (80:20 to 0:100), and sub-fraction 6 underwent purification on Sephadex and semi-prep HPLC with a MeOH and DIW mixture (1:1, isocratic) to yield compound **19** (300.8 mg).

Fraction VIII (5.5 g) underwent chromatography on silica gel. Subfractions 4, 5, 8, and 11 were subsequently chromatographed separately on Sephadex and semi-prep HPLC, following the previously mentioned protocol. This led to the isolation of compound **13** (8.4 mg) from sub-fraction 4, the compounds **6** (5.4 mg), **11** (10.8 mg), **12** (5.3 mg), and **18** (9.8 mg) from sub-fraction 5; compounds **5** (10.2 mg) and **15** (5.8 mg) from sub-fraction 8; and compounds **21** (4.4 mg) and **22** (25.2 mg) from sub-fraction 11.

4.3. *Compound* 11

Whitish yellow powder $[\alpha]_{25}^{D}$–18.5 (c 0.01, MeOH); UV (MeOH) λ_{max} 315, 277; FTIR (film) 3378, 1677, 1605, 1500, and 1463 cm^{-1}; ^{1}H NMR (DMSO-d_6, 400 MHz), and ^{13}C NMR (DMSO-d_6, 100 MHz), see Table 1; $C_{20}H_{18}O_5$ by its HRFABMS (positive mode). HRFABMS m/z 339.1232 [M+H]+ (calcd for $C_{20}H_{19}O_5$, 339.1227).

4.4. *Cell Culture and Treatments*

The human neuroblastoma SH-SY5Y cells were generously donated by the Blackburn Laboratory, University of Cape Town. Cells were grown in Dulbecco's Modified Eagle's medium (DMEM, Gibco, Life Technologies Corporation, Paisley, UK), supplemented with 10% fetal bovine serum (FBS, Gibco, Life Technologies Corporation, Paisley, UK), 100 U/mL penicillin, and 100 µg/mL streptomycin (Lonza Group Ltd., Verviers, Belgium). Cultures were incubated at 37 °C in humidified air with 5% CO_2 and cell growth medium was routinely changed every three days. Cells were sub-cultured when they attained 70 to 80 percent confluency, using a solution of 0.25% trypsin EDTA (Lonza Group Ltd., Verviers, Belgium).

4.5. *Treatments*

Stock solutions of 40 mg/mL and 10 mg/mL for total extract and compounds, respectively, were prepared in dimethyl sulfoxide (DMSO) (Sigma-Aldrich, St. Louis, MO, USA), from which final concentrations were made in cell growth media. To determine the optimum concentrations of licorice TE and compounds to be used for neuroprotection studies, SH-SY5Y cells were plated at a density of 10,000 cells/well and treated with concentrations of 12.5, 25, and 50 µg/mL of the TE, and 2.5, 5, and 10 µg/mL of the compounds. The vehicle-treated cells (cells treated with the same concentration of DMSO, similar to that of the highest concentration of extract) were used as control, and the treatments lasted 24 h. For MPP^+, 2000 mM was chosen as the concentration used to establish neurotoxicity, which is in accordance with our published works [27,53]. For neuroprotection experiments, cells were plated as above and pre-treated with optimized concentrations of licorice TE and compounds for 2 h prior to the addition of 2000 µM MPP^+. Treatments were incubated for 24 h, and the vehicle-treated cells served as control.

4.6. *Cell Viability Assays*

The MTT (Sigma-Aldrich, St. Louis, MO, USA) cell viability assay was used to determine the viability of cells following treatment with licorice TE- and compounds-only and the pre-treatment of cells with licorice TE and/or compounds and MPP^+. Cells were seeded in 96-well plates and treated as stated above, after which the MTT assay was performed. After treatment, 10 or 20 µL (depending on well volume) of the 5 mg/mL MTT solution in phosphate-buffered saline (PBS) (Lonza Group Ltd., Verviers, Belgium) was added to each well and left to incubate in the dark at 37 °C for 4 h. After incubation, the medium containing the MTT dye was discarded, and the MTT formazan was solubilized with 100 µL of DMSO for an absorbance reading using a microplate reader (BMG Labtech Omega® POLARStar, Offenburg, Germany) at a wavelength of 570 nm. Cell viability was calculated and expressed as a percentage of control.

4.7. *Adenosine Triphosphate Assay*

The Mitochondrial ToxGlo ATP assay kit (Promega, Madison, WI, USA) was used to investigate cell ATP levels. Briefly, cells were plated at a density of 10,000 cells per well in a white 96-well plate, and after attachment, cells were treated as per the neuroprotection assay above. After treatment, cells were processed according to the manufacturer's protocol by adding a volume of ATP detection reagent appropriate to the contents of each well and leaving the resulting mixture to incubate at 37 °C for 30 min. After incubation, luminescence intensity was read using the Promega GloMax® explorer multimode microplate reader, and luminescence values were expressed as percentages of control.

4.8. Caspase 3/7 Apoptosis Assay

To investigate apoptosis in the cells, the Caspase 3/7 assay kit (Promega, Madison, WI, USA) was used to estimate levels of caspase 3/7 activity in the cells, in a manner according with the manufacturer's instructions. Briefly, cells were plated in a white 96-well plate at a density of 10,000 cells per well and allowed to attach overnight, after which cells were pre-treated with licorice TE and compounds before the addition of 2000 μM MPP^+. Treatments lasted for 24 h, and at the end of the experiments, equal volumes of Caspase 3/7 assay mix were added to each well. The luminescence intensity was read with the Promega GloMax → explorer multimode microplate reader. Luminescence values of the treated cells were expressed as a multiple of the control.

4.9. Statistical Analysis

Data generated from this study were analyzed using GraphPad Prism 6 and expressed as means and standard error values of means of three independent experiments performed in quadruplicate wells. One-way analysis of variance (ANOVA) was used to compare treated cells to either control or MPP+ alone. The significance of difference $p < 0.05$ was determined using Tukey's multiple comparisons test and was indicated with * when comparing treatments to control or Φ when comparing licorice and TE and compounds to MPP^+ treated cells.

5. Conclusions

This study investigated the neuroprotective potentials of *G. glabra* TE and isolated compounds in an in vitro model of PD. The results show that some of the compounds were cytotoxic (including glabrol (**6**), abyssinone (**5**), liquiritin apioside (**4**), glabrocoumarin (**12**), isomedicarpin (**14**), and 3,11-dioxooleana-1,12-die-29-oic acid (**21**)), which might have implications for the treatment of cancer. However, some of the compounds (naringenin 4′-*O*-glucoside (**1**), isoliquiritin (**7**), 3′[*O*],4′-(2,2-dimethylpyrano)-3,7-dihydroxyflavanone (**11**), ononin (**16**), and neoliquiritin (**20**)) were further studied for their neuroprotective potentials. The protective effects were related not only to the inhibition of ATP degeneration, but also to the attenuation of MPP+-induced elevated caspase 3/7 activities. These results indicate that the compounds isolated from *G. glabra* may provide novel therapeutic strategies for the treatment of PD. One limitation of this study was that the biological characterization was only performed on cell lines; therefore, in the future, it would be interesting to see if these compounds would have similar effects on in vivo models of PD. In addition, we recommend that future studies further elucidate the mechanisms of action, with emphasis on the molecular and genetic events underpinning the actions of these compounds.

Supplementary Materials: The following supporting information can be downloaded at: https://www.mdpi.com/article/10.3390/ph17070852/s1, Table S1. ^{1}H and ^{13}C spectral data of compounds **1-22**, Figure S1. ^{1}H and ^{13}C spectra of compounds **1-22** and Scheme S1. The details of the isolation processes for compounds **1**–**22** from licorice.

Author Contributions: A.O.E.E., conceptualization; A.A.H., project researcher and supervisor; R.C.L., co-supervisor; S.I.O., investigation, formal analysis, and data curation; T.N.A., funding, investigation, reviewing of draft. All authors have read and agreed to the published version of the manuscript.

Funding: This work was supported by the National Research Foundation, South Africa (grant number 106055). CPUT and WITS are acknowledged for financial and infrastructural support. TNA acknowledges the Friedel Sellschop Fellowship Award and NRF CSUR funding.

Institutional Review Board Statement: Ethics waiver for this study was obtained from the Wits Human Research Ethics Committee with approval number W-CBP-221024-01.

Informed Consent Statement: Not applicable.

Data Availability Statement: The data associated with the isolated compounds, ^{1}H NMR, ^{13}C NMR spectra, and the biological data used to support the findings of this study are available from the corresponding author upon request.

Conflicts of Interest: The authors declare no conflicts of interest.

References

1. Lamptey, R.N.L.; Chaulagain, B.; Trivedi, R.; Gothwal, A.; Layek, B.; Singh, J. A Review of the Common Neurodegenerative Disorders: Current Therapeutic Approaches and the Potential Role of Nanotherapeutics. *Int. J. Mol. Sci.* **2022**, *23*, 1851. [CrossRef] [PubMed]
2. Kalia, L.V.; Lang, A.E. Parkinson's disease. *Lancet Neurol.* **2015**, *29*, 896–912. [CrossRef] [PubMed]
3. Postuma, R.B.; Berg, D.; Stern, M.; Poewe, W.; Olanow, C.W.; Oertel, W.; Obeso, J.; Marek, K.; Litvan, I.; Lang, A.E.; et al. MDS clinical diagnostic criteria for Parkinson's disease. *Mov. Disord.* **2015**, *30*, 1591–1601. [CrossRef]
4. Li, J.-L.; Lin, T.-Y.; Chen, P.-L.; Guo, T.-N.; Huang, S.-Y.; Chen, C.-H.; Lin, C.-H.; Chan, C.-C. Mitochondrial Function and Parkinson's Disease: From the Perspective of the Electron Transport Chain. *Front. Mol. Neurosci.* **2021**, *14*, 797833. [CrossRef]
5. Keane, P.; Kurzawa, M.; Blain, P.; Morris, C. Mitochondrial dysfunction in Parkinson's disease. *Park. Dis.* **2011**, *2011*, 716871. [CrossRef]
6. Nonnekes, J.; Post, B.; Tetrud, J.W.; Langston, J.W.; Bloem, B.R. MPTP-induced parkinsonism: An historical case series. *Lancet Neurol.* **2018**, *17*, 300–301.
7. Reeve, A.; Simcox, E.; Turnbull, D. Ageing and Parkinson's disease: Why is advancing age the biggest risk factor. *Ageing Res. Rev.* **2014**, *14*, 19–30. [CrossRef] [PubMed]
8. Thanvi, B.; Lo, N.; Robinson, T. Levodopa-induced dyskinesia in Parkinson's disease: Clinical features, pathogenesis, prevention and treatment. *Postgrad. Med. J.* **2007**, *83*, 384–388. [CrossRef]
9. Brahmachari, G. *Discovery and Development of Neuroprotective Agents from Natural Products*; Elsevier: Amsterdam, The Netherlands, 2017.
10. Abdolmaleki, A.; Akram, M.; Saeed, M.M.; Asadi, A.; Kajkolah, M. Herbal medicine as neuroprotective potential agent in human and animal models: A historical overview. *J. Pharm. Care* **2020**, *8*, 75–82. [CrossRef]
11. Bosch-Morell, F.; Villagrasa, V.; Ortega, T.; Acero, N.; Muñoz-Mingarro, D.; González-Rosende, M.E.; Castillo, E.; Sanahuja, M.A.; Soriano, P.; Martínez-Solís, I.P. Medicinal plants and natural products as neuroprotective agents in age-related macular degeneration. *Neural Regen. Res.* **2020**, *15*, 2207–2216.
12. Öztürk, M.; Altay, V.; Hakeem, K.; Akçiçek, E. *Liquorice: From Botany to Phytochemistry*; Springer: Berlin/Heidelberg, Germany, 2018.
13. Hayashi, H.; Hosono, N.; Kondo, M.; Hiraoka, N.; Ikeshiro, Y.; Shibano, M.; Kusano, G.; Yamamoto, H.; Tanaka, T.; Inoue, K. Phylogenetic relationship of six Glycyrrhiza species based on rbcL sequences and chemical constituents. *Biol. Pharm. Bull.* **2000**, *23*, 602–606. [CrossRef] [PubMed]
14. Hayashi, H.; Miwa, E.; Inoue, K. Phylogenetic relationship of Glycyrrhiza lepidota, American licorice, in genus Glycyrrhiza based on rbcL sequences and chemical constituents. *Biol. Pharm. Bull.* **2005**, *28*, 161–164. [CrossRef] [PubMed]
15. Avula, B.; Bae, J.-Y.; Chittiboyina, A.G.; Wang, Y.-H.; Wang, M.; Zhao, J.; Ali, Z.; Brinckmann, J.A.; Li, J.; Wu, C.; et al. Chemometric analysis and chemical characterization for the botanical identification of Glycyrrhiza species (*G. glabra*, *G. uralensis*, *G. inflata*, *G. echinata* and *G. lepidota*) using liquid chromatography-quadrupole time of flight mass spectrometry (LC-QTof). *J. Food Compos. Anal.* **2022**, *112*, 104679. [CrossRef]
16. Akhtar, N.; Ihsan-ul-Haq; Mirza, B. Phytochemical analysis and comprehensive evaluation of antimicrobial and antioxidant properties of 61 medicinal plant species. *Arab. J. Chem.* **2018**, *11*, 1223–1235. [CrossRef]
17. Sharma, V.; Katiyar, A.; Agrawal, R.C. Glycyrrhiza Glabra: Chemistry and Pharmacological Activity. In *Sweeteners*; Mérillon, J., Ramawat, K.G., Eds.; Springer: Cham, The Netherlands, 2018; pp. 87–100.
18. Jiang, M.; Zhao, S.; Yang, S.; Lin, X.; He, X.; Wei, X.; Song, Q.; Li, R.; Fu, C.; Zhang, J.; et al. An "essential herbal medicine" Licorice: A review of phytochemicals and its effects in combination preparations. *J. Ethnopharmacol.* **2020**, *249*, 112439. [CrossRef] [PubMed]
19. Hosseini, M.S.; Ebrahimi, M.; Samsampour, D.; Abadía, J.; Khanahmadi, M.; Amirian, R.; Ghafoori, I.N.; Ghaderi-Zefrehei, M.; Gogorcena, Y. Association analysis and molecular tagging of phytochemicals in the endangered medicinal plant licorice (*Glycyrrhiza glabra* L.). *Phytochemistry* **2021**, *183*, 112629. [CrossRef]
20. Chang, K.-H.; Chen, I.-C.; Lin, H.-Y.; Chen, H.-C.; Lin, C.-H.; Lin, T.-H.; Weng, Y.-T.; Chao, C.-Y.; Wu, Y.-R.; Lin, J.-Y.; et al. The aqueous extract of Glycyrrhiza inflata can upregulate unfolded protein response-mediated chaperones to reduce tau misfolding in cell models of Alzheimer's disease. *Drug Des. Dev. Ther.* **2016**, *10*, 885–896.
21. Chen, C.-M.; Weng, Y.-T.; Chen, W.-L.; Lin, T.-H.; Chao, C.-Y.; Lin, C.-H.; Chen, I.-C.; Lee, L.-C.; Lin, H.-Y.; Wu, Y.-R.; et al. Aqueous extract of Glycyrrhiza inflata inhibits aggregation by upregulating PPARGC1A and NFE2L2–ARE pathways in cell models of spinocerebellar ataxia 3. *Free Radic. Biol. Med.* **2014**, *71*, 339–350. [CrossRef] [PubMed]

22. Kong, Z.-H.; Chen, X.; Hua, H.-P.; Liang, L.; Liu, L.-J. The oral pretreatment of glycyrrhizin prevents surgery-induced cognitive impairment in aged mice by reducing neuroinflammation and Alzheimer's-related pathology via HMGB1 inhibition. *J. Mol. Neurosci.* **2017**, *63*, 385–395. [CrossRef]
23. Ravanfar, P.; Namazi, G.; Atigh, M.; Zafarmand, S.; Hamedi, A.; Salehi, A.; Izadi, S.; Borhani-Haghighi, A. Efficacy of whole extract of licorice in neurological improvement of patients after acute ischemic stroke. *J. Herb. Med.* **2016**, *6*, 12–17. [CrossRef]
24. Hasan, M.K.; Ara, I.; Mondal, M.S.A.; Kabir, Y. Phytochemistry, pharmacological activity, and potential health benefits of Glycyrrhiza glabra. *Heliyon* **2021**, *7*, 1–10. [CrossRef] [PubMed]
25. Yi, Y.; Zhang, M.; Xue, H.; Yu, R.; Bao, Y.-O.; Kuang, Y.; Chai, Y.; Ma, W.; Wang, J.; Shi, X.; et al. Schaftoside inhibits 3CLpro and PLpro of SARS-CoV-2 virus and regulates immune response and inflammation of host cells for the treatment of COVID-19. *Acta Pharm. Sin. B* **2022**, *12*, 4154–4164. [CrossRef] [PubMed]
26. Xiang, C.; Qiao, X.; Ye, M.; Guo, D. Classification and distribution analysis of components in Glycyrrhiza using licorice compounds database. *Acta Pharm. Sin.* **2012**, *47*, 1023–1030.
27. Omoruyi, S.I.; Ibrakaw, A.S.; Ekpo, O.E.; Boatwright, J.S.; Cupido, C.N.; Hussein, A.A. Neuroprotective activities of crossyne flava bulbs and amaryllidaceae alkaloids: Implications for parkinson's disease. *Molecules* **2021**, *26*, 3990. [CrossRef] [PubMed]
28. Egunlusi, A.O.; Malan, S.F.; Omoruyi, S.I.; Ekpo, O.E.; Palchykov, V.A.; Joubert, J. Open and rearranged norbornane derived polycyclic cage molecules as potential neuroprotective agents through attenuation of MPP+-and calcium overload-induced excitotoxicity in neuroblastoma SH-SY5Y cells. *Eur. J. Med. Chem.* **2020**, *204*, 112617. [CrossRef] [PubMed]
29. Oyama, K.-i.; Kondo, T. Total synthesis of apigenin 7, 4′-di-O-β-glucopyranoside, a component of blue flower pigment of Salvia patens, and seven chiral analogues. *Tetrahedron* **2004**, *60*, 2025–2034. [CrossRef]
30. Chen, K.; Hu, Z.-m.; Song, W.; Wang, Z.-l.; He, J.-b.; Shi, X.-m.; Cui, Q.-h.; Qiao, X.; Ye, M. Diversity of O-glycosyltransferases contributes to the biosynthesis of flavonoid and triterpenoid glycosides in Glycyrrhiza uralensis. *Am. Chem. Soc. Synth. Biol.* **2019**, *8*, 1858–1866. [CrossRef]
31. Wu, J.-Y.; Ding, H.-Y.; Wang, T.-Y.; Cai, C.-Z.; Chang, T.-S. Application of Biotransformation-Guided Purification in Chinese Medicine: An Example to Produce Butin from Licorice. *Catalysts* **2022**, *12*, 1–10. [CrossRef]
32. Tian, G.; Zhang, U.; Zhang, T.; Yang, F.; Ito, Y. Separation of flavonoids from the seeds of Vernonia anthelmintica Willd by high-speed counter-current chromatography. *J. Chromatogr. A* **2004**, *1049*, 219–222. [CrossRef]
33. Ji, S.; Li, Z.; Song, W.; Wang, Y.; Liang, W.; Li, K.; Tang, S.; Wang, Q.; Qiao, X.; Zhou, D.; et al. Bioactive Constituents of Glycyrrhiza uralensis (Licorice): Discovery of the Effective Components of a Traditional Herbal Medicine. *J. Nat. Prod.* **2016**, *79*, 281–292. [CrossRef]
34. Pastorino, G.; Cornara, L.; Soares, S.; Rodrigues, F.; Oliveira, M.B.P. Liquorice (*Glycyrrhiza glabra*): A phytochemical and pharmacological review. *Phytother. Res.* **2018**, *32*, 2323–2339. [CrossRef] [PubMed]
35. Park, J.-H.; Wu, Q.; Yoo, K.-H.; Yong, H.-I.; Cho, S.-M.; Chung, I.-S.; Baek, N.-I. Cytotoxic effect of flavonoids from the roots of Glycyrrhiza uralensis on human cancer cell lines. *J. Appl. Biol. Chem.* **2011**, *54*, 67–70. [CrossRef]
36. Asada, Y.; Li, W.; Yoshikawa, T. Biosynthesis of the dimethylallyl moiety of glabrol in *Glycyrrhiza glabra* hairy root cultures via a non-mevalonate pathway. *Phytochemistry* **2000**, *55*, 323–326. [CrossRef] [PubMed]
37. Nomura, T.; Fukai, T.; Akiyama, T. Chemistry of phenolic compounds of licorice (Glycyrrhiza species) and their estrogenic and cytotoxic activities. *Pure Appl. Chem.* **2002**, *74*, 1199–1206. [CrossRef]
38. Lee, J.E.; Lee, J.Y.; Kim, J.; Lee, K.; Choi, S.U.; Ryu, S.Y. Two minor chalcone acetylglycosides from the roots extract of Glycyrrhiza uralensis. *Arch. Pharmacal Res.* **2015**, *38*, 1299–1303. [CrossRef]
39. Wang, D.; Liang, J.; Zhang, J.; Wang, Y.; Chai, X. Natural chalcones in Chinese materia medica: Licorice. *Evid.-Based Complement. Altern. Med.* **2020**, *2020*, 3821248. [CrossRef] [PubMed]
40. Kaur, P.; Kaur, S.; Kumar, N.; Singh, B.; Kumar, S. Evaluation of antigenotoxic activity of isoliquiritin apioside from *Glycyrrhiza glabra* L. *Toxicol. Vitr.* **2009**, *23*, 680–686. [CrossRef] [PubMed]
41. Fu, B.; Li, H.; Wang, X.; Lee, F.S.C.; Cui, S. Isolation and Identification of Flavonoids in Licorice and a Study of Their Inhibitory Effects on Tyrosinase. *J. Agric. Food Chem.* **2005**, *53*, 7408–7414. [CrossRef] [PubMed]
42. Li, G.; Simmler, C.; Chen, L.; Nikolic, D.; Chen, S.-N.; Pauli, G.F.; van Breemen, R.B. Cytochrome P450 inhibition by three licorice species and fourteen licorice constituents. *Eur. J. Pharm. Sci.* **2017**, *109*, 182–190. [CrossRef]
43. Montoro, P.; Maldini, M.; Russo, M.; Postorino, S.; Piacente, S.; Pizza, C. Metabolic profiling of roots of liquorice (*Glycyrrhiza glabra*) from different geographical areas by ESI/MS/MS and determination of major metabolites by LC-ESI/MS and LC-ESI/MS/MS. *J. Pharm. Biomed. Anal.* **2011**, *54*, 535–544. [CrossRef]
44. Kinoshit, T.; Tamur, Y.; Mizutani, K. The Isolation and Structure Elucidation of Minor Isoflavonoids from Licorice of *Glycyrrhiza glabra* Origin. *Chem. Pharm. Bull.* **2005**, *53*, 847–849. [CrossRef]
45. Fukai, T.; Sheng, C.-B.; Horikoshi, T.; Nomura, T. Isoprenylated flavonoids from underground parts of *Glycyrrhiza glabra*. *Phytochemistry* **1996**, *43*, 1119–1124. [CrossRef]
46. Adesanya, S.; O'Neill, M.J.; Roberts, M.F. Structure-related fungitoxicity of isoflavonoids. *Physiol. Mol. Plant Pathol.* **1986**, *29*, 95–103. [CrossRef]
47. Piccinelli, A.L.; Fernandez, M.C.; Cuesta-Rubio, O.; Hernández, I.M.; Simone, F.D.; Rastrelli, L. Isoflavonoids Isolated from Cuban Propolis. *J. Agric. Food Chem.* **2005**, *53*, 9010–9016. [CrossRef]

48. Liaoa, W.C.; Linb, Y.-H.; Changc, T.-M.; Huang, W.-Y. Identification of two licorice species, *Glycyrrhiza uralensis* and *Glycyrrhiza glabra*, based on separation and identification of their bioactive components. *Food Chem.* **2012**, *132*, 2188–2193. [CrossRef]
49. Chintharlapalli, S.; Papineni, S.; Jutooru, I.; McAlees, A.; Safe, S. Structure-dependent activity of glycyrrhetinic acid derivatives as peroxisome proliferator–activated receptor γ agonists in colon cancer cells. *Mol. Cancer Ther.* **2007**, *6*, 1588–1598. [CrossRef] [PubMed]
50. Baltina, L.A.; Budaev, A.S.; Mikhailova, L.R.; Baltina, J.L.A.; Spirikhin, L.V.; Makara, N.S.; Zarudii, F.S. New stereoisomeric glycyrrhetic acid derivatives. *Chem. Nat. Compd.* **2014**, *50*, 1042–1046. [CrossRef]
51. Kuroda, M.; Mimakia, Y.; Honda, S.; Tanaka, H.; Yokota, S.; Mae, T. Phenolics from *Glycyrrhiza glabra* roots and their PPAR-c ligand-binding activity. *Bioorganic Med. Chem.* **2010**, *18*, 962–970. [CrossRef]
52. Hoglinger, G.U.; Carrard, G.; Michel, P.P.; Medja, F.; Lombès, A.; Ruberg, M.; Friguet, B.; Hirsch, E.C. Dysfunction of mitochondrial complex I and the proteasome:interactions between two biochemical deficits in a cellular modelof Parkinson's disease. *J. Neurochem.* **2003**, *86*, 1297–1307. [CrossRef]
53. Omoruyi, S.I.; Akinfenwa, A.O.; Ekpo, O.E.; Hussein, A.A. Aspalathin and linearthin from Aspalathus linearis (Rooibos) protect SH-SY5Y cells from MPP+-induced neuronal toxicity. *South Afr. J. Bot.* **2023**, *157*, 53–63. [CrossRef]
54. Kouli, A.; Torsney, K.M.; Kuan, W.-L. Parkinson's disease: Etiology, neuropathology, and pathogenesis. *Exon Publ.* **2018**, 3–26. [CrossRef]
55. Pang, S.Y.-Y.; Ho, P.W.-L.; Liu, H.-F.; Leung, C.-T.; Li, L.; Chang, E.E.S.; Ramsden, D.B.; Ho, S.-L. The interplay of aging, genetics and environmental factors in the pathogenesis of Parkinson's disease. *Transl. Neurodegener.* **2019**, *8*, 23. [CrossRef]
56. Massano, J.; Bhatia, K. Clinical approach to Parkinson's disease: Features, diagnosis, and principles of management. *Cold Spring Harb. Perspect. Med.* **2012**, *2*, a008870. [CrossRef] [PubMed]
57. HOhno; Araho, D.; Uesawa, Y.; Kagaya, H.; Ishihara, M.; Sakagami, H.; Yamamoto, M. Evaluation of Cytotoxiciy and Tumor-specificity of Licorice Flavonoids Based on Chemical Structure. *Anticancer Res.* **2013**, *33*, 3061–3068.
58. Goel, B.; Sharma, A.; Tripathi, N.; Bhardwaj, N.; Sahu, B.; Kaur, G.; Singh, B.; Jain, S.K. In-vitro antitumor activity of compounds from *Glycyrrhiza glabra* against C6 glioma cancer cells: Identification of natural lead for further evaluation. *Nat. Prod. Res.* **2021**, *35*, 5489–5492. [CrossRef] [PubMed]
59. Lee, C.S.; Kim, Y.J.; Lee, M.S.; Han, E.S.; Lee, S.J. 18β-Glycyrrhetinic acid induces apoptotic cell death in SiHa cells and exhibits a synergistic effect against antibiotic anti-cancer drug toxicity. *Life Sci.* **2008**, *83*, 481–489. [CrossRef] [PubMed]
60. Kowalska, A.; Kalinowska-Lis, U. 18β-Glycyrrhetinic acid: Its core biological properties and dermatological applications. *Int. J. Cosmet. Sci.* **2019**, *41*, 325–331. [CrossRef] [PubMed]
61. Tay, K.-C.; Tan, L.T.-H.; Chan, C.K.; Hong, S.L.; Chan, K.-G.; Yap, W.H.; Pusparajah, P.; Lee, L.-H.; Goh, B.-H. Formononetin: A Review of Its Anticancer Potentials and Mechanisms. *Front. Pharmacol.* **2019**, *10*, 820. [CrossRef] [PubMed]
62. Oh, J.-S.; Kim, T.-H.; Park, J.-H.; Lim, H.; Cho, I.-A.; You, J.-S.; Lee, G.-J.; Seo, Y.-S.; Kim, D.K.; Kim, C.S.; et al. Formononetin induces apoptotic cell death through the suppression of mitogen activated protein kinase and nuclear factor κB phosphorylation in FaDu human head and neck squamous cell carcinoma cells. *Oncol. Rep.* **2020**, *43*, 700–710. [CrossRef]
63. Jiang, D.; Rasul, A.; Batool, R.; Sarfraz, I.; Hussain, G.; Tahir, M.M.; Qin, Z.S.T.; Ali, M.; Li, J.; Li, X. Potential Anticancer Properties and Mechanisms of Action of Formononetin. *BioMed Res. Int.* **2019**, *2019*, 854315. [CrossRef]
64. Hsu, Y.-C.; Hsieh, W.-C.; Chen, S.-H.; Li, Y.-Z.; Liao, H.-F.; Lin, M.-Y.; Sheu, S.-M. 18β-glycyrrhetinic Acid Modulated Autophagy is Cytotoxic to Breast Cancer Cells. *Int. J. Med. Sci.* **2023**, *20*, 444–454. [CrossRef] [PubMed]
65. Han, X.; Ren, D.; Fan, P.; Shen, T.; Lou, H. Protective effects of naringenin-7-O-glucoside on doxorubicin-induced apoptosis in H9C2 cells. *Eur. J. Pharmacol.* **2008**, *581*, 47–53. [CrossRef] [PubMed]
66. Sugumar, M.; Sevanan, M.; Sekar, S. Neuroprotective effect of naringenin against MPTP-induced oxidative stress. *Int. J. Neurosci.* **2019**, *129*, 534–539. [CrossRef] [PubMed]
67. Hassan, H.M.; Elnagar, M.R.; Abdelrazik, E.; Mahdi, M.R.; Hamza, E.; Elattar, E.M.; ElNashar, E.M.; Alghamdi, M.A.; Al-Qahtani, Z.; Al-Khater, K.M.; et al. Neuroprotective effect of naringin against cerebellar changes in Alzheimer's disease through modulation of autophagy, oxidative stress and tau expression: An experimental study. *Front. Neuroanat.* **2022**, *16*, 1012422. [CrossRef] [PubMed]
68. Mansour, L.; Elshopakey, G.; Abdelhamid, F.; Albukhari, T.; Almehmadi, S.; Refaat, B.; El-Boshy, M.; Risha, E. Hepatoprotective and Neuroprotective Effects of Naringenin against Lead-Induced Oxidative Stress, Inflammation, and Apoptosis in Rats. *Biomedicines* **2023**, *11*, 1080. [CrossRef] [PubMed]
69. Li, Y.; Song, W.; Tong, Y.; Zhang, X.; Zhao, J.; Gao, X.; Yong, J.; Wang, H. Isoliquiritin ameliorates depression by suppressing NLRP3-mediated pyroptosis via miRNA-27a/SYK/NF-κB axis. *J. Neuroinflammation* **2021**, *18*, 1. [CrossRef] [PubMed]
70. Prajapati, R.; Seong, S.H.; Park, S.E.; Paudel, P.; Jung, H.A.; Choi, J.S. Isoliquiritigenin, a potent human monoamine oxidase inhibitor, modulates dopamine D1, D3, and vasopressin V1A receptors. *Sci. Rep.* **2021**, *11*, 23528. [CrossRef] [PubMed]
71. Qu, Z.; Chen, Y.; Luo, Z.-H.; Shen, X.-L.; Hu, Y.-J. 7-methoxyflavanone alleviates neuroinflammation in lipopolysaccharide-stimulated microglial cells by inhibiting TLR4/MyD88/MAPK signalling and activating the Nrf2/NQO-1 pathway. *J. Pharm. Pharmacol.* **2020**, *72*, 385–395. [CrossRef]
72. Pöltl, D.; Schildknecht, S.; Karreman, C.; Leist, M. Uncoupling of ATP-depletion and cell death in human dopaminergic neurons. *NeuroToxicology* **2012**, *33*, 769–779. [CrossRef]

73. Babu, V.; Khurana, N. A review on mitochondrial dysfunction and oxidative stress due to complex-i in Parkinson disease. *Res. J. Pharmacol. Pharmacodyn.* **2021**, *13*, 167–170. [CrossRef]
74. Dorszewska, J.D.P.; Kowalska, M.; Prendecki, M.; Piekut, T.; Kozłowska, J.; Kozubski, W. Oxidative stress factors in Parkinson's disease. *Neural Regen. Res.* **2021**, *16*, 1383–1391. [CrossRef] [PubMed]
75. Błaszczyk, J.W. Energy metabolism decline in the aging brain—Pathogenesis of neurodegenerative disorders. *Metabolites* **2020**, *10*, 450. [CrossRef] [PubMed]
76. Jiménez-Delgado, A.; Ortiz, G.G.; Delgado-Lara, D.L.; González-Usigli, H.A.; González-Ortiz, L.J.; Cid-Hernández, M.; Cruz-Serrano, J.A.; Pacheco-Moisés, F.P. Effect of Melatonin Administration on Mitochondrial Activity and Oxidative Stress Markers in Patients with Parkinson's Disease. *Oxidative Med. Cell. Longev.* **2021**, *2021*, 1–7. [CrossRef] [PubMed]
77. Zhou, Y.-z.; Li, X.; Gong, W.-x.; Tian, J.-s.; Gao, X.-x.; Gao, L.; Zhang, X.; Du, G.-h.; Qin, X.-m. Protective effect of isoliquiritin against corticosterone-induced neurotoxicity in PC12 cells. *Food Funct.* **2017**, *8*, 1235–1244. [CrossRef]
78. Abramov, A.; Angelova, P.R. Mitochondrial dysfunction and energy deprivation in the mechanism of neurodegeneration. *Turk. J. Biochem.* **2019**, *44*, 723–729. [CrossRef]

pharmaceuticals

Review

Natural Bioactive Compounds in the Management of Type 2 Diabetes and Metabolic (Dysfunction)-Associated Steatotic Liver Disease

Daniela Ciobârcă [1], Adriana Florinela Cătoi [2,*], Laura Gavrilaș [1], Roxana Banc [3], Doina Miere [3] and Lorena Filip [3,4]

[1] Department 2, Faculty of Nursing and Health Sciences, "Iuliu Hatieganu" University of Medicine and Pharmacy, 23 Gheorghe Marinescu Street, 400337 Cluj-Napoca, Romania; muresan.daniela@umfcluj.ro (D.C.); laura.gavrilas@umfcluj.ro (L.G.)

[2] Department of Pathophysiology, Faculty of Medicine, "Iuliu Hatieganu" University of Medicine and Pharmacy, 2-4 Victor Babes Street, 400012 Cluj-Napoca, Romania

[3] Department of Bromatology, Hygiene, Nutrition, Faculty of Pharmacy, "Iuliu Hatieganu" University of Medicine and Pharmacy, 6 Louis Pasteur Street, 400349 Cluj-Napoca, Romania; roxana.banc@umfcluj.ro (R.B.); dmiere@umfcluj.ro (D.M.); lfilip@umfcluj.ro (L.F.)

[4] Academy of Romanian Scientists (AOSR), 3 Ilfov Street, 050044 Bucharest, Romania

* Correspondence: adriana.catoi@umfcluj.ro; Tel.: +40-0744436820

Abstract: Type 2 diabetes (T2D) and metabolic (dysfunction)-associated steatotic liver disease (MASLD) affect a growing number of individuals worldwide. T2D and MASLD often coexist and substantially elevate the risk of adverse hepatic and cardiovascular clinical outcomes. Several common pathogenetic mechanisms are responsible for T2D and MASLD onset and progression, including insulin resistance, oxidative stress, and low-grade inflammation, among others. The latter can also be induced by gut microbiota and its derived metabolites. Natural bioactive compounds (NBCs) have been reported for their therapeutic potential in both T2D and MASLD. A large amount of evidence obtained from clinical trials suggests that compounds like berberine, curcumin, soluble fibers, and omega-3 fatty acids exhibit significant hypoglycemic, hypolipidemic, and hepatoprotective activity in humans and may be employed as adjunct therapy in T2D and MASLD management. In this review, the role of the most studied NBCs in the management of T2D and MASLD is discussed, emphasizing recent clinical evidence supporting these compounds' efficacy and safety. Also, prebiotics that act against metabolic dysfunction by modulating gut microbiota are evaluated.

Keywords: type 2 diabetes; metabolic (dysfunction)-associated steatotic liver disease; non-alcoholic fatty liver disease; gut dysbiosis; natural bioactive compounds; berberine; curcumin; soluble fibers; omega-3 fatty acids

1. Introduction

Type 2 diabetes (T2D), metabolic (dysfunction)-associated steatotic liver disease (MASLD), and obesity are cardiometabolic diseases (CMDs) that pose a substantial burden to global health due to their dramatically increased prevalence over the past decades [1,2]. T2D, which is closely linked to the obesity epidemic, remains a major public health issue and significantly enhances cardiovascular morbidity and mortality [3]. Globally, 415 million individuals have diabetes, of which >90% are diagnosed with T2D [4]. Individuals with T2D are at high risk for developing both micro- and macrovascular complications in the context of hyperglycemia and other components of metabolic syndrome (MS) [3]. Nearly

 https://doi.org/10.3390/ph18020279

two-thirds of deaths among T2D patients are related to cardiovascular diseases (CVDs), of which around 40% result from ischemic heart disease [5].

MASLD, previously known as non-alcoholic fatty liver disease (NAFLD), is a form of MS that manifests in the liver [6] and is strongly associated with both obesity and T2D. MASLD prevalence is rising alongside global trends in obesity and T2D [7], currently affecting 38% of adults globally [2] and between 70 and 80% of patients with T2D [8]. The spectrum of MASLD extends from simple steatosis (accumulation of lipids in hepatocytes) to steatohepatitis (steatosis, inflammation), cirrhosis, and hepatocellular carcinoma [6]. However, beyond the risk of hepatic complications, the main cause of mortality among patients with MASLD are CVDs [9]. The latter are responsible for approximately one-third of all deaths in patients with MASLD [10].

The relationship between T2D and MASLD is complex and bidirectional, in which one condition can precede or worsen the other [7]. This link is related to the roles of abdominal obesity and insulin resistance (IR), which are underlying traits of MS, in the pathogenesis of both T2D and MASLD [9]. In the last decade, gut microbiota has also been recognized as a potentially driving factor in the onset or progression of these diseases [11,12]. To emphasize its association with T2D, NAFLD has been recently redefined as MASLD, requiring the presence of at least one of five cardiometabolic risk factors (Table 1). Also, non-alcoholic steatohepatitis (NASH) has been reclassified as metabolic (dysfunction)-associated steatohepatitis (MASH) [6]. Since the MASLD/MASH terminology is applicable to populations initially diagnosed with NAFLD/NASH [13], this review adopts the updated MASLD nomenclature. Nevertheless, when referencing earlier clinical studies discussed in Sections 4 and 5, the original terminology will be retained.

Table 1. Cardiometabolic risk factors for MASLD diagnosis [14].

Cardiometabolic Criteria
BMI $\geq$ 25 kg/m^2 or WC > 94 cm (male) or 80 cm (female)
Fasting serum glucose $\geq$ 100 mg/dL or 2 h post-load glucose levels $\geq$ 140 mg/dL or HbA_{1c} $\geq$ 5.7% or T2D or T2D medication
Blood pressure $\geq$ 130/85 or hypertension medication
Plasma triglycerides $\geq$ 150 mg/dL or lipid-lowering medication
Plasma HDL-c $\leq$ 40 mg/dL (male) or $\leq$50 mg/dL (female) or lipid-lowering medication

Abbreviations: BMI = body mass index; WC = waist circumference; HbA_{1c} = glycosylated hemoglobin; HDL-c = high-density lipoprotein cholesterol.

Patients with T2D face more than double the risk of developing cirrhosis and liver cancer compared to the general population, such that international guidelines now recommend screening for MASLD-related liver fibrosis among patients with T2D [15]. The co-occurrence of MASLD in patients with T2D doubles the risk for the onset and development of CVDs compared to patients without T2D [16]. Owing to the tight interaction between T2D and MASLD, therapeutic agents targeting hyperglycemia, insulin sensitivity, and other cardiometabolic risk factors might contribute to the effective management of hepatic steatosis [17].

In recent years, various natural bioactive compounds (NBCs) and their derivatives have emerged as adjuvant alternatives, complementing a healthy lifestyle and conventional treatment, to help alleviate CMDs. The increasing research interest and growing popularity of NBCs with metabolic health benefits are important for several reasons. Firstly, natural entities, characterized by tremendous diversity and structural complexity, have been and continue to be a valuable source for drug discovery. Modern pharmacological therapies for the treatment of T2D are highly effective in improving glycemic control, but their use may be associated with certain adverse effects [18]. Moreover, conventional lipid-lowering treatments exhibit variable effectiveness in improving the blood lipid profile, and often residual cardiovascular risk persists [19]. For example, the prevalence of lipid abnormalities among T2D patients on statin-lowering therapy was found to be up to 50%, rendering them susceptible to increased residual cardiovascular risk [20]. On the other hand, statin intolerance, which manifests as statin-associated muscle symptoms, often leads to low treatment adherence, augmenting the risk for cardiovascular events [21]. Therefore, exploring NBCs from natural sources and their clinical applications could lead to the development of innovative medications with fewer side effects and improved efficacy [18]. Secondly, long-term adherence to lifestyle intervention, the first-line therapeutic approach for metabolic abnormalities, is often poor [22] and insufficient to reduce risk factors. Hence, multi-drug therapy is often required, which is also associated with reduced compliance, in addition to drug-drug interactions and adverse effects [23]. Thirdly, despite our extensive knowledge about MASLD pathogenesis, no pharmacological therapies have been approved so far [7]. For all these reasons, natural adjuvant therapy may be a promising strategy to help achieve treatment targets, improve outcomes, delay disease progression, and ultimately reduce cardiovascular risk.

The current review aims to describe the efficacy and safety profile of selective NBCs with hypoglycemic effects that also exhibit hypolipidemic and hepatoprotective properties, summarizing the scientific evidence from recent human clinical trials that supports the beneficial role of these compounds in improving glucose and lipid metabolism. We also address the role of prebiotics in managing T2D and MASLD via their impact on gut microbiota.

2. Methodology

A comprehensive literature search was conducted on Pubmed, Science Direct, and Google Scholar, using various keywords and medical subject headings (MeSH), such as T2D, fatty liver diseases—hepatic steatosis, NAFLD, NASH, MASLD, and MASH—as well as selected NBCs like berberine, curcumin (turmeric), resveratrol, anthocyanins, catechins, green tea, phenolic compounds, artichoke, carotenoids, lycopene, hesperidin, silymarin, cinnamon, fenugreek, soluble fibers/prebiotics, and omega-3 fatty acids.

The selection of articles was performed according to the following criteria: (i) articles written in English published in the last 25 years; (ii) studies focusing on adult human subjects, particularly randomized controlled trials, but also systematic reviews and meta-analyses of such trials, as well as narrative reviews; (iii) articles whose outcomes included glycemic control (fasting blood glucose, postprandial blood glucose, glycosylated hemoglobin, homeostasis model assessment for insulin resistance), blood lipid profile (total cholesterol, plasma triglycerides, LDL cholesterol, HDL cholesterol), liver-related parameters (alanine aminotransferase, aspartate aminotransferase, gamma-glutamyl transpeptidase or alkaline phosphatase, liver steatosis/fibrosis scores), inflammatory/anti-inflammatory markers (C-reactive protein, interleukin-6, interleukin-10, tumor necrosis factor α, adiponectin, etc.), antioxidant status (total antioxidant capacity, malondialdehyde, glutathione peroxidase, superoxide dismutase, etc.), and anthropometric indices (BMI, body weight, body fat percentage, waist circumference, waist-to-hip ratio). In vitro research, studies using animal models, and clinical studies with observational designs were excluded.

3. Pathogenetic Mechanisms Leading to T2D and MASLD

CMDs, such as obesity, T2D, or MASLD, encompass a cluster of processes that impair insulin sensitivity, glucose and lipid metabolism, and immune function. CMDs frequently occur concomitantly, appear to share common pathogenetic mechanisms, and are associated with an increased risk of disability and premature death [24]. They also possess a complex genetic [25] and environmental etiology [3]. Although many aspects of these clinical entities are not fully elucidated, it is believed that IR, inflammation, and oxidative stress are the most common pathogenetic mechanisms underlying their onset and progression [26] (Figure 1).

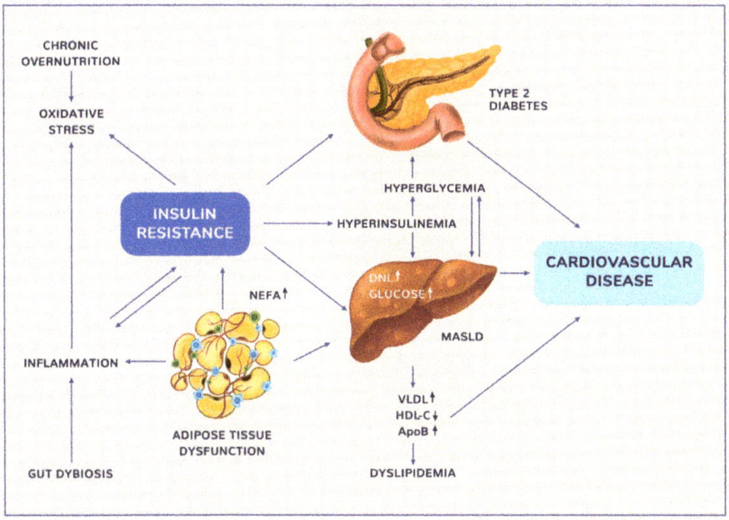

Figure 1. IR as a central mechanism in the pathogenesis of T2D and MASLD [27,28]. ApoB, apolipoprotein B; DNL, de novo lipogenesis; NEFA, non-esterified plasma free fatty acids; HDL-c, high-density lipoproteins; VLDL, very low-density lipoproteins.

3.1. Insulin Resistance

IR is a clinical condition in which insulin produces a lower-than-expected biological response [29] to suppress hepatic glucose production, stimulate glucose disposal in skeletal muscle, inhibit lipolysis, and promote glycogen synthesis [3]. The IR state requires increased insulin secretion to compensate, leading to high levels of fasting plasma insulinemia. Chronic overnutrition in the context of IR causes hyperinsulinemia, which further exacerbates IR, leading to β-cell failure [30] and liver cell injury [31] due to the toxic effects of excessive glucose and lipids (gluco- and lipotoxicity) [30,31].

T2D mainly results from progressively impaired insulin secretion by β-cells in the context of pre-existing liver, skeletal muscle, and adipose tissue IR, often a consequence of obesity. In the liver, IR and insulin deficiency, in the setting of hyperglucagonemia, increased glucagon sensitivity, and the supply of gluconeogenic substrates (fatty acids, glycerol, lactate, and amino acids), stimulate gluconeogenesis, which results in fasting hyperglycemia [3]. Since endogenous glucose production increases in a state of impaired fasting glucose accompanied by hyperinsulinemia, hepatic IR is the main defect promoting hyperglycemia in the early and intermediate stages of T2D [32]. In skeletal muscle, IR affects insulin's ability to stimulate glucose disposal [33] by altering glucose transporter type 4 (GLUT4) translocation to the cell surface in response to insulin [34]. Because of its major role in postprandial glucose uptake (up to 80%), skeletal muscle is recognized as a key factor in systemic IR [33]. Factors responsible for skeletal muscle IR include defective insulin signaling, altered glucose transport or glucose phosphorylation, and decreased mitochondrial oxidative capacity. IR in adipose tissue accelerates lipolysis, leading to increased non-esterified plasma free fatty acids (NEFA) levels, which further exacerbate IR in the liver and muscle [3].

IR affects not only the liver, muscle, and adipose tissue but also the kidneys, vasculature, and brain. Increased renal glucose reabsorption and an elevation of the renal threshold for glucose also contribute to fasting hyperglycemia. IR in the vascular endothelium causes metabolic stress by altering the vasodilator action of insulin and subsequently decreases the supply of glucose, as well as insulin itself [3]. In the brain, IR is associated with a decrease or absence of regulatory signals that modulate peripheral metabolism, particularly in the postprandial state. Hence, certain peripheral metabolic responses, including endogenous glucose synthesis, cellular glucose uptake, liver energy metabolism, and pancreatic insulin secretion, are compromised in the state of IR [35]. In summary, T2D is caused by multi-organ IR coupled with a progressive decline in insulin secretion [36].

Adipose tissue IR is characterized by an increased NEFA flux to the liver, which promotes intrahepatic fat accumulation. Excessive NEFA can either be oxidized, reassembled into triglycerides (TGs) and stored in hepatocyte lipid droplets, or released as large very low-density lipoproteins (VLDL) into circulation. Overproduction of VLDL-cholesterol leads to atherogenic dyslipidemia, characterized by increased levels of triglycerides and apolipoprotein B particles, as well as decreased concentrations of HDL-cholesterol. Dyslipidemia is frequently associated with the extent of liver fat accumulation (Figure 1) [37]. Hepatic TG assembly is generally coordinated with VLDL production and stored intracellular TGs. Hence, hepatic fat accumulation occurs when the equilibrium between lipid storage and clearance in the liver becomes disrupted [9]. In addition to lipid overflow due to excessive peripheral lipolysis, de novo lipogenesis (DNL) and increased hepatic uptake of chylomicron remnants and intrahepatically generated VLDL also contribute to liver steatosis [9]. In MASLD, insulin fails to suppress gluconeogenesis and glucose output from the liver, yet continues to increase lipid synthesis, leading to hyperglycemia and hypertriglyceridemia. This process is known as selective IR. It is estimated that, in the setting of both hyperglycemia and hyperinsulinemia, DNL accounts for around 38% of liver triglycerides (TGs), compared to 11% in lean subjects [38].

Mitochondrial dysfunction contributes to MASLD pathogenesis due to the role that mitochondria play in gluco- and lipogenesis, as well as fatty acid oxidation. In IR states, particularly obesity or T2D, hepatic mitochondrial oxidative activity is initially increased to adapt to elevated lipid availability. However, the oxidative capacity of the mitochondria in the liver has been shown to decrease over time in individuals with steatosis, leading to oxidative stress, mitochondrial alterations, and worsening of MASLD [35].

The accumulation of TGs in the liver is believed to be a protective mechanism to prevent endoplasmic reticulum stress, reactive oxygen species synthesis, and lipid intermediate formation [35]. While the storage of lipids as TGs in hepatocytes is relatively benign, the accumulation of cholesterol, phosphatidylcholines, diacylglycerol, and certain saturated fatty acids accentuates lipotoxicity, leading to local IR and inflammation. Chronic adipose tissue-related inflammation and lipotoxicity from excessive fat accumulation in the liver trigger stress-activated signaling pathways that lead to liver cell apoptosis. The liver initiates a healing response, including proliferation and fibrosis, which can eventually progress to more severe conditions, such as cirrhosis or cancer [39].

Molecular Mechanisms Underlying IR

Insulin elicits its biological effects by binding to its receptor (INSR) and subsequently activating specific proteins, including insulin receptor substrates (IRSs, particularly IRS-1 and IRS-2) and insulin receptor tyrosine kinase. In turn, phosphorylated IRS proteins trigger major intracellular signaling pathways, such as phosphatidylinositol 3-kinase (PI3K) and

RAS-mitogen-activated protein kinase (MAPK). PI3K is responsible for the translocation of GLUT4 to the cell membrane, thereby stimulating glucose uptake in skeletal muscle [3]. The MAPK pathway modulates the mitogenic and proliferative effects of insulin [28]. Defective phosphorylation of IRS proteins (e.g., increased serine and decreased tyrosine phosphorylation) promotes IR [3]. In obesity and T2D, the tyrosine phosphorylation of IRS-1 is inhibited, leading to altered IRS-1 signaling and subsequent skeletal muscle IR [40]. Other potential triggering mechanisms of IRS serine phosphorylation include ectopic lipid accumulation, endoplasmic reticulum stress, mitochondrial dysfunction, and inflammation [3].

3.2. Inflammation and Oxidative Stress

Adipose tissue produces various anti-inflammatory and proinflammatory molecules, whose abnormal expression is involved in the development of metabolic dysfunction [41]. Obesity is characterized by a proinflammatory state that decreases the plasma concentration of anti-inflammatory mediators, such as adiponectin (APN) [41] and interleukin (IL) 10 [42]. APN stimulates muscle glucose disposal and fatty acid oxidation while promoting the suppression of hepatic gluconeogenesis [41]. Decreased APN levels have been associated with inflammation markers in obesity-related disorders [43].

Since it was discovered that adipocytes secrete inflammatory mediators and that obesity is characterized by an increased number of macrophages in adipose tissue, adipose tissue inflammation has been considered the primary cause of IR [36]. Highly proinflammatory macrophages, together with adipocytes, produce abnormal cytokine synthesis [e.g., tumor necrosis factor-α (TNF-α), IL-1, and IL-6], increased acute-phase reactants, and mediators, as well as activate inflammatory signaling pathways such as JNK and IKKβ, leading to impaired insulin action [44]. JNK modulates the serine phosphorylation of IRS-1, contributing to the TNF-α-related impairment of insulin signaling [45]. IKKB activates the nuclear transcription factor kappa B (NF-kB), which, in turn, augments the expression of proinflammatory molecules. Inflammasomes, multi-protein complexes activated by intracellular nutrients (e.g., glucose, free fatty acids), are also components of the low-grade inflammation process [46]. In addition to impaired insulin signaling, cytokines and proinflammatory mediators produced by adipocytes and macrophages lead to β-cell failure, impaired vascular flow, and endothelial dysfunction by upregulating various inflammatory pathways [47].

Oxidative stress (OS) is a significant upstream event for inflammation, as it promotes macrophage activation, increased cytokine production, and the inflammatory response, leading to IR, T2D [48], and MASLD [49]. Glucotoxicity leads to an increase in ROS in β-cells [32], causing mitochondrial damage, negative effects on insulin secretion, cellular death, and tissular damage [50]. Moreover, chronically elevated levels of glucose and NEFA exert synergistic harmful effects and maximize β-cell toxicity [51]. ROS derived from dysfunctional mitochondria have been associated with NLRP3 inflammasome activation [52], which controls the secretion of proinflammatory cytokines IL-1β and IL-18 [53]. IL-1β is considered responsible for the development of chronic complications in T2D [54].

Excessive fat accumulation in the liver due to hepatic lipid overflow results in lipotoxicity, with subsequent mitochondrial dysfunction, endoplasmic reticulum stress, and ROS formation. The overproduction of ROS causes mitochondrial injury, hepatic cellular death, and lipid oxidation, leading to inflammation and fibrogenesis [49].

3.3. Gut Microbiota-Related Inflammation

Beyond adipose tissue and the liver, the gastrointestinal tract may also be a source of inflammation due to its altered microbiota (dysbiosis), causing IR and metabolic dysfunction. Studies in both animal models and humans have shown that T2D [11] and MASLD [12] are associated with gut microbiota (GM) function and composition abnormalities, although conflicting evidence regarding the specific dysbiotic profiles in these conditions has emerged [11,12].

A large body of evidence highlights the role of the gut–liver axis in the pathogenesis and management of both T2D [11] and MASLD [12]. The gut–liver axis is a bidirectional pathway of communication between the intestine and liver [55] that plays a central role in maintaining energy homeostasis [56]. This bidirectional crosstalk is facilitated, on one hand, by the portal vein, which carries gut-derived products to the liver. In addition, immune cells activated by nutrients or gut metabolites enter lymphatic vessels, influencing immune responses in distal organs. On the other hand, the liver responds to the gut by releasing bile acids (BAs) and other metabolites into the biliary tract and systemic circulation. BAs possess antimicrobial activity, controlling unrestricted bacterial overgrowth. This is crucial for maintaining the normal function of the gut–liver axis. Also, BAs regulate multiple metabolic processes by activating nuclear receptors [55].

Various genetic and environmental factors may disrupt the complex interplay among the GM, intestinal barrier, immune system, and liver, leading to CMDs [57]. Gut barrier dysfunction manifests as increased intestinal permeability, which enables the translocation of microbes and their metabolites [endotoxins, particularly lipopolysaccharide (LPS)] to distal organs through the portal circulation, causing inflammation [55] and IR [58]. Gut dysbiosis is also linked to a reduced number of short-chain fatty acid (SCFA)-producing bacteria, the induction of an immune response against LPS, high levels of ethanol-producing bacteria, and subsequent increased ethanol synthesis, as well as the conversion of choline to trimethylamine and abnormal levels and composition of plasma BAs [59]. The overgrowth of ethanol-producing bacteria may accelerate MASLD progression to more severe forms of liver disease [60].

4. Natural Bioactive Compounds for T2D and MASLD Treatment

NBCs are small molecules found in various plant parts or foods that can provide health benefits [61] due to their modulatory effects on metabolic pathways (e.g., cholesterol-lowering or anti-inflammatory activity) [62]. To date, numerous NBCs have been discovered, each possessing its own distinct pharmacologic effects and health benefits. As such, NBCs exert powerful antioxidant, anti-inflammatory, and antimicrobial effects [63], which exhibit hypoglycemic, hepatoprotective, hypolipidemic, hypotensive, and cardioprotective properties [64].

NBCs have a wide range of natural sources and possess strikingly diverse chemical structures and biological activities [63]. They are either primary or secondary metabolites of plants or nutritional components [62], such as polyphenols, flavonoids, alkaloids, tannins, carotenoids, etc. These compounds are found in various parts of plants, such as leaves, bark, and roots, or may naturally occur in foods [61]. For example, fruits, vegetables, grains, seeds, nuts, legumes, herbs, and spices are valuable sources of NBCs. Several NBCs, however, originate from animal sources and have been extensively researched for their functional benefits on human health (e.g., omega-3 PUFA) [62]. In addition to fresh foods, NBCs are common ingredients in nutraceuticals and dietary supplements [64].

In this section, we will discuss in detail the clinical evidence supporting the efficacy and safety of specific NBCs with antidiabetic, hypolipidemic, and hepatoprotective activity. The selected NBCs used in the management of both T2D and MASLD are summarized in Figure 2.

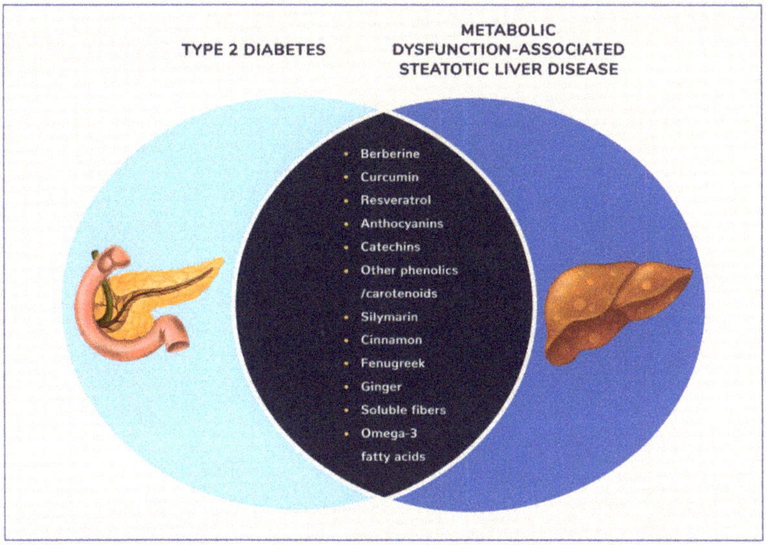

Figure 2. NBCs with potential therapeutic roles in T2D and MASLD.

4.1. Berberine

Berberine (BBR) is an alkaloid extracted from *Rhizoma coptidis* (Huanglian) that has been traditionally used in the management of T2D [65]. BBR's antidiabetic activity was first reported in 1986, and subsequent in vivo studies confirmed its role in improving glucolipid metabolism [66]. Other reported pharmacological effects of BBR include anti-inflammatory, anti-carcinogenetic [65], antibacterial, anti-platelet aggregation, and cardioprotective properties [67].

Clinical evidence in T2D. The glucose- and lipid-lowering effects of BBR were confirmed by multiple randomized clinical trials (RCTs) in patients with T2D (Table 2). Yin et al. (2008) compared the efficacy of BBR monotherapy with metformin monotherapy (1500 mg daily for 3 months) in patients with newly diagnosed T2D (n = 31). Results showed significant improvements in fasting blood glucose (FBG), postprandial blood glucose (PBG), and HbA_{1c} in both groups. BBR's glucose-lowering effect was compared to that of metformin. In a second study involving 43 patients with poorly controlled T2D, the authors showed that BBR significantly lowered FBG, PBG, and HbA_{1c} levels, along with fasting insulin (FI) plasma concentration and homeostasis model assessment for insulin resistance (HOMA-IR) levels. In addition, BBR supplementation exhibited positive effects on the blood lipid profile in both studies, significantly decreasing plasma total cholesterol (TC) and TGs, as well as TC and LDL-c levels [68].

Zhang et al. (2010) also demonstrated that BBR (1 g/day for 2 months) significantly lowered FBG, HbA_{1c}, insulin, and TG levels in patients with T2D (n = 50). BBR exhibited a similar efficacy in improving glycemic control as metformin (n = 26) and rosiglitazone (n = 21) [69].

Another RCT by Gu et al. (2010) analyzed the effects of either BBR or placebo on glucolipid metabolism and indicated that BBR (1 g/day) improved glucose and lipid metabolism parameters in patients with T2D (n = 60). After 3 months, BBR significantly decreased FBG, 2 h PBG, HbA_{1c}, TC, TGs, and LDL-c levels compared to placebo. The authors demonstrated that BBR mainly modulated the metabolism of free fatty acids in T2D patients [70].

Table 2. Summary of RCTs investigating the hypoglycemic, hypolipidemic, and anti-steatosis effects of BBR.

Disease	Participants (Total)	Intervention	Control	Duration	Main Outcomes */**	References
T2D	Study A: n = 31 Study B: n = 43	BBR 1500 mg/day BBR 1500 mg/day + T2D treatment	Metformin 1500 mg/day -	3 months	Study A: ↓ FBG, PBG, HbA_{1c} **, TGs, TC * Study B: ↓ FBG, PBG, HbA_{1c}, HOMA-IR, FI, TC, LDL-c **	[68]
T2D	n = 97	BBR 1 g/day	Metformin 1.5 g/day RSG 4 mg/day	2 months	↓ FBG, HbA_{1c}, TGs **	[69]
T2D	n = 60	BBR 1 g/day	Placebo	3 months	↓ FBG, PBG, HbA_{1c}, TGs, TC, LDL-c *	[70]
T2D	n = 63	BBR + SLM (1000/210 mg/day)	BBR 1000 mg/day	4 months	↓ HbA_{1c} *	[71]
T2D	n = 45	BBR + SLM + statins BBR + SLM + ezetimibe	BBR + SLM (1000/210 mg/day)	12 months	↓ FBG, HbA_{1c}, TC, LDL-c **	[72]
T2D	n = 69	BBR 300 mg/day	Standard treatment	24 months	↓ CRP, MDA, ↑ HMW-APN, GSH-Px, SOD, TAC *	[73]
NAFLD	n = 155	BBR 1.5 g/day + LSI	LSI	16 weeks	↓ HFC, BW, HOMA-IR, TC, TGs *	[74]
NAFLD	n = 80	BBR 1.5 g/day + LSI	LSI	16 weeks	↓ HFC, TC, TGs, BMI, BW, WC *	[75]
NASH/T2D	n = 88	BUDCA 2000 mg/day	Placebo	18 weeks	↓ HFC, HbA_{1c}, ALT, GGT, BW *	[76]
MAFLD	n = 63	BBR 1500 mg/day	Placebo	12 weeks	↓ ALT, AST/ALT ratio, TC *	[77]

* Statistically significant between groups ($p < 0.05$); ** Statistically significant from baseline ($p < 0.05$); "↓", decreased; "↑", increased. Abbreviations: ALT, alanine aminotransferase; AST, aspartate aminotransferase; BBR, berberine; BW, body weight; BUDCA, berberine ursodeoxycholate; CRP, C-reactive protein; FBG, fasting blood glucose; GGT, gamma-glutamyl transpeptidase; GSH-Px, glutathione peroxidase; HbA_{1c}, glycosylated hemoglobin; HOMA-IR, homeostatic model assessment of insulin resistance; HFC, hepatic fat content; HMW-APN, high molecular weight adiponectin; LDL-c, low-density lipoprotein cholesterol; LSI, lifestyle intervention; PBG, postprandial blood glucose; SLM, silymarin; SOD, superoxide dismutase; TC, total cholesterol; TAC, total antioxidant capacity; TGs, triglycerides; WC, waist circumference.

A 2013 RCT demonstrated that equal doses of BBR (1 g/day) and BBR in combination with silymarin (BBR 1 g/day and SML 210 mg/day) were capable of significantly decreasing FBG, TC, TG, and liver enzyme levels [alanine aminotransferase (ALT) and aspartate transferase (AST]) in patients with T2D and suboptimal glycemic control (n = 63). Moreover, BBR-SLM was proven to be more effective than BBR alone in reducing HbA_{1c} concentration. LDL-c also declined significantly only in the BBR-SLM-supplemented patients, but there were no differences between groups. It was proposed that in combination with SLM, BBR has increased bioavailability, as the former may act as a potential antagonist of P-glycoprotein. The latter mediates the extrusion of BBR from gut cells and promotes its extensive biliary excretion [71].

In clinical practice, most patients on statin-lowering therapy do not reach their LDL-c goal due to statin intolerance [21] or refractory hypercholesterolemia [78], among other factors. Hence, a non-statin hypolipidemic treatment or a lipid-lowering combination therapy is often recommended [21,78]. Recent studies have demonstrated the beneficial effects of proprotein convertase subtilisin/kexin type 9 (PCSK9) inhibitors on lowering LDL-c and cardiovascular risk [79]. Notably, BBR directly inhibits PCSK9 expression [80]. In 2015, a combined therapy of BBR and SLM was administered to patients with T2D and statin intolerance (n = 45). Patients enrolled in the study were divided into three groups receiving a low statin dose (n = 15), ezetimibe (n = 15), or no treatment at all (n = 15). Results showed that BBR and SLM, either as monotherapy or as add-on therapy to statins and ezetimibe, significantly reduced TGs and LDL-c in all patients after 12 months. Also, significant improvements were reported in FBG and HbA_{1c} levels [72].

Dai et al. reported that 300 mg of BBR (n = 36) administered alongside hypoglycemic and hypotensive medication led to a significant decrease in C-reactive protein (CRP) and malondialdehyde (MDA) levels, as well as a significant increase in high molecular weight APN, glutathione peroxidase (GSH-Px), superoxide dismutase (SOD) activity, and total antioxidant capacity (TAC) in T2D patients. However, FBG and HbA_{1c} concentrations did not differ significantly between groups at the end of the study period [73].

More recently, a 2022 systematic review and meta-analysis (SRMA) by Xie et al. reported statistically significant improvements in FBG, HbA_{1c}, and 2 h PBG following BBR supplementation in patients with T2D (n = 3048). BBR's glucose-lowering effect was associated with baseline mean FBG and HbA_{1c} levels. BBR dosages ranged from 0.9 g to 2.4 g/day, while intervention durations varied from 14 days to 6 months [67].

Clinical evidence in MASLD. In addition to being a robust oral hypoglycemic and hypolipidemic agent, BBR also exerts positive effects on liver function (Table 2). Yan et al. (2015) performed an RCT involving 155 NAFLD patients who randomly received lifestyle intervention (LSI) alone or in combination with BBR (0.5 g three times daily) or pioglitazone (15 mg/day) for 16 weeks. BBR and LSI significantly lowered hepatic fat content (HFC) compared to LSI alone. Also, significant improvements in blood lipid profiles, HOMA-IR, and body weight (BW) were also observed. BBR was superior to pioglitazone in improving lipid profile levels and BW. Liver enzyme levels declined in all three groups at the end of the study period, but there were no significant differences between the groups [74].

Chang et al. (2016) showed that in patients with NAFLD (n = 80) treated with LSI alone or in combination with BBR (0.5 g three times daily), HFC, TC, and TGs levels were significantly decreased in the intervention group after 16 weeks. However, liver enzyme concentrations, specifically, ALT, AST, and gamma-glutamyl transpeptidase (GGT), did not differ significantly between the BBR and LSI groups at the end of the follow-up period. More significant improvements in anthropometric indices (BMI, BW, WC) were also observed in the intervention group compared to the control group. The lipid-lowering effect of BBR was mediated by the downregulation of circulating ceramides [75].

Harrison et al. (2021) reported that berberine ursodeoxycholate (1 g twice daily for 18 weeks) was more effective than a placebo in decreasing HFC in patients with presumed NASH and T2D (n = 88). Significant decreases in liver enzyme levels (ALT, GGT), HbA_{1c}, and BW were also observed in the treatment group compared to the control group [76].

Koperska et al. (2024) demonstrated that, after 12 weeks of treatment, patients with metabolic dysfunction-associated fatty liver disease (MAFLD) (n = 63) receiving BBR (1.5 g/day) showed a statistically significant decrease in ALT, ALT/AST ratio, and TC levels compared to placebo recipients. No other significant differences regarding glucose and lipid parameters between the groups were found [77].

Finally, a 2024 SRMA of 10 RCTs (n = 811), mainly conducted in China, showed that BBR used as an adjunct therapy can significantly improve liver enzyme levels, IR, dyslipidemia, and body weight, with minimal adverse effects. In 7 out of 10 RCTs, patients also presented with comorbid T2D. However, certain results showed increased heterogeneity, highlighting the need for further research. The doses of BBR administered varied between 0.6 and 6.35 g/day, while the study durations ranged from 7 to 24 weeks [81].

Safety. BBR has a high safety profile, with fewer side effects than conventional antidiabetic agents [67]. Commonly reported adverse effects include constipation, diarrhea, abdominal pain, and flatulence. In combination therapy with antidiabetic medication, a dose of 300 mg three times daily is well tolerated [68]. BBR carries a low risk of hypoglycemia [67].

Summary. BBR is a promising regulator of glucose and lipid parameters in patients with metabolic dysfunction. According to clinical evidence, BBR's has proven efficient in alleviating glycemic control in patients with T2D is similar to that of metformin and rosiglitazone. In addition, BBR appears to improve several characteristics of MASLD.

4.2. Curcumin

Curcumin (CRM) is an NBC derived from the rhizome of *Curcuma longa* (turmeric) that has been extensively studied due to its numerous pharmacological effects. CRM is the main active constituent of turmeric, along with other structurally related curcuminoids. Studies conducted in vitro and in vivo have shown that CRM possesses hypoglycemic, antioxidant, and anti-inflammatory properties, as well as cardio- and hepatoprotective activity. Nevertheless, CRM has low bioavailability, which restrains its clinical use [82]. Therefore, most studies have evaluated different bioavailability-enhanced CRM formulations (e.g., phytosomal, nano-micellar CRM) or CRM in combination with other compounds, e.g., piperine [83] and omega-3 fatty acids [84], which significantly improve CRM absorption or reduce its metabolization [82].

Clinical evidence in T2D. According to current evidence, CRM may improve glycemic control and blood lipid profiles in patients with T2D (Table 3). A 2012 RCT conducted by Na et al. involving T2D patients (n = 50) who received 300 mg of curcuminoids daily for 3 months, along with conventional treatment, showed that patients in the interventional group experienced significantly decreased FBG, HbA_{1c}, and HOMA-IR levels compared to placebo recipients (n = 50). In addition, in the CRM-treated group, a significant reduction in total free fatty acids and TG levels was observed [85].

Table 3. Summary of RCTs investigating the hypoglycemic, hypolipidemic, and anti-steatosis effects of CRM.

Disease	Participants (Total)	Intervention	Control	Duration	Main Outcomes */**	References
T2D	n = 100	CRMs 300 mg/day	Placebo	3 months	↓ FBG, HbA_{1c}, HOMA-IR, TGs *	[85]
T2D	n = 70	CRM 80 mg/day	Placebo	3 months	↓ FBG, HbA_{1c}, BMI *	[86]
T2D	n = 100	CRM 1000 mg/day + piperine 10 mg/day	Placebo	12 weeks	↓ TC, ↑ HDL-c *	[83]
T2D	n = 95	nano-CRM + EPA	Placebo	12 weeks	↓ insulin, hs-CRP, ↑ TAC *	[84]
T2D	n = 229	CRM 1500 mg/day	Placebo	12 months	↓ FBG, HbA_{1c}, HOMA-IR, ↑ APN *	[87]
T2D	n = 227	CRM 1500 mg/day	Placebo	12 months	↓ LDL-c, ApoB, hs-CRP, IL-6, TNF-α *	[88]
NAFLD	n = 77	CRM 500 mg/day	Placebo	8 weeks	↓ HFC, ALT, AST, FBG, HbA_{1c}, TC, TGs, LDL-c *	[89]
NAFLD	n = 48	CRM 1500 mg/day	Placebo	12 weeks	↓ ALT, AST, hs-CRP, TNF-α, BMI, BW, WC, steatosis/fibrosis **	[90]
NAFLD	n = 50	CRM 1500 mg/day + LSI	Placebo + LSI	12 weeks	↓ FLI, FLS **	[91]
NAFLD	n = 60	CRM 500 mg/day + piperine 5 mg/day	Placebo	12 weeks	↓ ALT, AST, TC, LDL-c, FBG, WC *	[92]

* Statistically significant between groups ($p < 0.05$); ** Statistically significant from baseline ($p < 0.05$); "↓", decreased; "↑", increased. Abbreviations: ALT, alanine aminotransferase; APN, adiponectin; ApoB, apolipoprotein B; AST, aspartate aminotransferase; BMI, body mass index; BW, body weight; FBG, fasting blood glucose; FLI, fatty liver index; FLS, fatty liver score; HbA_{1c}, glycosylated hemoglobin; HDL-c, high-density lipoprotein cholesterol; HOMA-IR, homeostatic model assessment of insulin resistance; hs-CRP, high-sensitivity C-reactive protein; HFC, hepatic fat content; IL-6, interleukin-6; LDL-c, low-density lipoprotein cholesterol; LSI, lifestyle intervention; TC, total cholesterol; TGs, triglycerides; TNF-α, tumor necrosis factor α; WC, waist circumference.

An HbA_{1c}-lowering effect was also reported by Rahimi et al. (2016) following supplementation with nano-CRM (nano-micelle 80 mg/day for 3 months) versus placebo in 70 patients with T2D. Also, between-group comparisons revealed significant differences in FBG and BMI following supplementation, but no changes were observed in the lipid profile.

However, in the nano-CRM-treated patients, significant improvements in the levels of FBG, HbA_{1c}, TC, TGs, LDL-c, HDL, as well as in BMI, were observed after the intervention [86].

In another RCT (2017) involving curcuminoids (1000 mg/day, along with piperine 10 mg/day) or a placebo with conventional T2D treatment (n = 100) for 12 weeks, TC, non-HDL-c and lipoprotein (a) levels were significantly reduced in the CRM group at the end of the study. A significant elevation in HDL-c concentration was also reported in CRM-treated patients, although no significant changes in TG and LDL-c levels were observed between the groups [83].

A 2023 updated SRMA involving 28 studies in patients with T2D and MS revealed that CRM supplementation led to significant post-intervention improvements in the levels of FBG, HbA_{1c}, LDL-c, HDL-c, and serum insulin. No significant reductions were reported for TC or TG concentrations [93].

Asghari et al. (2024) investigated the effects of nano-CRM, eicosapentaeneoic acid (EPA), and their combination on various metabolic parameters in T2D patients (n = 95). Although significant improvements in insulin, high-sensitivity C-reactive protein (hs-CRP) levels, and TAC were reported after 12 weeks of supplementation with nano-CRM and EPA compared to the placebo, no meaningful differences were observed in FBG, HOMA-IR, quantitative insulin sensitivity check index (QUICKI), and HbA_{1c} levels among the four groups. Nevertheless, HOMA-IR decreased significantly in all treatment groups, while the QUICKI index increased significantly only in the EPA plus nano-CRM group. In addition, HbA_{1c} and TG levels decreased significantly following supplementation with nano-CRM, with or without EPA. The consumption of both EPA and nano-CRM also led to notable improvements in TC and HDL-c levels. In addition, LDL-c decreased non-significantly in all intervention groups [84].

In contrast to these results, Yaikwawong et al. (2024) reported a significant glucose-lowering effect, as evidenced by FPG and HbA1c levels, after CRM supplementation (1500 mg/day) versus placebo for 12 months in T2D patients (n = 227). In addition, CRM-treated patients exhibited significantly lower levels of HOMA-IR and a higher APN concentration [87].

Finally, CRM was proven effective in enhancing vascular health, which, in conjunction with its lipid-modulating potential, decreases cardiovascular risk in T2D patients. According to a 2024 RCT, CRM supplementation (250 mg curcuminoids six times daily for 12 months) exhibited significant reductions in ApoB, LDL-c, small-dense LDL-c, and pulse wave velocity levels, as well as in various proinflammatory cytokines (hs-CRP, IL-6, TNF-α) in T2D patients (n = 227) compared to placebo recipients [88].

Clinical evidence in MASLD. CRM represents a promising therapeutic approach for NAFLD patients (Table 3). Rahmani et al. (2016) demonstrated that compared to placebo, CRM intake (500 mg/day of dispersion formulation for 8 weeks) was associated with a significant decrease in HFC in NAFLD patients (n = 77). Also, a significant reduction in FBG, HbA_{1c}, TC, TGs, LDL-c, ALT, and AST levels was reported in CRM-treated patients [89].

Improvements in liver fibrosis scores were observed in NAFLD patients supplemented with CRM (500 mg/day, three times daily) in a 2019 RCT. In addition, hepatic steatosis, liver enzymes (ALT, AST), hs-CRP and TNF-α levels, as well as anthropometric indices (BW, BMI, WC), decreased significantly in both groups, but not significantly, suggesting that CRM is not superior to lifestyle modifications in improving inflammation in NAFLD patients [90].

Comparable results were reported by a 2022 RCT involving a similar number of patients with NAFLD and doses of CRM. The findings indicated that, compared to LSI, CRM supplementation did not significantly improve steatosis scores [fatty liver index (FLI) and fatty liver score (FLS)] or adipose tissue-related markers, providing no additional benefits for cardiometabolic health. Nevertheless, the number of patients with severe fatty liver and MS was significantly lower in the CRM group after the intervention compared to the placebo group [91].

CRM supplementation, in combination with piperine (500 mg/day plus 5 mg/day for 3 months) (n = 30), versus a placebo (n = 30) was also not shown to reduce hepatic steatosis and fibrosis in patients with moderate to high NAFLD, but it may be used to improve blood glucose, the lipid profile, anthropometric variables, and liver function [92].

Finally, a 2023 umbrella meta-analysis of patients with NAFLD comprising 11 meta-analyses of 99 RCTs (n = 5546) revealed that CRM was effective in significantly improving levels of ALT, AST, TGs, and HOMA-IR. Also, CRM supplementation has proven effective in reducing obesity [94].

Safety. Various animal and human studies have reported the safety and tolerability of CRM, even at high doses (up to 12 g/day via oral administration) [82]. So far, no adverse effects on blood sugar levels have been observed. However, CRM may cause gastrointestinal side effects, such as gastric irritation, flatulence, stimulation of bile flow, and potential cholangitis. In combination with piperine, CRM's cholecystokinetic effect is amplified, and it may increase the risk of hepatotoxicity [95].

Summary. CRM has considerable potential for improving glycemic control, lipid profile, and inflammation status in T2D, with minimal side effects. Although its efficacy in ameliorating MASLD traits is less conclusive, CRM could be recommended as a complementary therapy for these patients.

4.3. Resveratrol

Resveratrol (RSV) is a natural polyphenolic compound initially extracted from the roots of white melon and later identified in many other plants. RSV is considered to possess a broad spectrum of biological activities related to health, exhibiting antidiabetic, anti-obesity, antioxidant, anti-inflammatory, cardioprotective, and antitumor properties, among others [96].

Clinical evidence in T2D. Currently, only a small body of RCTs has investigated the effects of RSV supplementation in T2D (Table 4). In a 2012 open-label RCT, it was shown that RSV supplementation (250 mg/day for 3 months), in combination with hypoglycemic medication, led to improvements in HbA_{1c} and TC. However, no significant changes in BW, LDL-c, and HDL-c levels were observed [97].

In another crossover RCT (2016), Thazhath et al. also failed to detect any significant improvements in the glycemic control (FBG, PBG) and BW of diet-controlled T2D patients (n = 14) after 1000 mg RSV/day for two 5-week intervention periods [98].

Timmers et al. (2016) investigated whether RSV intake (150 mg/day) could improve insulin sensitivity in patients with T2D (n = 17). After 30 days of treatment, no changes were reported in hepatic and peripheral insulin sensitivity. The authors argued that the lack of insulin-sensitizing effects following RSV supplementation could be explained by the interaction between RSV and Metformin. Liver fat content also remained unchanged after RSV supplementation, although a negative correlation between plasma RSV levels and intrahepatic lipid content was reported [99].

Similarly, Bo et al. (2016) supplemented T2D patients (n = 179) with two different RSV dosages (500 and 40 mg/day) and a placebo for 6 months but observed no significant improvements in anthropometric indices (body weight, BMI, WC), glucose metabolism parameters (FBG, HbA_{1c}, HOMA-IR, insulin), lipid profile (TC, TGs, LDL-c, HDL-c), inflammatory markers (IL-6, APN), or liver enzyme levels (AST, ALT, GGT) between the interventional and control groups. However, a decrease in CRP levels was observed in both RSV-treated arms, although this was not significantly different compared to the placebo.

Moreover, a subgroup analysis revealed a decline in CRP levels among patients with a shorter history of T2D following 40 mg/day RSV supplementation. In addition, TC and TG levels were shown to increase modestly in the 500 mg/day RSV-treated patients [100].

By contrast, Hoseini et al. (2019) performed a RCT involving 56 patients with T2D and coronary heart disease, using 500 mg of RSV/day (n = 28) or a placebo for 4 weeks. FBG, IR, and the TC/HDL-c ratio significantly decreased after RSV intake, whereas marked improvements were reported in HDL-c levels, insulin sensitivity, and several biomarkers of oxidative damage. However, RSV supplementation did not alter the IL-1 and TNF-α gene expression [101].

Table 4. Summary of RCTs investigating the hypoglycemic, hypolipidemic, and anti-steatosis effects of RSV.

Disease	Participants (Total)	Intervention	Control	Duration	Main Outcomes */**	References
T2D	n = 57	RSV 250 mg/day	T2D medication	3 months	↓ HbA_{1c}, TC **	[97]
T2D	n = 14	RSV 1000 mg/day	Placebo	5 weeks	no significant changes	[98]
T2D	n = 17	RSV 150 mg/day	Placebo	30 days	no significant changes	[99]
T2D	n = 179	RSV 500 mg or 40 mg/day	Placebo	6 months	no significant changes	[100]
T2D + CHD	n = 56	RSV 500 mg/day	Placebo	4 weeks	↓ FBG, HOMA-IR, ↑ HDL-c, QUICKI, TAC, ↓ MDA **	[101]
T2D	n = 110	RSV 200 mg/day	Placebo	24 weeks	FBG, HbA_{1c}, HOMA-IR, FI, hs-CRP, TNF-α, IL-6 **	[102]
NAFLD	n = 20	RSV 3000 mg/day	Placebo	8 weeks	no significant changes	[103]
NAFLD	n = 50	RSV 500 mg + LSI	Placebo	12 weeks	↓ ALT *, AST BMI **	[104]
NAFLD	n = 60	RSV 600 mg/day	Placebo	3 months	↓ ALT, AST, glucose, HOMA-IR, TC, LDL-c, TNF-α, CK18-M30, ↑ APN *	[105]
NAFLD	n = 26	RSV 1500 mg/day	Placebo	6 months	no significant changes	[106]

* Statistically significant between groups ($p < 0.05$); ** Statistically significant from baseline ($p < 0.05$). "↓", decreased; "↑", increased. Abbreviations: ALT, alanine aminotransferase; APN, adiponectin; AST, aspartate aminotransferase; BMI, body mass index; CK18-M30, cytokeratin 18 M30; FBG, fasting blood glucose; FI, fasting insulin; HbA_{1c}, glycosylated hemoglobin; HDL-c, high-density lipoprotein cholesterol; HOMA-IR, homeostatic model assessment of insulin resistance; hs-CRP, high-sensitivity C-reactive protein; IL-6, interleukin-6; LDL-c, low-density lipoprotein cholesterol; MDA, malondyladehyde; QUICKI, quantitative insulin sensitivity check index; TAC, total antioxidant capacity; TC, total cholesterol TNF-α, tumor necrosis factor.

Finally, a significant glucose-lowering effect (FBG, HbA_{1c}, HOMA-IR, FI) was reported by Mahjabeen et al. (2022) in T2D patients (n = 110) supplemented with 200 mg RSV/day (n = 55) for 24 weeks compared to a placebo (n = 55). RSV treatment also led to a significantly improved anti-inflammatory status (hs-CRP, TNF-α, IL-6), but no considerable effects were observed on the lipid profile (TC, TGs, HDL-c, and LDL-c) between the two groups [102].

Clinical evidence in MASLD. Research on animal models indicates that RSV alleviates fibrosis and inflammation associated with NAFLD [107], but clinical study results are inconclusive (Table 4). Chachay et al. (2014) reported a negative result regarding the antisteatotic effects of RSV. In this study, a large dosage of RSV (3000 mg/day) was administered to patients with NAFLD (n = 10) compared to a placebo (n = 10). No significant improvements were observed in hepatic (AST, ALT), metabolic (FBG, HOMA-IR, insulin, TC, TGs, HDL-c, LDL-c), and antioxidant-related markers following 8 weeks of RSV intake. Moreover, levels of liver enzymes (ALT, AST) increased significantly until week 6 in the RSV-treated group. Nevertheless, RSV was well tolerated. A slight decrease in IL-6 concentration was reported, although repeated measurements at various time points did not reflect significant changes. Other inflammation markers, such as CRP or TNF-α, remained unchanged [103].

In 2015, Faghihzadeh et al. conducted a RCT involving NAFLD patients (n = 50) for 12 weeks using either 500 mg of RSV/day or a placebo, along with lifestyle modifications. ALT levels, as well as hepatic steatosis, decreased significantly in the RSV-treated patients, whereas AST and BMI decreased significantly in both groups, but there was no significant difference between them. Lipid profile and glucose metabolism markers did not differ significantly between the RSV- and placebo-supplemented patients [104].

In contrast to previous results, a consistent reduction in ALT and AST, as well as in glucose, HOMA-IR, TC, and LDL-c levels, was reported after 600 mg RSV/day supplementation (n = 30) for 3 months versus placebo (n = 30) in patients with NAFLD. Inflammation status significantly improved in the RSV-treated patients, as shown by significant changes in TNF-α and APN levels. Cytokeratin 18 M30 (CK18-M30) concentration also declined significantly after RSV intake relative to placebo [105]. However, in a longer-term RCT (2016) involving patients (n = 13) treated with high doses of RSV (1500 mg/day) for 6 months, Heebøll et al. failed to detect any significant effects in attenuating NAFLD-related clinical or histological markers compared to placebo recipients (n = 13) [106].

A lack of antisteatotic effects following RSV supplementation in NAFLD was also reported by a 2021 SRMA, despite significant improvements in inflammatory markers, such as hs-CRP and TNF-α [107].

Finally, a 2021 umbrella review of meta-analyses showed that although RSV supplementation exerts some beneficial effects on glucolipid metabolism in patients with T2D and on inflammation status in patients with NAFLD, the currently existing evidence does not recommend its use in the management of these diseases [108].

Safety. Currently, the potential deleterious effects of RSV are not well characterized due to insufficient research. High doses of RSV (2–5 g/day) may cause nausea, hypersensitivity, anal pruritus, and light or mild diarrhea. However, these adverse effects may be insignificant in the healthy state, posing an increased risk particularly for individuals with pathological conditions [109].

Summary. The effectiveness of RSV in managing T2D and MASLD has yielded controversial results, making it difficult to reach a conclusion about its therapeutic benefits. However, RSV may alleviate chronic inflammation in patients with metabolic dysfunction. More RCTs with larger samples and longer durations are needed to explain the clinical effects of RSV on glucolipid metabolism parameters.

4.4. Anthocyanins

Anthocyanins (ACNs) are a subclass of polyphenols that provide red, purple, and blue colors to fruits and vegetables. ACNs have been reported to exhibit a plethora of therapeutic benefits, including antidiabetic, anti-obesity, anticancer, anti-inflammatory, and antioxidant effects. The latter effects are attributed to the colored pigments found in blackcurrants, berries, and other blue or red fruits [110].

Clinical evidence in T2D. ACNs have been found to improve glycemic control and blood lipid profiles in patients with T2D (Table 5) [111]. In 2013, Kianbakht et al. conducted a RCT in T2D patients (n = 37) using ACNs (whortleberry fruit extract, 350 mg every 8 h for 2 months) in combination with antidiabetic medication. At the end of the study, FBG, 2 h PBG, and HbA_{1c} levels significantly decreased in the ACN-treated patients. In addition to ACNs, whortleberry also contains myricetin and chlorogenic acid, which may potentiate its antihyperglycemic effects [112].

Table 5. Summary of RCTs investigating the hypoglycemic, hypolipidemic, and anti-steatosis effects of ACNs.

Disease	Participants (Total)	Intervention	Control	Duration	Main Outcomes */**	References
T2D	n = 37	ACNs 350 mg every 8 h	Placebo	2 months	↓ FBG, 2h-PBG, HbA_{1c} *	[112]
T2D	n = 58	ACNs 320 mg/day	Placebo	24 weeks	↓ FBG, HOMA-IR, TGs, LDL-c *, ↑ HDL-c, APN *	[113]
Prediabetes/T2D	n = 138	ACNs 320 mg/day	Placebo	12 weeks	↓ FBG, ↑ APN * (only in TD2)	[114]
T2D	n = 52	22 g freeze-dried blueberries	Placebo	8 weeks	↓ HbA_{1c}, TGs, AST, ALT *	[115]
T2D	n = 20	1.4 g bilberry extract/day	Placebo	4 weeks	No significant changes	[116]
Prediabetes/T2D	n = 40	ACNs 320 mg/day	-	4 weeks	↓ IL-6, TNF-α *	[117]
NAFLD	n = 36	HS extract 2700 mg/day	Placebo	12 weeks	↓ WC, WHR, BF, FFA *	[118]
NAFLD	n = 74	ACNs 320 mg/day	Placebo	12 weeks	↓ ALT, CK18-M30, MPD *	[119]
NAFLD	n = 40	CMFE 20 mL/day	Placebo	12 weeks	No significant changes	[120]
MAFLD	n = 108	CMFP 30 g/day + diet	Diet	8 weeks	↓ AST, ALT, GGT, FBG, HbA_{1c}, HOMA-IR, TC, TGs, LDL-c, BW, BF, WC, CRP **	[121]

* Statistically significant between groups ($p < 0.05$); ** Statistically significant from baseline ($p < 0.05$); "↓", decreased; "↑", increased. Abbreviations: ACNs, anthocyanins; ALT, alanine aminotransferase; APN, adiponectin; AST, aspartate aminotransferase; BF, body fat; BW, body weight; CMFE, *Cornus mas* L. fruit extract; CMFP, *Cornus mas* L. fruit powder; CK18-M30, cytokeratin 18 M30; CRP, C-reactive protein; FFA, free fatty acids; FBG, fasting blood glucose; HbA_{1c}, glycosylated hemoglobin; GGT, gamma-glutamyl transpeptidase; HDL-c, high-density lipoprotein cholesterol; HOMA-IR, homeostatic model assessment of insulin resistance; HS, *Hibiscus sabdariffa*; IL-6, interleukin-6; LDL-c, low-density lipoprotein cholesterol; MPD, myeloperoxidase; 2-h PBG, 2-h postprandial blood glucose; TC, total cholesterol; TGs, triglycerides; TNF-α, tumor necrosis factor; WC, waist circumference; WHR, waist-to-hip ratio.

Positive effects following pure ACNs supplementation (160 mg twice daily for 24 weeks) were also reported in T2D patients (n = 29) by Li et al. (2015). Compared to placebo (n = 29), ACNs-treated patients experienced lowered FBG, HOMA-IR, TGs, LDL-c, apolipoprotein (apo) B-48, and apo C III levels, as well as increased HDL-c and APN concentrations [113]. Also, purified ACNs supplements administered for 12 weeks were shown to be effective in reducing FBG and serum APN levels relative to placebo in patients with newly diagnosed T2D (n = 62), but not in those with prediabetes (n = 76) [114].

In 2020, Stote et al. conducted an RCT using either 22 g of freeze-dried blueberries or a placebo in 52 patients with T2D. In agreement with previous trials, cardiometabolic parameters, including HbA_{1c}, TGs, AST, and ALT, were significantly lower in the experimental group (n = 26), but no significant changes between groups were observed regarding FBG, serum insulin, body weight, LDL-c, HDL-c, and CRP levels [115].

As opposed to the findings mentioned so far, short-term bilberry extract supplementation was not found to be associated with significant improvements in glycemic control, lipid profile, or antioxidant and anti-inflammatory markers in patients with T2D. As such, Chan et al. (2021) reported that the administration of 1.4 g/day of bilberry extract for two 4-week periods did not significantly alleviate cardiometabolic markers (FBG, HbA_{1c}, lipid profile, CRP) in ACNs-treated patients compared to placebo recipients [116].

An open-label RCT investigated the effects of a daily intake of 320 mg of ACNs over the course of 4 weeks in T2D patients (n = 12), individuals with prediabetes (n = 14), and healthy individuals (n = 14). Compared to healthy individuals, patients with T2D experienced significant improvements in IL-6 and TNF-α levels. However, the trial did not employ a placebo, and the T2D participants followed an anti-inflammatory diet, which might have enhanced the effects of ACNs [117].

A 2023 SRMA by Mao et al. involving patients with T2D analyzed 13 RCTs (n = 703) and concluded that an average intake of 320 mg of ACNs, either from fruit extracts or pure supplements, over approximately 8 weeks led to significant reductions in FBG, 2 h PBG, HbA_{1c}, TG, and LDL-c levels. Nevertheless, no significant effects were observed regarding HOMA-IR, FI, TC, HDL-c, or blood pressure levels in patients with T2D. Notably, compared to pure supplements, ACNs derived from fruit extracts or powders exhibited a more pronounced effect on HbA_{1c} levels [111].

Clinical evidence in MASLD. Several RCTs (Table 5) demonstrated a significant reduction in liver enzyme levels following ACNs intake in patients with NAFLD [119]; however, other human studies found no beneficial effects of ACNs on these parameters [120]. Chang et al. reported in 2014 that *Hibiscus sabdariffa* extract consumption for 12 weeks had some beneficial effects on liver steatosis, mainly through improvements in anthropometric indices and free fatty acid levels. The latter decreased significantly in the intervention group compared to the placebo at the end of the follow-up period. The fatty liver score improved in both groups but did not differ significantly between HSE- and placebo-treated patients after 12 weeks. Also, no significant changes between groups were observed regarding ALT and AST levels, glucose concentration, or lipid profile [118].

In 2015, Zhang et al. showed that compared to a placebo, purified ACN intake (320 mg/day for 12 weeks) led to a significant reduction in plasma ALT concentration and 2 h glucose loading test levels in patients with NAFLD. Improvements in FBG, HOMA-IR, TGs, and HDL-c were also shown, but mean percentage changes were not significantly different from controls. ACN supplementation did not affect AST, FBG, plasma insulin, TC, and LDL-c levels or anthropometric indices. However, the ACN-treated patients exhibited significant decreases in cytokeratin-18 M30 fragment (CK18-M30) levels, which is a predictor of NAFLD progression, and myeloperoxidase concentration, which is an inflammation- and oxidative stress-related enzyme, as well as a tendency toward improvement in the NAFLD fibrosis score [119].

Sangsefidi et al. (2021) tested the effects of *Cornus mas* L. fruit extract (20 mL daily for 12 weeks) on several NAFLD-related markers. The authors failed to detect any significant differences within or between the intervention group (n = 22) and the placebo controls (n = 18) regarding ALT and AST levels or steatosis scores. Despite a significant decrease in CK18-M30 concentration in the ACN-supplemented NAFLD patients, no significant difference between groups was found at the end of the study period [120].

Another RCT (2024) involving 87 patients with metabolic dysfunction-associated fatty liver disease (MAFLD) reported that lyophilized *Cornus mas* L. fruit powder (CMFP), with/without diet therapy, led to statistically significant decreases in liver enzyme levels glycemic indices, lipid profile and anthropometric variables from baseline to the end of the study period. CRP levels also decreased significantly at the end of the follow-up period (8 weeks) in the groups treated with CMFP and diet therapy, and only diet therapy. Notably, no significant differences in anthropometric, biochemical, and inflammatory parameters were reported at the end of the study between the CMFP with diet therapy group and the diet therapy alone group [121].

Finally, Khan et al. concluded in their 2024 SRMA that there is currently no evidence that ACN supplementation could significantly improve liver function in patients with NAFLD [122]. These results are in line with another 2024 SRMA, which found no significant effects on liver function following supplementation with *Cornus mas* L. in individuals at high risk [123].

Safety. So far, no adverse effects associated with ACNs consumption have been reported. In various human studies, most subjects tolerated a dosage of 160 mg of ACNs extract administered twice daily for 2 months. Only 4% of participants experienced side effects, which consisted of eczema and gastrointestinal distress [124].

Summary. RCTs investigating the effects of ACNs supplementation on cardiometabolic risk factors in patients with T2D or MASLD are scarce. While ACNs may play a role in the management of T2D via improvements in glycemic indices, lipid profiles, or chronic inflammation, there is a lack of evidence regarding the extension of these effects to patients with MASLD.

4.5. Catechins

Catechins are a type of natural phenolic compound found in high concentrations, particularly in green tea, but also in black and oolong tea. The main catechins in green tea extracts include epigallocatechin gallate (EGCG), epigallocatechin, epicatechin gallate, and epicatechin. Among these, EGCG is the most abundant catechin (50–80%) [125] and is often studied due to its antioxidant, anti-inflammatory, antimutagenic [126], and cardioprotective properties [125].

Clinical evidence in T2D. Research outcomes regarding catechins' ability to improve glycemic control and blood lipid levels are heterogeneous (Table 6). In 2009, green tea enriched with either 582.8 mg of catechins (experimental group, n = 23) or 96.3 mg of catechins/day (control group, n = 20) was administered to patients with T2D. After 12 weeks, a significant decrease in HbA_{1c} levels was observed in the catechin group patients receiving insulinotropic agents compared to controls. Also, in these patients (approximately 77%), insulin levels significantly increased at the end of the study period, suggesting catechins' capacity to stimulate insulin secretion. The catechin-rich beverage intake led to a decrease in abdominal obesity, as evidenced by a significantly lower WC in patients assigned to the intervention group after 12 weeks. Similarly, APN levels increased significantly in the intervention group from baseline to the end of the study, although there was no significant difference between groups [127].

Human RCTs have not always demonstrated the benefits of catechin supplementation in the management of glycemic control and lipid profiles. A double-blind, placebo-controlled trial (2011) reported that in T2D patients with obesity, a daily dose of decaffeinated green tea (GTE) extract (856 mg EGCG) for 16 weeks led to no statistically significant improvement between groups in markers of glucolipid metabolism. However, a significant within-group reduction of 0.4% in HbA_{1c} level was observed in supplemented patients at the end of the follow-up period. GTE-treated patients also experienced a significant decrease in HOMA-IR and WC [128].

In a 2013 2-month trial, patients with T2D (n = 63) were randomly assigned to three groups with daily intakes of green tea as follows: four cups (n = 24), two cups (n = 25), and a control group (n = 14). Except for BW, BMI and WC, which significantly decreased in the four cups of green tea group, no significant changes in glucolipid or oxidative stress parameters were detected in the other two groups or between groups [129].

In 2014, Liu et al. performed an RCT involving 92 patients with T2D and lipid disturbances, who received either 500 mg of GTE three times daily (n = 39) or a placebo (n = 38) for 16 weeks. GTE consumption significantly decreased TG and HOMA-IR levels while increasing HDL-c concentration at the end of the intervention. APN increased pronouncedly in both groups, without showing a statistically significant difference between them. In addition, between-group comparisons only revealed a decreasing tendency for TG levels, with no statistically significant differences after 16 weeks of GTE versus the placebo [125].

In a double-blind, placebo-controlled RCT (2020), 44 patients with T2D were supplemented with either two tablets of EGCG (n = 25) or a placebo for 2 months. A significant reduction in the mean levels of TC and TGs was observed in the EGCG-treated patients. Also, compared to the placebo group, the mean changes in TC and total antioxidant capacity were significantly different in the intervention group. No other statistically significant differences were found in the lipid profile between the two groups. IL-6 levels remained unchanged [130].

In 2023, an RCT was performed involving patients with T2D and nephropathy to investigate the effects of green tea infusion on metabolic parameters. Patients were randomly divided into three groups: one receiving three cups of green tea/day (n = 22), another receiving two cups of green tea/day (n = 22), and a control group (n = 20). Results showed that, compared to the control group, patients consuming three cups of green tea daily presented significant improvements in HbA_{1c}, TC, and HDL-c levels after 12 weeks [131].

Finally, an SRMA performed by Asbaghi et al. (2020) involving 14 RCTs concluded that green tea supplementation exerted no effects on FBG, FI, HbA_{1c}, and HOMA-IR in patients with T2D. Study participants were supplemented with green tea, GTE, or EGCG in doses ranging from 300 to 10,000 mg/daily for 8–16 weeks. However, subgroup analysis indicated that green tea intake for more than 8 weeks significantly decreased FBG, while supplementation for 8 weeks or less led to a significant decrease in HbA_{1c}. An improved glycemic response after green tea intake was reported exclusively by RCTs performed in Asia, while those conducted on other populations did not show significant outcomes. Inter-ethnic differences may be explained by a genetic polymorphism responsible for a slower metabolism of green tea among Asian individuals, which enhances its glucose-lowering effect [132].

Clinical evidence in MASLD. In a 2013 randomized double-blind study, green tea rich in catechins (700 mL/day containing > 1 g catechins), green tea low in catechins, or a placebo were administered to patients with NAFLD (n = 17). After 12 weeks, ALT levels and body fat percentage (BF%) significantly decreased in the green tea rich in catechins group compared to the other two groups. Also, HFC was significantly improved in the green tea rich in catechins group compared with the low-density catechin and placebo groups, as indicated by the liver-to-spleen attenuation ratio [133].

Table 6. Summary of RCTs investigating the hypoglycemic, hypolipidemic, and anti-steatosis effects of catechins.

Disease	Participants (Total)	Intervention	Control	Duration	Main Outcomes */**	References
T2D	n = 43	Catechins 582.8 mg/day	Catechins 96.3 mg/day	12 weeks	↓ HbA_{1c}, WC, ↑ insulin *	[127]
T2D	n = 68	GTE 1500 mg/day	Placebo	16 weeks	↓ HbA_{1c}, HOMA-IR, WC **	[128]
T2D	n = 63	Green tea 2 or 4 cups/day	No green tea	2 months	↓ BMI, BW, WC **	[129]
T2D	n = 92	GTE 1500 mg/day	Placebo	16 weeks	↓ HOMA-IR, TGs, ↑ HDL-c, APN **	[125]
T2D	n = 44	EGCG 300 mg/day	Placebo	2 months	↓ TC, ↑ TAC *	[130]
T2D	n = 64	Green tea 3 or 2 cups/day	No green tea	12 weeks	↓ HbA_{1c}, TC, ↑ HDL-c *	[131]
NAFLD	n = 17	High-density catechins- green tea	Placebo	12 weeks	↓ BF, ALT, HFC *	[133]
NAFLD	n = 71	GTE 500 mg/day	Placebo	90 days	↓ BW, BMI, ALP *	[134]
NAFLD	n = 45	GTE 550 mg/day + diet	Placebo	3 months	↓ BW, AST, FBG *	[135]
NAFLD	n = 80	GTE 1000 mg/day	Placebo	12 weeks	↓ BW, BMI, ALT, AST, TC, TGs, LDL-c, HDL-c, HOMA-IR, hs-CRP, APN *	[136]

* Statistically significant between groups ($p < 0.05$); ** Statistically significant from baseline ($p < 0.05$); "↓", decreased; "↑", increased. Abbreviations: ALT, alanine aminotransferase; ALP, alkaline phosphatase; APN, adiponectin; AST, aspartate aminotransferase; BMI, body mass index; BF, body fat; BW, body weight; FBG, fasting blood glucose; GTE, green tea extract; HbA_{1c}, glycosylated hemoglobin; HDL-c, high-density lipoprotein cholesterol; HFC, hepatic fat content; HOMA-IR, homeostatic model assessment of insulin resistance; hs-CRP, high-sensitivity C-reactive protein; LDL-c, low-density lipoprotein cholesterol; TAC, total antioxidant capacity; TC, total cholesterol; TGs, triglycerides; WC, waist circumference.

Later, in 2016, Pezeshki et al. demonstrated that GTE (500 mg/day for 12 weeks) led to significant improvements in ALT, AST, and ALP levels in patients with NAFLD (n = 35). In the placebo group (n = 36), ALT and AST also declined, but to a lesser extent, while ALP showed a significant reduction at the end of the study. Notably, BW decreased significantly in both groups after 90 days, but the mean weight change was significantly greater in the GTE group compared to the placebo group [134].

Similarly, following 550 mg GTE intake and diet therapy for 3 months, patients with NAFLD (n = 21) experienced significant improvements in BMI, AST, and FBG levels, as well as in BW, compared to placebo recipients (n = 24). However, no significant differences between groups were observed regarding ALT and HOMA-IR levels [135].

Compared to placebo (n = 40), GTE administration (1000 mg/day for 12 weeks) to patients with NAFLD and DLD (n = 40) was found to be effective in improving BW, BMI, ALT, AST, TC, TGs, LDL-c, HDL-c, and HOMA-IR. Also, GTE significantly improved inflammatory markers, specifically hs-CRP and APN, and fatty liver grading [136].

A 2020 SRMA including 15 RCTs reported that although the overall effect of green tea on liver enzymes was not significant, the subgroup analysis revealed that it may decrease liver enzyme levels in NAFLD patients. However, in healthy subjects, a modest but significant increase in hepatic enzyme concentration was observed [137].

Safety. Green tea intake raises liver-related safety concerns due to the potential risk of hepatotoxicity [138]. According to the European Food Safety Authority (EFSA), the intake of doses equal to or above 800 mg EGCG/day as a food supplement may cause a significant increase in serum transaminase levels [139]. A 2016 SRMA concluded that liver-related adverse effects after green tea extract intake are expected to be rare [138].

Summary. Green tea exerts important anti-inflammatory and antioxidant effects that may benefit patients with T2D and MASLD. Nevertheless, the evidence regarding the effectiveness of green tea in improving glycemic control and liver steatosis is not conclusive.

4.6. Other Phenolic Compounds and Carotenoids

Intake of dietary phenols and carotenoids derived from artichokes, tomatoes, and citrus fruits has been shown to exert various biological effects, particularly hypoglycemic [140–142], hypolipidemic [141], and hepatoprotective [143] effects.

Artichoke (*Cynara cardunculus* var. *scolymus* L.) has long been used as an herbal remedy with powerful therapeutic properties. Artichoke leaf extract (ALE) mainly consists of phenolic acids, sesquiterpene lactones, and flavonoids [140]. Lycopene (LYC), a lipophilic carotenoid, is found naturally in red-colored fruits such as tomatoes, red grapefruit, and watermelon. LYC's antioxidant capacity is twice as effective as that of ß-carotene and 100 times more efficient than that of α-tocopherol [142]. Citrus flavonoids (hesperidin) are abundant in phenolic compounds with enhanced antioxidant activity that can improve glucolipid parameters [144].

Clinical evidence in T2D. There are limited published data linking artichoke or ALE to glycemic control (Table 7). In 2012, Fallah Huseini et al. performed an RCT involving 72 patients with T2D who were supplemented with either free-fiber ALE (1200 mg/day) (n = 36) or a placebo (n = 36) for 2 months, along with their standard anti-T2D medication. ALE was found to be efficient in alleviating certain lipid profile markers (TC, LDL-c) compared to placebo, but did not lead to significant changes in glycemic parameters (FBG, 2 h PBG, HbA_{1c}), liver enzymes (ALT, AST), or other lipids. The authors suggested that dietary fibers may be responsible for improving glycemic control in patients with T2D [145].

Table 7. Summary of RCTs investigating the hypoglycemic, hypolipidemic, and anti-steatosis effects of phenolic compounds and carotenoids.

Disease	Participants (Total)	Intervention	Control	Duration	Main Outcomes */**	References
T2D	n = 72	ALE 1200 mg/day	Placebo	2 months	↓ TC, LDL-c *	[145]
MS	n = 68	ALE 1800 mg/day	Placebo	12 weeks	↓ TGs *	[140]
T2D	n = 52	Tomato juice 500 mL/day	Placebo	4 weeks	↑ resistance to LDL oxidation **	[146]
T2D	n = 64	HES 500 mg/day	Placebo	6 weeks	↓ TNF-α, IL-6, hs-CRP *	[147]
MS	n = 49	HES 1000 mg/day + LSI	Placebo	12 weeks	↓ FBG, TGs, TNF-α *	[148]
NASH	n = 60	AE 2700 mg/day	Placebo	2 months	↓ ALT, AST, TC, TGs *	[149]
NAFLD	n = 90	ALE 600 mg/daily	Placebo	2 months	↓ ALT, AST, TC, TGs, LDL-c, HDL-c *	[143]
T2D/ NAFLD	n = 80	Cyc + BPF 300 mg/day	Placebo	16 weeks	↓ ALT, AST, GGT, ALP, TNF-α *	[150]
NAFLD	n = 49	HES 1 g/day + LSI	Placebo	12 weeks	↓ ALT, GGT, TC, TGs, hs-CRP, TNF-α *	[151]
NAFLD	n = 92	HES 1 g/day + LSI Flaxseeds 30 g/day + LSI HES + flaxseeds + LSI	LSI	12 weeks	↓ FBG, HOMA-IR, ALT, FLI *	[152]

* Statistically significant between groups ($p < 0.05$); ** Statistically significant from baseline ($p < 0.05$); "↓", decreased; "↑", increased. Abbreviations: ALE, artichoke leaf extract; ALT, alanine aminotransferase; ALP, alkaline phosphatase; AST, aspartate aminotransferase; BPF, bergamot phenolic fraction; Cyc, *Cynara cardunculus*; FLI, fatty liver index; FBG, fasting blood glucose; GGT, gamma-glutamyl transpeptidase; HES, hesperidin; HDL-c, high-density lipoprotein cholesterol; HOMA-IR, homeostatic model assessment of insulin resistance; hs-CRP, high-sensitivity C-reactive protein; IL-6, interleukin-6; LDL-c, low-density lipoprotein cholesterol; LSI, lifestyle intervention; TC, total cholesterol; TGs, triglycerides; TNF-α, tumor necrosis factor α.

More recently, Ebrahimi-Mameghani et al. also failed to detect significant differences in glucolipid parameters (FBG, HOMA-IR, TC, LDL-c, HDL-c), except for TGs, following ALE supplementation (1800 mg/day for 12 weeks) compared to a placebo in patients with MS. However, ALE led to a significant decline in HOMA-IR and insulin levels in a subgroup of patients with MS and TCF7L2 polymorphism (n = 10). The latter is associated with an increased risk of developing T2D and could explain the variation in metabolic benefits of ALE among different subjects [140].

In a 2000 RCT, 52 patients with well-controlled T2D who supplemented with placebo for 4 weeks were randomly assigned to receive tomato juice (n = 15), vitamin E (n = 12), vitamin C (n = 12), or placebo (n = 15) for another 4 weeks. Results showed that levels of LYC increased significantly (almost three-fold) following supplementation with tomato juice. Also, these patients exhibited an increased resistance to LDL oxidation (~42%), similar to that observed in the vitamin E-treated patients (54%). However, plasma CRP levels remained unchanged after tomato juice supplementation, while they declined significantly among patients receiving vitamin E. No significant changes were reported regarding BMI, FBG, and TC levels after tomato juice consumption [146].

However, Homayouni et al. (2018) demonstrated that 500 mg/day HES supplementation is effective in improving the inflammation status of patients with T2D. As such, oral HES intake led to significant changes in the mean percent changes of TNF-α, IL-6, and hs-CRP levels in patients with T2D (n = 32) compared to placebo recipients (n = 32) after 6 weeks [147].

In a 2020 RCT, 49 patients with MS were randomly assigned to receive either HES (1000 mg/day) or a placebo, along with lifestyle modifications. After 12 weeks, changes in lifestyle led to a significant reduction in BW in both groups. In addition, FBG, TG, and TNF-α levels decreased significantly in the HES group (n = 24) compared to the placebo group (n = 25). Compared to baseline, hs-CRP, glucose, insulin, TC, LDL, and TG concentrations declined significantly after HES supplementation [148].

Finally, a group-specific meta-analysis involving 152 patients with T2D (2022) showed that LYC supplementation is effective in improving FBG [142]. However, a 2019 SRMA that included six RCTs (n = 318) investigating the effect of HES supplementation on glycemic control failed to detect any significant improvement in glycemic indices [FBG, HbA_{1c}, HOMA-IR, quantitative insulin sensitivity check index (QUICKI), or insulin] in healthy overweight individuals or subjects with either prediabetes or T2D [153].

Clinical evidence in MASLD. Phenolic compounds have also demonstrated therapeutic potential in individuals with MASLD/MASH (Table 7). In 2016, 60 patients with NASH were enrolled in an RCT to receive either *Cynara scolymus* extract (2700 mg/day) or a placebo for 2 months. Compared to the placebo, significant improvements in ALT, AST, TC, and TG levels were reported at the end of the study [149].

Panahi et al. (2018) showed that, compared to placebo (n = 41), supplementation with ALE in patients with NAFLD (n = 49) led to a significant reduction in serum ALT and AST, as well as improvements in the ALT/AST ratio, portal vein diameter, hepatic vein flow, and liver size. Also, between-group comparisons revealed that ALE-treated individuals experienced significantly lower levels of TC, LDL-c, TGs, and HDL-c. Notably, ALE supplementation had no significant effect on glycemic control (FBG, HbA_{1c}, insulin) [143].

Cynara cardunculus (Cyc) has also been found to exert anti-steatosis effects, particularly in combination with bergamot phenolic fraction (BPF). The beneficial influence of bergamot polyphenol extract against NAFLD was demonstrated in a previous in vitro study [154]. In a 2020 RCT, 80 patients with T2D and NAFLD were randomly allocated into four groups to receive Cyc—300 mg/day (n = 20); BPF—300 mg/day (n = 20); Cyc plus BPF (50/50%)—300 mg/day (n = 20); or a placebo (n = 20). Supplementation with both Cyc and BPF resulted in improvements in liver imaging profiles and several markers of liver fibrosis in NAFLD associated with T2D. Also, compared to placebo, Cyc + BPF significantly decreased serum concentrations of ALT, AST, GGT, ALP, and TNF-α, as well as markedly improved several markers of oxidative stress, such as GSH-Px, SOD, and MDA [150].

In addition, a 2021 SRMA that included eight RCTs concluded that artichoke supplementation significantly reduced liver enzyme levels compared to placebo, particularly in individuals with NAFLD. The doses of artichoke ranged from 100 to 2700 mg/day, whereas the study duration varied from 4 to 12 weeks [155].

The hepatoprotective effect of HES was investigated in a 2019 RCT involving 49 NAFLD patients who received either HES (1 g/day) (n = 24) or a placebo (n = 25) for 12 weeks. All participants were instructed to follow lifestyle changes during the study duration. At the end of the study, reductions in ALT, GGT, TC, TGs, hs-CRP, TNF-α, and the steatosis score were significantly improved in the HES-treated group compared to the placebo group. FBG decreased significantly in the interventional group, but this change was not significantly different from that in the placebo group. HES supplementation alongside lifestyle adjustments has proven superior to lifestyle changes alone in alleviating NAFLD [151].

In line with these results, Yari et al. demonstrated in a 2020 open-label RCT that HES in combination with flaxseeds ameliorates hepatic steatosis, glucolipid metabolism, and inflammation in patients with NAFLD. Study participants were divided into four groups, with three groups receiving either HES (1 g daily) (n = 22), flaxseeds (30 g daily) (n = 24), or HES in combination with flaxseeds (1 g HES and 30 g flaxseeds daily) (n = 25), and one group receiving no supplementation (n = 21). All participants were given lifestyle recommendations. Liver steatosis declined significantly in all groups at the end of the study, with no difference in the mean reduction of the controlled attenuation parameter score (CAP). Liver fibrosis decreased significantly among flaxseed-supplemented patients, with or without HES. Lifestyle modifications and dietary supplements were more effective in reducing HFC than LSI alone, as evidenced by significant differences in the fatty liver score. ALT and GGT levels reduced significantly in all groups, but not in the control group. The lipid profile (TC, TGs, and LDL-c) improved significantly in all intervention groups compared to baseline, while glycemic control (FBG, HOMA-IR, insulin) was significantly ameliorated in the flaxseed groups, with or without HES, compared to the control group. Finally, hs-CRP and TNF-α decreased significantly within the HES groups, alone or in combination with flaxseeds, after 12 weeks [152].

Safety. When used in recommended amounts or as a standardized extract, ALE is well tolerated with minimal side effects. Moderate transient mild effects, such as increased flatulence, were reported by 1 out of 100 participants in a study investigating its safety [156]. LYC, consumed either through supplements or diet, has also been shown to be safe and well tolerated at different concentrations [157]. Finally, HES is considered a generally safe NBC, even when administered at very high doses, but more research is needed to evaluate its safety in clinical settings [158].

Summary. Currently, there is limited clinical evidence supporting the therapeutic role of ALE, LYC, and HES in patients with T2D. More large-scale, well-designed RCTs are needed to validate their clinical effectiveness, particularly for LYC, where a significant shortage of RCTs exists. The addition of dietary fibers to phenolic compounds may enhance their hypoglycemic effects observed in both T2D and MASLD. ALE may also help mitigate liver steatosis, inflammation, and oxidative stress.

4.7. Silymarin

Milk thistle fruits contain a blend of four major flavonolignans collectively referred to as silymarin (SLM) [159], with silybin (or silibinin) as the primary component [160]. SLM has been shown to possess a wide range of biological activities, encompassing antioxidant, anti-inflammatory, lipid-lowering, antitumor, immunomodulating [159], anti-fibrotic, antidiabetic, choleretic, and liver-regenerating properties [160].

Clinical evidence in T2D. Currently, only a few RCTs are available involving individuals with T2D, most of which show that SLM, in combination with standard treatment or aerobic training, improved glucolipid metabolism parameters (Table 8). Huseini et al. (2006) conducted an RCT with 51 patients aged between 40 and 65 years who had a history of T2D for more than 2 years. Patients assigned to the experimental group (n = 25) received 200 mg SLM three times daily, in addition to standard treatment, for 4 months. The results showed that SLM intake, compared to both baseline and placebo, led to significant reductions in FBG, HbA_{1c}, TC, TGs, LDL-c, ALT, and AST levels [161].

Ebrahimpour-Koujan et al. investigated the effects of SLM extract supplements in 40 subjects with T2D in 2015 and again in 2018. In both triple-blinded RCTs, patients with T2D received either 140 mg of SLM thrice daily (n = 20) or a placebo (n = 20) for 45 days. The results of the first study showed that SLM supplementation led to a significant decrease in anti-inflammatory and oxidative stress markers. Specifically, hs-CRP significantly decreased, while GPX and SOD activity, as well as TAC, significantly increased in the SLM-supplemented patients compared to the placebo group. MDA declined significantly compared to baseline following SLM consumption [162].

The second RCT revealed that compared to placebo, SLM significantly improved FBG, serum insulin, HOMA-IR, TGs, HDL-c, and QUICKI levels. Also, in the experimental group, a significant decrease from baseline was observed in TC and LDL-c levels [163].

Table 8. Summary of RCTs investigating the hypoglycemic, hypolipidemic, and anti-steatosis effects of SLM.

Disease	Participants (Total)	Intervention	Control	Duration	Main Outcomes */**	References
T2D	n = 51	SLM 600 mg/day	Placebo	4 months	↓ FBG, HbA_{1c}, TC, TGs, LDL-c, ALT, AST *	[161]
T2D	n = 40	SLM 420 mg/day	Placebo	45 days	↓ hs-CRP, ↑ GPx, SOD, TAC *	[162]
T2D	n = 40	SLM 420 mg/day	Placebo	45 days	↓ FBG, SI, HOMA-IR, TGs, ↑ QUICKI, HDL-c *	[163]
T2D	n = 60	SLM 140 mg/kg/day SLM + AT AT	Placebo	8 weeks	↓ FBG, SI, HOMA-IR, ALT, AST, ALP *	[164]
T2D	n = 48	SLM 420 mg/day + diet	Diet	12 weeks	no changes	[165]
NAFLD	n = 36	SLM 1080.6 mg/day + Vitamin E 36 mg/day + LSI	LSI	3 months	↓ GGT, BW, WC **	[166]
NAFLD	n = 150	SLM 140 mg/day Metformin 500 mg/day Pioglitazone 15 mg/day Vitamin E 400 UI/day	Placebo + LSI	3 months	↓ ALT, AST, TGs, LDL-c **	[167]
NASH	n = 99	SLM 2100 mg/day + LSI	Placebo + LSI	48 weeks	↓ TGs *	[168]
MASLD	n = 83	SLM 103.2 mg/day	Placebo	24 weeks	↓ GGT, LSM, ApoB *	[169]

* Statistically significant between groups ($p < 0.05$); ** Statistically significant from baseline ($p < 0.05$); "↓", decreased; "↑", increased. Abbreviations: ALT, alanine aminotransferase; ALP, alkaline phosphatase; ApoB, apolipoprotein B; AST, aspartate aminotransferase; AT, aerobic training; BW, body weight; FBG, fasting blood glucose; GGT, gamma-glutamyl transpeptidase; GPx, glutathione peroxidase; HDL-c, high-density lipoprotein cholesterol; HbA_{1c}, glycosylated hemoglobin; HOMA-IR, homeostatic model assessment of insulin resistance; hs-CRP, high-sensitivity C-reactive protein; LDL-c, low-density lipoprotein cholesterol; LSI, lifestyle intervention; LSM, liver stiffness measurement; QUICKI, quantitative insulin sensitivity check index; SI, serum insulin; SLM, silymarin; SOD, superoxide dismutase; TC, total cholesterol; TAC, total antioxidant capacity; TGs, triglycerides; WC, waist circumference.

In 2020, Ghalandari et al. performed a RCT involving 60 men with T2D, who were randomly assigned to four groups: one receiving 140 mg/kg SLM daily, one receiving 140 mg/kg SLM daily plus aerobic training (AT), one receiving AT plus a placebo, and one receiving a placebo. The AT protocol included three training sessions per week, with a duration of 20–45 min at an intensity of 60–80% of the heart rate reserve. Results showed that FBG, insulin, and HOMA-IR levels were significantly reduced at the end of the study in all intervention groups, except the control group. SLM and AT were significantly more effective in reducing FBG levels than SLM alone. AST, ALT, and ALP levels declined significantly in all three experimental groups compared to baseline and the control group. The reduction of AST was significantly lower in the SLM plus AT group compared to the SLM group. BW and weight-to-hip ratio (WHR) decreased significantly compared to baseline in the SLM plus AT and AT groups. [164].

In contrast to these results, a 2024 open-label RCT conducted by Ferdowsi et al. involving 48 patients with T2D indicated that the intake of 140 mg SLM (three capsules daily) plus diet for 12 weeks failed to significantly decrease the levels of FBG, HbA_{1c}, and blood lipid markers. The comparison intervention was diet [165].

Clinical evidence in MASLD. SLM has traditionally been used for its potential to alleviate liver diseases. However, RCTs investigating its efficacy in NAFLD management are scarce and have yielded inconclusive results, especially when SLM is used as monotherapy [169]

(Table 8). Aller et al. (2015) investigated the effects of SLM in combination with vitamin E (n = 36) and lifestyle modification on glucolipid metabolism markers, liver enzyme levels, several noninvasive NAFLD parameters, and anthropometric indices before and after the intervention. The results showed that, after the intervention, glucose, HOMA-IR, and ALT levels declined significantly compared to baseline only in the control group. However, a significant decrease in GGT level was observed in both groups. No changes were reported in the levels of TGs. Both groups experienced significantly improved liver function tests (FLI and noninvasive NAFLD index) and anthropometric measurements (BW, WC). Notably, patients in the intervention group who failed to lose 5% of BW still exhibited decreased GGT levels and improvements in liver function, while patients in the control group who did not lose 5% of their weight displayed no changes in metabolic status [166].

In agreement with these results, in another RCT (2019), 150 patients with NAFLD were assigned to five groups: SLM 140 mg/day (n = 30), metformin 500 mg/day (n = 30), pioglitazone 15 mg/day (n = 30), vitamin E 400 IU/day (n = 30), and lifestyle plus a placebo (n = 30). All patients were given lifestyle advice during the study duration. ALT, AST, TGs, and LDL-c declined significantly in all treatment groups. Also, significant improvements in FBG, TC, BMI, and WC were reported in all groups after 3 months. Between-group comparisons revealed that ALT and AST improved significantly in the pioglitazone, metformin, and SLM groups compared to the other two groups, while TC decreased significantly in the placebo and vitamin E groups compared to the other three groups [167].

However, in a 2017 RCT involving 99 patients with NASH, which is a more severe form of NAFLD, an SLM intake of 700 mg three times daily for 48 weeks (n = 49) did not achieve a significant reduction in the NAS score (the sum of scores for steatosis, lobular inflammation, and ballooning) compared to the placebo (n = 50). However, there was a significant reduction in liver fibrosis in the SLM-treated group compared to the placebo. Also, a significantly greater percentage of individuals in the interventional group experienced improvements in liver fibrosis and stiffness compared to placebo recipients. Within-group comparisons showed that SLM-treated patients displayed a significant decline in ALT, AST, GGT, HbA_{1c}, and TGs. Except for TGs, other parameters did not change significantly in the interventional group compared to placebo. HDL-c concentration also increased significantly in the SLM group, whereas a significant reduction in ALT levels was reported in the placebo controls [168].

In a 2024 RCT, Jin et al. demonstrated that, compared to placebo (n = 41), SLM supplementation (103.2 mg/day) significantly decreased liver fibrosis (assessed by liver stiffness measurement), GGT, and ApoB levels, but it had no significant effect on liver steatosis (as measured by CAP), fibrosis index, aminotransferases, glucolipid parameters, anthropometric indices, hs-CRP, and SOD levels in patients with MASLD (n = 42) [169].

Finally, a meta-analysis involving six RCTs concluded that although SLM supplementation significantly reduced the levels of AST and ALT in NAFLD patients, the results were clinically irrelevant. No significant change in GGT levels was observed following SLM supplementation [170].

Safety. SLM utilization has proven to be generally safe and well tolerated, with minimal adverse effects in both T2D [171] and MASLD/MASH [170].

Summary. The effect of SLM supplementation in patients with T2D remains inconclusive, although it appears to improve glycemic parameters. SLM seems effective in decreasing liver enzyme levels in MASLD, but these findings warrant cautious interpretation, particularly in clinical practice.

4.8. Cinnamon

Cinnamon (CNM) has long been a popular spice, with four of the 250 species belonging to the genus Cinnamomum used for this purpose. CNM is available in many forms, such as sticks (bark), pulverized stick powder, and extracts derived from the powder, each with a different phytochemical composition and bioavailability. Currently, it is not clear which bioactive compounds are responsible for CNM's biological effects, making standardized formulation difficult to develop [172]. It has been shown that CNM has hypoglycemic, hypolipidemic, anti-inflammatory, antioxidant, and antihypertensive properties [173].

Clinical evidence in T2D. Oral supplementation of CNM supplements has been suggested to be effective in improving glycemic control and lipid profile, possibly providing a potential adjuvant for the treatment of T2D. However, RCT results are conflicting, particularly regarding CNM's lipid-lowering properties (Table 9). In a 2003 placebo-controlled RCT, Khan et al. reported that following supplementation with 1, 3, or 6 g of CNM/day for 40 days, patients with T2D receiving sulfonylureas (n = 30) experienced a significant reduction in serum glucose, TGs, and TC levels. A significant change was also observed in LDL-c concentration in patients consuming 3 and 6 g of CNM [174].

Table 9. Summary of RCTs investigating the hypoglycemic, hypolipidemic, and anti-steatosis effects of CNM.

Disease	Participants (Total)	Intervention	Control	Duration	Main Outcomes */**	References
T2D	n = 60	CNM 1, 3 or 6 g/day	Placebo	40 days	↓ glucose, TC, TGs **	[174]
T2D	n = 58	CNM 2 g/day	Placebo	12 weeks	↓ HbA_{1c} *	[175]
T2D	n = 66	CNM 120 mg/day or 360 mg/day	Placebo	3 months	↓ FBG, HbA_{1c} **	[176]
T2D	n = 37	CNM 3 g/day	Placebo	8 weeks	↓ FBG, HbA_{1c}, TGs, BW, BMI, BF **	[177]
T2D	n = 138	CNM 1 g/day	Placebo	3 months	↓ FBG, 2-h PBG, HOMA-IR, FI, TC, LDL-c, ↑ HDL-c	[178]
T2D	n = 39	CNM 3 g/day	Placebo	8 weeks	no significant changes	[179]
NAFLD	n = 45	CNM 1.5 g/day +LSI	Placebo + LSI	12 weeks	↓ ALT, AST, GGT, TC, TGs, FBG, HOMA-IR, QUICKI, hs-CRP *	[180]

* Statistically significant between groups ($p < 0.05$); ** Statistically significant from baseline ($p < 0.05$); "↓", decreased; "↑", increased. Abbreviations: ALT, alanine aminotransferase; AST, aspartate aminotransferase; BF, body fat; BMI, body mass index; BW, body weight; CNM, cinnamon; FBG, fasting blood glucose; FI, fasting insulin; GGT, gamma-glutamyl transpeptidase; HDL-c, high-density lipoprotein cholesterol; HbA_{1c}, glycosylated hemoglobin; HOMA-IR, homeostatic model assessment of insulin resistance; hs-CRP, high-sensitivity C-reactive protein; LDL-c, low-density lipoprotein cholesterol; LSI, lifestyle intervention; QUICKI, quantitative insulin sensitivity check index; 2-h PBG, 2-h postprandial blood glucose; TC, total cholesterol; TGs, triglycerides.

Akilen et al. (2010) demonstrated that, compared to placebo (n = 28), 2 g of CNM for 12 weeks led to a significant decrease in mean HbA_{1c} in patients with poorly controlled T2D (n = 30). In addition, a significant reduction in FBG, BMI, and WC was observed in the interventional group compared to baseline, but CNM supplementation had no effects on blood lipid parameters (TC, TGs, HDL-c, LDL-c), either within or between the groups [175].

Lu et al. randomly assigned 66 patients with T2D into three groups: one receiving 120 mg of CNM/day (n = 23), another receiving 360 mg of CNM/day (n = 23), and a placebo group (n = 20). All patients were treated with gliclazide throughout the trial. After 3 months, FBG and HbA_{1c} were significantly reduced in the CNM-treated patients. TG levels also decreased significantly in the group receiving 120 mg of CNM/day. TC, LDL-c, HDL-c, and liver enzyme levels (ALT, AST) remained unchanged in all patients at the end of the follow-up period [176].

Vafa et al. (2010) tested the effects of CNM supplementation (3 g/day for 8 weeks) compared to a placebo in 37 patients with T2D. Compared to baseline, levels of FBG, HbA_{1c}, and TGs, as well as anthropometric indices (BMI, BW, BF%), significantly improved in the CNM-supplemented group. However, no significant differences were observed between the groups regarding glucolipid or anthropometric parameters [177].

In 2019, Zare et al. conducted a triple-blind, placebo-controlled RCT involving 138 patients with T2D, divided into four groups based on their BMI (>/< 27 kg/m^2) and intervention (1 g of CNM/day or placebo for 3 months). The results showed that CNM improved glycemic (FBG, 2 h PBG, HOMA-IR, FI) and lipid (TC, LDL-c, HDL-c) measurements, except for TG levels. In addition, anthropometric indices (BMI, BF%, visceral fat) also significantly ameliorated in the CNM-supplemented patients. Improvements were significantly greater in patients with BMI > 27 kg/m^2, except for TC and LDL-c [178].

Another RCT (2020) involving 39 patients with T2D (intervention, n = 20 and placebo, n = 19) investigated the effect of CNM supplementation on inflammation status. No beneficial impact was observed on plasma levels of hs-CRP, IL-6, or TNF-α following CNM consumption. Moreover, a significant within-group reduction in hs-CRP was reported in the placebo controls at the end of the study [179].

Finally, a review analyzing 11 RCTs (n = 694) concluded that CNM supplementation, in addition to hypoglycemic medication and lifestyle changes, has only modest effects on glycemic control (FBG and HbA_{1c}) in patients with T2D [172]. Another clinical review reported that supplementation with 1 to 6 g of CNM seemed to be beneficial in alleviating glucose metabolism parameters [181]. In addition, a 2025 SRMA including 28 RCTs (n = 3054) reported, with significant heterogeneity, that CNM appears to improve BMI, glycemic, and lipid parameters in patients with T2D, especially when administered in capsule form at a daily dosage of $\leq$2 g [182].

Clinical evidence in MASLD. CNM's hepatoprotective effects in patients with NAFLD were investigated in a single double-blind, placebo-controlled RCT (2014) (n = 45). All patients followed lifestyle recommendations throughout the study. The authors reported that CNM supplementation (1.5 g/day for 12 weeks) led to significant improvements in ALT, AST, GGT, TC, and TG levels compared to placebo. No changes were reported regarding HDL-c concentration. In addition, significant reductions in FBG, HOMA-IR, QUICKI, and hs-CRP concentrations were observed in the intervention group compared to the control group. LDL-c decreased significantly in both groups. BMI and WC remained unchanged during the study [180].

Safety. CNM appears to be well tolerated, without adverse effects, and may improve health status as an adjunct treatment for T2D. However, further high-quality studies are needed to firmly establish its risk potential and safety profile [183].

Summary. CNM may be employed as an add-on phytotherapy to standard medication in T2D, particularly due to its glucose-lowering effect. However, RCTs have not always shown positive outcomes, and it seems that CNM's therapeutic potential in glycemia regulation is rather modest. Regarding MASLD, there is currently insufficient clinical evidence to recommend the use of CNM in its management.

4.9. Fenugreek (Trigonella Foenum-Graecum)

Trigonella foenum-graecum (TFG), or fenugreek, has been widely used for its antidiabetic properties, primarily derived from its seeds. The hypoglycemic effect of TFG is attributed to several NBCs, including trigonelline, diosgenin, soluble fibers, and 4-hydroxyisoleucine. In addition, TFG has demonstrated anti-hyperlipidemic, anti-obesity, anti-inflammatory, antioxidant, and anticancer effects [184].

Clinical evidence in T2D. In recent years, multiple RCTs have investigated the role of TFG in T2D management (Table 10). In 2001, Gupta et al. performed a double-blind placebo-controlled RCT in newly diagnosed patients with T2D (n = 25), testing TFG supplementation (1 g/day of hydroalcoholic extract for 2 months, n = 12) on glycemic parameters. Although the results failed to show a significant difference between groups regarding FBG and 2 h PBG levels, TFG supplementation has proven effective in improving insulin resistance, as well as TG and HDL-c levels [185].

Table 10. Summary of RCTs investigating the hypoglycemic, hypolipidemic, and anti-steatosis effects of TFG.

Disease	Participants (Total)	Intervention	Control	Duration	Main Outcomes */**	References
T2D	n = 25	TFG extract 1 g/day	Placebo + LSI	2 months	↓ HOMA-IR, TGs, ↑ HDL-c *	[185]
T2D	n = 69	TFG extract 6.3 g/day + LSI	Placebo + LSI	12 weeks	↓ FBG, 2-h PBG, HbA_{1c} *	[186]
T2D	n = 88	TFG seeds 10 g/day	Placebo	8 weeks	↓ FBG, HbA_{1c}, SI, HOMA-IR, TC, TGs, ↑ APN *	[187]
T2D	n = 9	TFG 2 g/day + Metformin	Glibenclamide 5 mg/day + Metformin	12 weeks	↑ SI, HDL/LDL ratio **	[188]
T2D	n = 95	TFG seed powder solution 50 g/day	Metformin	1 month	↓ TC, TGs, HDL-c, LDL-c *	[189]
T2D	n = 48	TFG seed powder 15 g/day + LSI	LSI	8 weeks	↓ FBG, ALT, ALP *	[190]
T2D	n = 43	TFG extract 1005 mg/day	Placebo	8 weeks	↑ HDL-c *	[191]
NAFLD	n = 24	TFG extract 1 g/day + LSI	Placebo + LSI	3 months	no changes	[192]

* Statistically significant between groups ($p < 0.05$); ** Statistically significant from baseline ($p < 0.05$); "↓", decreased; "↑", increased. Abbreviations: ALT, alanine aminotransferase; ALP, alkaline, phosphatase; APN, adiponectin; FBG, fasting blood glucose; HDL-c, high-density lipoprotein cholesterol; HbA_{1c}, glycosylated hemoglobin; HOMA-IR, homeostatic model assessment of insulin resistance; LDL-c, low-density lipoprotein cholesterol; LSI, lifestyle intervention; 2-h PBG, 2-h postprandial blood glucose; SI, serum insulin; TC, total cholesterol; TGs, triglycerides.

In 2008, Lu et al. evaluated the effectiveness of TFG extract combined with sulfonylureas (SU) for managing T2D in 69 patients with insufficiently controlled T2D using SU alone. Patients received either TFG (n = 46) or placebo (n = 23) daily for 12 weeks in conjunction with SU. All participants were instructed to maintain lifestyle recommendations throughout the study. At the end of the follow-up period, TFG-treated patients experienced a significant reduction in FBG, 2 h PBG, and HbA_{1c} compared to both baseline and placebo. No improvements in BMI levels were observed in either group [186].

Similar results were reported by Rafraf et al. (2014) in a triple-blind RCT involving 88 patients with T2D. After 8 weeks of supplementation with TFG (10 g/day of powdered seeds), FBG, HbA_{1c}, serum insulin, HOMA-IR, TC, TG, and APN levels significantly improved in the interventional group compared to the placebo. No changes were observed in LDL and HDL-c levels [187].

In a 12-week open-label trial involving nine patients with T2D who were not adequately controlled with metformin, participants consumed either TFG (2 g/day) or glibenclamide (5 mg/day). It was shown that TFG led to a significant increase in FI concentration and the HDL/LDL ratio, but did not significantly affect FBG, HbA_{1c}, HOMA-IR, TG, or LDL-c levels. However, compared to TFG, glibenclamide significantly lowered HOMA-IR and HbA_{1c} levels. Notably, HbA_{1c} levels were lower at baseline in the glibenclamide-treated group compared to the TFG-supplemented group [188].

Geberemeskel et al. (2019) investigated the effect of TFG supplementation (25 g of seed powder solution twice daily) versus metformin on the lipid profile in patients with newly diagnosed T2D (n = 95). After 1 month, in TFG-treated patients (n = 49), significant improvements in TC, TG, and HDL and LDL cholesterol levels were observed compared to both baseline and the control group. Blood lipid levels in the control group remained unchanged [189].

Hadi et al. (2020) reported that, in patients receiving standard T2D medication, supplementation with TFG (15 g/day for 8 weeks, n = 24) resulted in a significant reduction in FBG, ALT, and ALP levels compared to a placebo (n = 24). Also, compared to baseline, the levels of AST decreased significantly in the intervention group [190].

More recently, however, Chehregosha et al. (2024) failed to detect significant changes in glycemic indices, the lipid profile, or the prooxidant/antioxidant balance in patients with T2D (n = 23) following supplementation with TFG (335 mg of TFG dry seed extract three times daily for 8 weeks). TFG only improved HDL-c levels in the intervention group (n = 20) compared to baseline and the placebo group [191].

Finally, a 2024 SRMA of 19 RCTs (n = 1612) involving patients with T2D investigating the efficacy of TFG supplementation showed that TFG led to significant improvements in FBG, HbA_{1c}, HOMA-IR, BMI, TC, LDL-c, and HDL-c concentrations. No effects were observed on FI, TG level, or BW in the overall analysis. Consistent heterogeneity was reported among the included clinical trials. Dosages of TFG (extract or powder) ranged from 25 to 50,000 mg/day, while the duration of interventions varied from 4to 24 weeks. In addition, TFG's natural compounds may seem to act as powerful anti-inflammatory and antioxidant molecules to alleviate insulin signaling, but these findings are primarily based on preclinical studies [184].

Clinical evidence in MASLD. Evidence of the effect of TFG supplementation on liver function and histology in human subjects is limited (Table 10). A sole triple-blind controlled pilot clinical trial investigating the effect of TFG supplementation on the liver in patients with NAFLD was performed by Babaei et al. Thirty patients with NAFLD were randomly assigned to two groups, receiving either hydroalcoholic extract TFG (1 g/day for 3 months) (n = 13) or a placebo (n = 11). At baseline, all patients were given lifestyle advice. At the end of the study, some improvements in liver steatosis percentage and CAP score were observed among TFG-treated patients, but these changes were not statistically significant compared to those in the placebo group. In addition, no significant differences in ALT and AST levels were detected between the two groups. Anthropometric indices (BMI, BW, WHR) remained unchanged in both groups [192].

Safety. TFG supplementation is generally well tolerated. The most commonly reported adverse effects include nausea, diarrhea, dyspepsia, and flatulence, affecting up to 20% of study participants. Some subjects may also experience allergic reactions, probably due to TFG's high protein antigen content. In addition, coumarin compounds in TFG have raised concerns regarding possible hepatotoxicity and anticoagulant effects; however, there is currently no evidence from clinical trials indicating these risks at standard therapeutic dosages [184].

Summary. To date, clinical research findings indicate that TFG has some beneficial effects on glycemic control and lipid profile in patients with T2D, but the study outcomes are inconsequential. The limited availability of RCTs investigating TFG's therapeutic value in MASLD highlights the importance of further large, high-quality studies to confirm its potential clinical efficacy.

4.10. Ginger

Ginger (GGR) is derived from the rhizomes of the plant *Zingiber officinale* Roscoe and has been utilized for its antitumor, immunomodulatory, and antiemetic properties. The main functional compound of GGR is gingerol, which has been acknowledged as a potent anti-inflammatory molecule [193]. Other non-volatile components of GGR include shogaols, zingerones, and paradols [194]. According to clinical studies, ginger also exhibits hypoglycemic, hypolipidemic [194], and hepatoprotective activity [195].

Clinical evidence in T2D. Several RCTs have investigated the effects of GGR on glycemic control (Table 11). The first clinical study was performed in 2013 by Mahluji et al. and involved 58 patients with T2D who were administered GGR (n = 28) or a placebo (n = 30) for 2 months. The results showed that GGR supplementation led to significantly improved levels of HOMA-IR, QUICKI, insulin, LDL-c, and TGs relative to the placebo. However, no significant changes were observed concerning FBG, HbA_{1c}, TC, and HDL-c concentrations or regarding BW [194].

Table 11. Summary of RCTs investigating the hypoglycemic, hypolipidemic, and anti-steatosis effects of GGR.

Disease	Participants (Total)	Intervention	Control	Duration	Main Outcomes */**	References
T2D	n = 58	GGR 2 g/day	Placebo	2 months	↓ HOMA-IR, insulin, LDL-c, TGs, ↑ QUICKI *	[194]
T2D	n = 81	GGR 3 g/day	Placebo	8 weeks	↓ FBG, HbA_{1c}, ↑ QUICKI *	[196]
T2D	n = 63	GGR 1600 mg/day	Placebo	12 weeks	↓ glucose, HbA_{1c}, HOMA-IR, insulin, TC, TGs, CRP *	[197]
T2D	n = 45	GGR 3 g/day	Placebo	3 months	↓ glucose, HbA_{1c}, insulin, HOMA-IR, hs-CRP, MDA, ↑ TAC *	[198]
T2D	n = 45	GGR 2000 mg/day	Placebo	10 weeks	↓ FBG, HbA_{1c} *	[199]
T2D	n = 103	GGR 1.2 g/day	Placebo	90 days	↓ FBG, TC *	[200]
NAFLD	n = 44	GGR 2 g/day + LSI	Placebo	12 weeks	↓ ALT, GGT, CAP, HOMA-IR, hs-CRP, TNF-α *	[201]
NAFLD	n = 46	GGR 1500 mg/day + LSI	Placebo	12 weeks	↓ ALT, FBG, HOMA-IR, TC, LDL-c, hs-CRP *	[195]
T2D/NAFLD	n = 72	GGR 2000 mg/day	Placebo	3 months	↓ HOMA-IR, insulin, ↑ HDL-c **	[202]

* Statistically significant between groups ($p < 0.05$); ** Statistically significant from baseline ($p < 0.05$); "↓", decreased; "↑", increased. Abbreviations: ALT, alanine aminotransferase; CAP, controlled attenuation parameter score; CRP, C-reactive protein; FBG, fasting blood glucose; GGR, ginger; GGT, gamma-glutamyl transpeptidase; HDL-c, high-density lipoprotein cholesterol; HbA_{1c}, glycosylated hemoglobin; HOMA-IR, homeostatic model assessment of insulin resistance; hs-CRP, high-sensitivity C-reactive protein; LDL-c, low-density lipoprotein cholesterol; LSI, lifestyle intervention; MDA, malondialdehyde; QUICKI, quantitative insulin sensitivity check index; TAC, total antioxidant capacity; TC, total cholesterol; TGs, triglycerides; TNF-α, tumor necrosis factor.

Significantly improved glycemic control was reported by Khosravi et al. (2014) among patients with T2D treated with hypoglycemic agents and either GGR (n = 40) or placebo (n = 41) for 8 weeks. During the intervention, all patients were encouraged to maintain their usual diet and perform no physical activities. At the end of the study, GGR-supplemented patients exhibited a significant reduction in FBG and HbA_{1c} levels, as well as a significantly greater increase in the QUICKI index compared to the placebo group. HOMA-IR decreased significantly in both groups, but no significant differences between the groups were observed. On the other hand, BMI did not differ significantly between the groups either before or after the intervention [196].

Consistent with these findings, another 2014 RCT showed that, compared to placebo (n = 30), GGR (1600 mg) administered daily for 12 weeks was effective in improving several glucolipid and inflammatory markers in patients with T2D (n = 33). Study participants were asked to maintain their lifestyle habits during the trial. Significant decreases in plasma glucose, HbA_{1c}, HOMA-IR, insulin, TC, TGs, and CRP levels were detected following GGR supplementation. There was no significant difference between groups regarding TNF-α concentration. BW and BMI remained unchanged in both groups [197].

Similar results were reported following GGR supplementation with 3 g of GGR for 3 months in 45 patients with T2D. After the intervention, a significant decrease in serum glucose, HbA_{1c}, insulin, HOMA-IR, and hs-CRP was observed in the GGR-treated participants. Also, they exhibited increased TAC and reduced MDA levels compared to the control group [198].

Makhdoomi Arzati et al. also confirmed GGR's hypoglycemic effect in a 2017 RCT involving patients with T2D. GGR intake significantly reduced FBG and HBA_{1c} levels after 10 weeks compared to placebo. The ratio of LDL-c/HDL-c also decreased after GGR supplementation, although no other changes in the blood lipid profile were reported [199].

In 2020, Nunes Carvalho et al. demonstrated that GGR consumption improved both FBG and TC levels in T2D. The study participants were supplemented with either GGR (n = 47) or a placebo (n = 56) for 90 days. HbA_{1c} concentration declined more substantially in the intervention group compared to the control group, although this change was not statistically significant. Notably, LDL-c levels exhibited a greater reduction in the placebo control group [200].

A 2022 SRMA including 10 RCTs (n = 597) concluded that GGR consumption was effective in alleviating FBG and HbA_{1c} levels in patients with T2D. Nevertheless, in patients older than 50 years, no significant effect of GGR supplementation on HbA_{1c} levels was found. In addition, GGR intake failed to improve the blood lipid profile. GGR dosages ranged from 1200 to 3000 mg/day, whereas study durations varied from 8 to 13 weeks [203].

Clinical evidence in MASLD. RCTs investigating GGR's effects in MASLD are scarce (Table 11). In 2016, Rahimlou et al. conducted a clinical trial involving 44 patients with NAFLD who were supplemented with GGR (2 g/day) or a placebo for 12 weeks. All study participants received lifestyle recommendations. Compared to the placebo, GGR intake was superior in improving ALT, GGT, HOMA-IR, hs-CRP, and TNF-α levels. Also, significant changes compared to the placebo were reported regarding liver steatosis grade. Nevertheless, GGR did not significantly affect AST levels or fibrosis score. Anthropometric parameters reduced significantly in both groups, but only the reduction in hip circumference was significantly different between the intervention and control groups [201].

Rafie et al. (2020) found that GGR (1500 mg/day) intake for 12 weeks led to a significant reduction in ALT, FBG, HOMA-IR, TC, LDL-c, and hs-CRP levels compared to placebo in patients with NAFLD. No significant differences between the two groups were observed concerning GGT, AST, FLI score, fatty liver grade, FI, HDL-c, TGs, TNF-α, APN, TAC, or BW. All patients followed a diet and physical activity regimen during the clinical trial [195].

Finally, a 2024 RCT reported that GGR supplementation may alleviate some metabolic dysfunction characteristics. Seventy-two patients with T2D and NAFLD were administered either GGR (2000 mg/day) or a placebo for 3 months. At the end of the study, no significant effects on liver steatosis and fibrosis scores were observed. Liver enzyme levels (AST, ALT, GGT) and anthropometric indices (BW, BMI, WC) decreased in both groups, without significant differences between them. HOMA-IR, HDL-c, and serum insulin levels improved compared to baseline in the GGR-treated patients [202].

Safety. GGR is recognized as safe by the Food and Drug Administration and has good tolerability with minimal side effects [204]. Reported adverse effects across RCTs include transient heartburn [201,202], dyspepsia, and nausea [202].

Summary. GGR consumption demonstrates promising potential as an adjuvant in T2D and MASLD management. Nevertheless, despite its hypoglycemic effects, GGR does not appear to significantly influence the blood lipid profile in T2D. In addition, GGR's role in MASLD, particularly in T2D with MASLD, requires more in-depth investigation.

4.11. Soluble Fibers

Dietary fibers have long been recognized for their role in managing metabolic dysfunction. However, since modest improvements in glycemic control require unrealistic intake levels of dietary fibers (>50 g/zi), many fiber supplements have been developed, with extensive research highlighting their efficacy and ease of use [205]. Viscous, gel-forming fibers, such as psyllium, inulin-type fructans (ITFs), or guar gum, are among the most studied fibers that may be effective in alleviating metabolic dysfunction in patients with T2D [205–207] and MASLD [208] (Table 12).

Soluble fibers are often regarded as prebiotics due to their ability to promote the growth of beneficial gut microbial communities while reducing harmful bacteria [209]. The prebiotic effect of soluble fiber on GM-related outcomes in patients with T2D and NAFLD will be discussed in the next subsection.

Clinical evidence in T2D. A 2009 RCT evaluated the effect of psyllium (10.5 g/day) compared to placebo on glycemic control and lipid profiles in 40 patients with T2D treated with sulfonylureas and diet. Patients in both groups exhibited significantly lower FBG, HbA_{1c}, BMI, and WC values after 2 months compared to baseline. However, TG concentration significantly decreased in the psyllium-treated group, but not in the control group (diet alone). The postprandial lipoprotein profile remained unchanged between the two groups [210].

Psyllium. Significant improvements in glucose metabolism parameters were reported by Feinglos et al. in a 2013 RCT assessing the dose–response effects of psyllium on metabolic control in 37 patients with T2D receiving conventional treatment. The patients were supplemented with either 6.8 or 13.6 g of psyllium/day or a placebo for 12 weeks. Both psyllium doses led to significantly lower FBG at weeks 4, 8, and 12. Moreover, HbA_{1c} levels significantly decreased compared to placebo at week 8 following supplementation with 13.6 g of psyllium and at week 12 with both dosages [211].

A 2015 SRMA of studies involving individuals with euglycemia, dysglycemia, and T2D concluded that in patients with T2D, psyllium was beneficial in significantly reducing the levels of FBG and HbA_{1c}. Psyllium's glycemic benefits were proportional to the baseline value of FBG, with no significant effects in normoglycemia, modest effects in prediabetes, and significant effects in T2D [212].

More recently, Abutair et al. (2018) also reported that compared to the control group (regular diet, n = 18), psyllium supplementation (10.5 g/day for 8 weeks) led to significant reductions in FBG, TC, TGs, and WC in newly diagnosed patients with T2D (regular diet, n = 18). The LDL-c level declined in both groups, but not significantly [213].

Psyllium has also been shown to have some beneficial effects on improving inflammation status. As such, a 2018 open RCT showed that patients with T2D following a moderate carbohydrate diet supplemented with psyllium (n = 20) exhibited significantly reduced fasting TNF-α and FI levels compared to baseline and to individuals receiving a low-carbohydrate diet and placebo (n = 17). It should be noted that these changes took place irrespective of weight changes since no significant variations in BW were reported between the two groups. No significant changes within groups or differences between groups were observed regarding FBG, PBG, and postprandial insulin. Postprandial TNF-α concentrations were significantly reduced compared to baseline in the intervention group, but there was no significant difference when compared to placebo controls [214].

Table 12. Summary of RCTs investigating the hypoglycemic, hypolipidemic, and anti-steatosis effects of soluble fibers.

Disease	Participants (Total)	Intervention	Control	Duration	Main Outcomes */**	References
T2D	n = 40	Psyllium 10.5 g/day + diet	Diet	2 months	↓ FBG, HbA_{1c}, BMI, WC **	[210]
T2D	n = 37	Psyllium 6.8 or 13.6 g/day	Placebo	12 weeks	↓ HbA_{1c} *	[211]
T2D	n = 36	Psyllium 10.5 g/day	Regular diet	8 weeks	↓ FBG, TC, TGs, WC *	[213]
T2D	n = 37	Psyllium 7 g/day	Placebo	2 weeks	↓ fasting TNF-α, FI *	[214]
T2D	n = 49	Inulin 10 g/day	Placebo	2 months	↓ FBG, HbA_{1c}, BMI, BW, MDA, ↑ TAC, SOD *	[215]
T2D	n = 49	Inulin 10 g/day	Placebo	8 weeks	↓ FBG, HbA_{1c}, HOMA-IR, FI, hs-CRP, TNF-α *	[216]
T2D	n = 52	Inulin 10 g/day	Placebo	8 weeks	↓ FBG, HbA_{1c}, IL-6, TNF-α *	[217]
T2D	n = 49	Inulin (chicory) 10 g/day	Placebo	2 months	↓ FBG, HbA_{1c}, ALP *	[218]
T2D	n = 44	PHGG 10 g/day	Placebo	6 weeks	↓ HbA_{1c}, WC **	[219]
T2D	n = 79	Whey protein 17 g GG 5 g	Flavored placebo	12 weeks	↓ PBG, HbA_{1c} *	[220]
NASH	n = 7	Inulin 16 g/day	Placebo	8 weeks	↓ AST *	[221]
NAFLD	n = 75	Psyllium 10 g/day +LSI	Ground wheat 10 g/day + LSI	10 weeks	↓ ALT, BMI, BW, BF, WC *	[222]
NAFLD	n = 70	PP 10 g/day OB 10 g/day PP + OB 10 g/day	Placebo	12 weeks	no changes	[223]

* Statistically significant between groups ($p < 0.05$); ** Statistically significant from baseline ($p < 0.05$); "↓", decreased; "↑", increased. Abbreviations: ALT, alanine aminotransferase; ALP, alkaline phosphatase; AST, aspartate aminotransferase; BMI, body mass index; BF, body fat; BW, body weight; FBG, fasting blood glucose; CRP, C reactive protein; GG, guar gum; FI, fasting insulin; HbA_{1c}, glycosylated hemoglobin; HOMA-IR, homeostatic model assessment of insulin resistance; IL-6, interleukin 6; LSI, lifestyle intervention; MDA, malondialdehyde; OB, *Ocimum basilicum;* PBG, postprandial blood glucose; PHGG, partially hydrolyzed guar gum; PP, *Plantago psyllium*; SOD, superoxide dismutase; TC, total cholesterol; TAC, total antioxidant capacity; TGs, triglycerides; TNF-α, tumor necrosis factor α; WC, waist circumference.

Finally, a 2024 SRMA of 19 RCTs (n = 962) revealed that, compared to placebo, psyllium significantly decreased FBG, HbA_{1c}, and HOMA-IR, but not serum insulin. Psyllium's effect on FBG was effective at dosages both below and above 10 g/day with interventions lasting longer than 50 days. No significant changes in HbA_{1c} were observed with psyllium intake below 10 g/day. HOMA-IR and insulin levels showed no significant differences with psyllium consumption either below or above 10 g/day [224].

Inulin. Three RCTs involving women with T2D and overweight (n = 49, n = 49, n = 52) showed that supplementation with 10 g of inulin or oligofructose-enriched inulin versus placebo for 8 weeks was effective in significantly [215–217] improving glycemic control, anthropometric indices, oxidant and inflammation status. As such, Gargari et al. observed significant changes in FBG, HbA_{1c}, MDA, TAC, and SOD after inulin consumption (n = 24) compared to the placebo (n = 25). No significant difference was observed regarding HOMA-IR between the two groups. Both BMI and BW decreased significantly in the inulin-treated patients relative to placebo controls after 2 months [215]. In another RCT, between-group comparisons showed a significant decline in FBG, HbA_{1c}, HOMA-IR, FI, hs-CRP, and TNF-α in the inulin group (n = 24) compared to the placebo group (n = 25). IL-10 also increased in the inulin-treated patients, but this change was not significant. BW and BMI significantly decreased after 2 months in the intervention group, but not in the control group [216].

Finally, the third study reported significant improvements in FBG, HbA_{1c}, IL-6, and TNF-α after inulin supplementation (n = 27) compared to the placebo (n = 25). Changes in hs-CRP and IL-10 levels were also noted in the intervention group, but these changes were not statistically significant. At the end of the study, both BMI and BW declined significantly after inulin consumption, while remaining unchanged following placebo intake [217].

A 2015 SRMA by Liu et al. involving healthy individuals, individuals with DLD, and those with overweight/obesity and T2D (n = 607) reported that ITF supplementation may decrease LDL-c levels in all studied populations. In addition, according to the T2D subgroup analysis (three RCTs), inulin supplementation was positively correlated with decreased FBG and FI levels, as well as increased HDL-c concentration [207].

In 2016, Farhangi et al. tested the effects of enriched chicory inulin supplementation (10 g/day) versus placebo on glucose parameters and liver enzymes in female patients with T2D (n = 49). After 2 months, significant reductions in FBG and HbA_{1c} were reported in the intervention group (n = 27) compared to baseline and placebo recipients (n = 22). AST levels also decreased significantly compared to baseline in the chicory-treated patients, while ALP concentration declined significantly in the intervention group compared to both baseline and controls. No significant changes were observed in ALT levels [218].

Finally, Wang et al. (2019) conducted an SRMA involving 33 RCTs (n = 1346) in healthy individuals and patients with obesity or T2D supplemented with ITFs. The results showed that overall, prebiotics were effective in reducing FBG, HbA_{1c}, FI, and HOMA-IR levels, particularly in individuals with prediabetes and T2D. Glycemic control improved following supplementation of $\geq$10 g of ITFs/day for 6 weeks or longer [225].

Partially hydrolyzed guar gum. Dall'Alba et al. (2013) investigated the effects of supplementation with partially hydrolyzed guar gum (PHGG, 10 g/day for 6 weeks) versus placebo on cardiovascular risk factors in patients with T2D and MS (n = 44). PHGG-treated patients (n = 23) experienced a significant reduction in HbA_{1c} levels and WC after 4 and 6 weeks compared to baseline. No changes were observed in FBG, the blood lipid profile, or CRP in either group [219].

A 12-week trial by Watson et al. (2019) reported that supplementation with 150 mL of a flavored drink containing either 17 g of whey protein and 5 g of guar gum (n = 37) versus a placebo (n = 42), taken 15 min before breakfast and dinner daily, led to a significant reduction in gastric emptying and PBG compared to a placebo. The rate of gastric emptying was correlated with the degree of blood glucose decrease. Also, a modest but significant decline in HbA_{1c} levels was observed at the end of the study in the interventional group compared to the control group. There were no differences in BW between the two groups [220].

Pooled data from 14 RCTs included in a 2023 SRMA showed that guar gum is effective in reducing HbA_{1c} levels, without influencing FBG concentrations or BW. However, according to a subgroup analysis, an intake above 15 g/day of guar gum was shown to significantly improve FBG levels in patients with T2D [226]. Guar gum was also reported to significantly reduce TC and LDL-c concentrations in patients with T2D at a dosage ranging from 5 to 30 g/day. TG levels also decreased following supplementation of $\geq$ 20 g of guar gum/day. No effect on HDL-c concentration was observed [206].

Clinical evidence in MASLD. An overview of the RCTs discussed in this subsection is provided in Table 12. In 2005, a pilot study on the effects of soluble fiber in patients with NASH (n = 7) was performed by Daubioul et al. After 8 weeks of supplementation with 16 g of inulin/day, a significant decrease in plasma levels of AST was observed, but not in ALT, ALP, or GGT. No changes were reported in glucose and lipid metabolism parameters [221].

A 2015 trial involving patients with NAFLD (n = 75) who were supplemented with either 10 g of psyllium (n = 38) or ground wheat (n = 37) daily for 10 weeks, in addition to diet and increased physical activity, reported that fiber intake led to a significant reduction in BMI, WC, BF%, and serum ALT levels. The reduction in AST was not significant [222].

A four-arm, parallel, single-blind RCT (2016) compared the impact of psyllium *(Plantago psyllium*, PP) versus basil (*Ocimum basilicum*, OB) supplementation on anthropometric indices in patients with NAFLD (n = 70). Participants were allocated to four groups, each receiving one of the following supplementations: 10 g of PP/day; 10 g of OB/day; a combination of psyllium and OB at 10 g/day; or a placebo. After 12 weeks, the results failed to show any significant differences in BMI, BW, or body composition-related parameters between the intervention and control groups. The authors argued that the ineffectiveness of PP and OB supplementation could be explained by the low dosage of fibers administered [223].

However, a 2020 SRMA (n = 242) investigating the metabolic outcomes in NAFLD patients following soluble fiber intake reported that supplementation at a dosage of 10–16 g/day for 10 to 12 weeks results in favorable effects on anthropometric (BMI), metabolic (HOMA-IR, FI), and liver-related parameters (ALT, AST) [208].

Safety. Soluble fibers have proven efficient and are well tolerated in the management of CMDs. However, excessive intake may cause gastrointestinal symptoms, such as abdominal cramps, flatulence, constipation, or diarrhea [227].

Summary. Soluble fiber supplements may represent a viable and safe strategy to improve glycemic control, lipid profile, and hepatic steatosis in patients with T2D and MASLD. In addition, soluble fibers may have beneficial effects on anthropometric parameters, which also help enhance the metabolic health outcomes of these patients.

4.12. Omega-3 Fatty Acids

Omega-3 fatty acids (ω-3 PUFA) of marine origin are polyunsaturated fatty acids that exist in two forms: eicosapentaenoic acid (EPA) and docosahexaenoic acid (DHA) [228]. Research suggests that ω-3 PUFA exert cardioprotective benefits, although their effects on the plasma lipid profile are rather modest [229]. ω-3 PUFA are also associated with hypoglycemic activity [228], anti-steatosis effects [230], and body composition improvements [229].

Clinical evidence in T2D. An in-depth meta-analysis regarding the effects of ω-3 PUFA in T2D (n = 1533) was published in 2009. Hartweg et al. reported that compared to placebo, long-term supplementation with marine-derived ω-3 PUFA was effective in reducing TG levels, highlighting a potential dose–response effect. TG levels decreased with the administration of higher doses of ω-3 PUFA (>2 g/day). Also, a small but significant increase in LDL-c concentration was observed following supplementation. Other cardioprotective effects associated with ω-3 PUFA, such as attenuated fibrinogen and platelet aggregation, were also reported in this review [231].

In 2012, Crochemore et al. performed a single-blind trial involving 41 women with T2D who were given 2.5 g of fish oil/day (n = 14), 1.5 g of fish oil/day (n = 14), or a placebo (n = 13) for 30 days (Table 13). Study participants were encouraged to maintain their lifestyle habits throughout the trial. Patients receiving the lower dose of ω-3 PUFA experienced a greater decrease in BW and WC than patients supplemented with a higher dose. Also, among patients taking the lower dose of ω-3 PUFA, more frequent reductions in FBG, HbA_{1c}, and TC levels were observed, as well as an increase in HDL-c concentration. Moreover, the higher dose of ω-3 PUFA showed a tendency to reduce insulin sensitivity. Since the lower dose of ω-3 PUFA was more effective in improving the study's outcomes, the authors concluded that ω-3 PUFA supplementation is not essential for women with T2D treated with oral hypoglycemics to improve BW, body composition, or the lipid profile [229].

Table 13. Summary of RCTs investigating the hypoglycemic, hypolipidemic, and anti-steatosis effects of ω-3 PUFA.

Disease	Participants (Total)	Intervention	Control	Duration	Main Outcomes */**	References
T2D	n = 41	ω-3 PUFA 2.5 g/ ω-3 PUFA 1.5 g	Placebo	30 days	↓ BW, WC *	[229]
T2D	n = 84	ω-3 PUFA 2.7 g/day	Placebo	8 weeks	↓ IL-2, TNF-α *	[232]
T2D	n = 166	ω-3 PUFA 2 g/day ALA 2.5 g/day	Placebo	180 days	↓ HbA_{1c}, TC, TGs, TC/HDL, LDL-c *	[233]
T2D	n = 99	ω-3 PUFA 2.4 g	Placebo	6 months	↓ TGs, ↑ HDL-c *	[234]
T2D	n = 54	ω-3 PUFA 520 mg/day	Placebo	24 weeks	↓ serum glucose, WC, TGs **	[235]
T2D	n = 70	ω-3 PUFA 1 g/day	Placebo	12 weeks	↓ FBG, HbA_{1c}, HOMA-IR, TC, TGs, LDL-c,* ↑ HDL-c *	[236]
NAFLD	n = 36	ω-3 PUFA 2 g/day	Diet	6 months	↓ ALT, GGT, TGs, HOMA-IR, BMI, TNF-α **, ↑ HDL-c **	[237]
NAFLD	n = 70	ω-3 PUFA 4 g/day	Placebo	3 months	↓ glucose, TC, TGs, ApoB, ALT GGT, TNF-α, CK18-M30, ↑ APN *	[238]
NASH	n = 243	EPA-E 1800 mg/day 2700 mg/day	Placebo	12 months	↓ TGs *	[239]
NASH/T2D	n = 37	ω-3 PUFA 3.6 g + LSI	Placebo + LSI	48 weeks	↑ FBG, HOMA-IR **	[240]
NAFLD	n = 60	ω-3 PUFA 3.6 g + LSI	Placebo	1 year	↓ GGT *	[241]

* Statistically significant between groups ($p < 0.05$); ** Statistically significant from baseline ($p < 0.05$); "↓", decreased; "↑", increased. Abbreviations: ALA, alpha-linolenic acid; ALT, alanine aminotransferase; ApoB, apolipoprotein B; APN, adiponectin; BMI, body mass index; BW, body weight; CK18-M30, cytokeratin 18 M30; EPA-E, ethyl-eicosapentanoic acid; FBG, fasting blood glucose; GGT, gamma-glutamyl transpeptidase; HbA_{1c}, glycosylated hemoglobin; HDL-c, high-density lipoprotein cholesterol; HOMA-IR, homeostatic model assessment of insulin resistance; IL-2, interleukin 2; LDL-c, low-density lipoprotein cholesterol; LSI, lifestyle intervention; ω-3 PUFA, ω-3 poliunsaturated fatty acids; TC, total cholesterol; TGs, triglycerides; TNF-α, tumor necrosis factor α; WC, waist circumference.

Short-term ω-3 PUFA supplementation may enhance the anti-inflammatory status of patients with T2D. In a 2012 RCT, Malekshahi et al. (2012) demonstrated that patients supplemented with 2.7 g of ω-3 PUFA/day (n = 42) exhibited significantly different levels of interleukin 2 and TNF-α after 8 weeks compared to placebo recipients (n = 42). No changes were observed in CRP concentration at the end of the study, which is likely the result of a small sample size [232].

In a 2016 double-blind RCT, 166 patients with T2D were randomized to receive either fish oil (2 g of ω-3 PUFA/day, n = 58), flaxseed oil (2.5 g of alpha-linolenic acid/day, n = 53), or corn oil (control, n = 65) for 180 days. Supplementation with ω-3 PUFA led to significant improvements in HbA_{1c}, TC, TC/HDL, and TG levels compared to the control group. No changes were observed regarding FBG, HOMA-IR, or FI. Flaxseed oil intake did not significantly influence any of the abovementioned parameters [233].

Wang et al. (2017) administered either 2.4 g/day of ω-3 PUFA or a placebo (corn oil) to 99 patients with T2D. After 6 months, significant improvements in TGs and HDL-c levels were observed in the ω-3 PUFA group (n = 49) compared to the placebo group (n = 50), although FBG, HbA_{1c}, HOMA-IR, insulin, TC, and LDL-c levels remained unchanged [234].

ω-3 PUFA anti-inflammatory activity was also investigated by Jacobo-Cejudo et al. (2017) in a RCT involving 54 patients with T2D. All study participants maintained a regular diet and medication during the 24-week trial. Results showed that glucose, TGs, and WC declined significantly only in the ω-3 PUFA group, while HbA_{1c} decreased significantly in both groups at the end of the study. In contrast, HOMA-IR and insulin levels increased significantly in all study participants. No significant changes were observed in other anthropometric indices (BMI, BW, WHR, BF%) or APN levels in either group [235]. In 2018, O'Mahoney et al. conducted the largest meta-analysis and meta-regression assessing the impact of ω-3 PUFA supplementation in T2D. This review, involving 45 RCTs (n = 2674), showed that ω-3 PUFA intake was associated with significant reductions in HbA_{1c}, LDL, and TG levels. In addition, ω-3 PUFA exhibited anti-inflammatory effects by decreasing both TNF-α and IL-6 concentrations. However, other markers related to glycemic control, lipid profile, and inflammatory status did not change following supplementation. The doses of ω-3 PUFA ranged from 0.4 to 18 g, while the duration of the intervention varied from 2 to 104 weeks [242].

Finally, a 2023 RCT involving patients with T2D treated with glimepiride led to significant improvements in FBG, HbA_{1c}, HOMA-IR, TC, TGs, LDL-c, and HDL-c levels following 12 weeks of ω-3 PUFA consumption (n = 35) compared to a placebo (n = 35) [236].

Clinical evidence in MASLD. Numerous RCTs and several SRMAs have evaluated the effects of ω-3 PUFA supplementation on liver function in patients with NAFLD (Table 13). In 2008, Spadaro et al. performed a RCT involving 36 patients with NAFLD who were treated with either 2 g of ω-3 PUFA/day and an American Heart Association (AHA) recommended diet (n = 18) or an AHA regular diet (n = 18). After 6 months, both groups experienced significant weight loss. In addition, significant decreases in levels of ALT, GGT, TGs, HOMA-IR, and TNF-α were observed in the ω-3 PUFA group, but not in the diet group. HDL concentration also improved after ω-3 PUFA intake. Full reversal of steatosis was observed in over one-third of the supplemented patients, while half of them exhibited an overall decrease in the severity of NAFLD. However, no complete regression of hepatic fat accumulation was noted with diet alone, although some improvements in the steatosis score occurred in almost 30% of participants [237].

In a 2012 SRMA of nine studies (n = 355), Parker et al. reported beneficial effects on liver fat and AST levels following ω-3 PUFA supplementation. ALT levels were not significantly decreased. Notably, when RCT data were considered, only the efficacy of ω-3 PUFA on liver fat content remained significant. The median dose of ω-3 PUFA was 4 g/day (0.8–13.7 g/day), and the median duration of treatment was 6 months (8 weeks–12 months) [243].

Seventy patients with NAFLD associated with hyperlipidemia were randomly allocated to consume ω-3 PUFA (n = 36, 4 g/d) or a placebo (n = 34) for 3 months in a 2015 double-blind RCT. ω-3 PUFA led to significant reductions in the levels of glucose, TC, TGs, ApoB, and the liver enzymes ALT and GGT compared to placebo recipients. Significant improvements in inflammation-related markers, specifically APN, TNF-α, and CK18-M30, were also observed after ω-3 PUFA supplementation. No significant differences between groups were noted regarding anthropometric indices, HOMA-IR, LDL, HDL-c, and hs-CRP levels [238].

A phase 2 RCT conducted in 2014 assessed the efficacy of ethyl-eicosapentanoic acid (EPA-E), a synthetic PUFA, in patients with NASH and significant NAFLD (n = 243). Study participants were administered a low dose of EPA-E (1800 mg/day), a high dose of EPA-E (2700 mg/day), or a placebo for 12 months. Results failed to show any significant improvements in NASH-related histopathology, liver enzymes, glycemic control, BW, hs-CRP, or APN levels. Nevertheless, TG concentrations were significantly reduced compared to the placebo group following high-dose EPA-E treatment [239].

In line with these results, Dasarathy et al. (2015) demonstrated that a daily intake of 3.6 g of ω-3 PUFA for 48 weeks led to no significant changes in BW, body composition, or liver enzyme levels in patients with well-controlled T2D and NASH. Moreover, at the end of the study period, ω-3 PUFA worsened glucose control and histological parameters compared to the placebo [240].

However, in their 2016 SRMA of seven RCTs involving 442 patients with NAFLD/NASH, He et al. showed that ω-3 PUFA supplementation is effective in improving the lipid profile, particularly TGs, but also TC and HDL-c levels, as well as ALT concentration. The doses of ω-3 PUFA used in the included trials varied between 0.83 and 6.4 g/day, and the duration of the studies ranged from 6 to 18 months [244].

Finally, one year of ω-3 PUFA treatment (3.6 g/day) led to a significant decrease in GGT levels in 30 patients with NAFLD and MS compared to placebo recipients (n = 30). Moreover, ω-3 PUFA seemed to promote liver fat reduction in patients who also experienced weight loss. According to the study's results, a significant association between BW decrease and liver fat reduction was observed, but only among the ω-3 PUFA-treated patients. However, BW or HFC did not change significantly in either group at the end of the intervention. Similarly, no changes in noninvasive NASH-related parameters or liver fibrosis scores were observed [241].

Safety. ω-3 PUFA intake has an excellent safety profile, with minimal to no long-term side effects, particularly following supplementation with a dose below the highest approved. Both the U.S. Food and Drug Administration and the EFSA consider ω-3 PUFA supplementation safe at doses up to 5 g/day [228]. However, doses greater than 3 g/day are likely to increase LDL-c levels, particularly in patients with hypertriglyceridemia [245].

Summary. Clinical evidence suggests that ω-3 PUFA may be an effective therapeutic adjuvant in T2D, as they exhibit a modest yet beneficial influence on glucose and lipid parameters. In MASLD, improvements in liver steatosis-related parameters and lipid profiles, particularly TGs, were also reported following ω-3 PUFA supplementation. However, its effectiveness in alleviating MASH features remains uncertain.

5. NBCs for GM Modulation in T2D and MASLD

A reduced Bacteroidetes-to-Firmicutes ratio has long been proposed as a marker for dysbiosis in individuals with obesity. However, this ratio may not adequately reflect the metabolic dysfunction in patients with T2D, since its increase was positively associated with reduced glucose tolerance [11,246]. The GM profile of patients with T2D exhibits a higher abundance of pathogenic and opportunistic Gram-negative microbes, including *Enterobacteriaceae, Clostridiales, E. coli, Bacteroides caccae, Prevotella copri,* and *Bacteroides vulgates.* Gram-negative bacteria (e.g., Bacteroidetes) are associated with high levels of LPS [11]. Moreover, several genera have been reported to have a consistent negative correlation with T2D, specifically *Bifidobacterium, Bacteroides, Faecalibacterium, Roseburia,* and *Akkermansia,* while *Ruminococcus, Fusobacterium,* and *Blautia* have been found to be increased in patients with T2D [246].

Compared to healthy individuals, patients with MASLD display increased levels of Proteobacteria, Enterobacteriaceae, *Escherichia,* and *Dorea* and decreased levels of Rikenellaceae, Ruminococaceae, *Faecalibacterium, Eubacterium,* and *Prevotella* [247]. Notably, there is a partial overlap between the MASLD-related GM profile and the GM dysbiotic signature described in T2D. For example, Proteobacteria has a higher prevalence in both T2D and MASLD patients [11,247], whereas low levels of *Faecalibacterium prausnitzii* are also reported in patients with T2D or obesity [248]. In addition, *Bacteroides vulgates,* which is reportedly increased in T2D, severe obesity, and IR, has also been shown to be abundant in patients with liver fibrosis [248].

GM acts as a key modulator of the host's physiology, partly through certain metabolites, such as SCFAs and LPS [58]. Altered levels of SCFAs (acetate, propionate, and butyrate) are pivotal in the onset and development of CMDs. For instance, a reduction in butyrate-producing species (*Roseburia intestinalis, Faecalibacterium prausnitzii*) is involved in the pathogenesis of T2D [11]. Elevated levels of LPS, a major outer wall component of Gram-negative bacteria, result in metabolic endotoxemia, triggering a state of low-grade inflammation and IR [58]. In the setting of endotoxemia, LPS promotes liver lipogenesis and augments intrahepatic inflammation [249].

LPS-binding protein (LPB) is an acute-phase protein that forms a complex with LPS and facilitates its binding to cellular receptors (TLR4/CD14), with the subsequent initiation of inflammatory signaling pathways. As such, LBP is involved in the regulation of immune responses by modulating inflammatory reactions induced by LPS. Whereas the role of LPS in the development of CMDs is well-known, the effects of LPB are not clear [249]. Some studies have reported increased circulating levels of LPB in obesity and obesity-related diseases, including T2D and MASLD [58,250,251], while others have not confirmed these findings [249].

Prebiotics

Prebiotics are nondigestible carbohydrates, polyunsaturated fatty acids, or polyphenols that can be converted to SCFAs [11]. SCFAs influence metabolic health by reducing IR, curbing appetite, decreasing lipolysis, and enhancing energy expenditure (Figure 3) [252].

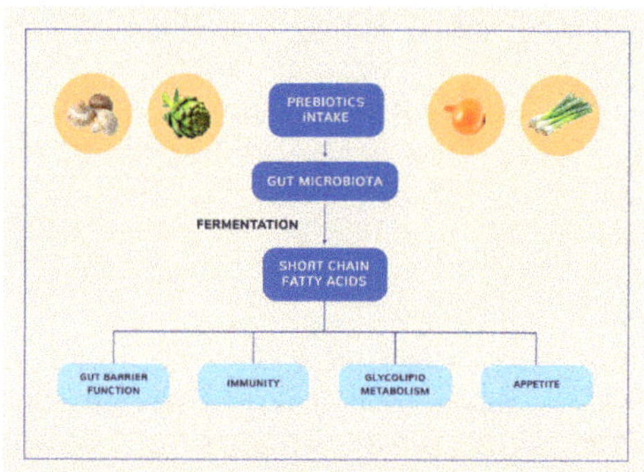

Figure 3. Impact of prebiotics on metabolic function via SCFAs [252].

The carbohydrate prebiotics include inulin, fructooligosaccharides (FOS), and galactooligosaccharides (GOS). Inulin and FOS are collectively known as ITFs. Prebiotics beneficially influence GM by increasing the number of *Lactobacillus* and/or *Bifidobacterium* species [253]. Indeed, studies on healthy adults have shown an increased bifidogenic effect at doses as low as 5 g of ITFs/day, with an optimal dose of 10 g/day [254]. However, in T2D, there is a complex interplay between prebiotics and GM, which is influenced not only by the dysbiosis that accompanies this condition but also by the effects of antidiabetic medication. Metformin, for instance, has antibiotic-like properties, altering GM independently of prebiotic intake and consequently confounding the results of clinical trials assessing the composition of gut bacteria in T2D [253]. Currently, only a limited number of interventional trials in T2D and MASLD have included GM-specific outcome measures following prebiotic supplementation (Table 14).

A 2014 study involving female patients with T2D demonstrated that compared to placebo, inulin supplementation (10 g/day for 8 weeks, n = 24) was effective in improving glycemic control and reducing plasma LPS levels [216]. In a second study by the same authors involving 52 women with T2D, 8 weeks of prebiotic supplementation (10 g/day of oligofructose-enriched inulin, n = 27) led to significant reductions in glucose metabolism parameters and inflammatory markers, including LPS, compared to placebo recipients [217].

Table 14. Summary of RCTs investigating the hypoglycemic, hypolipidemic, and anti-steatosis effects of prebiotics.

Disease	Participants (Total)	Intervention	Control	Duration	Main Outcomes */**	References
T2D	n = 49	Inulin 10 g/day	Placebo	8 weeks	↓ LPS *	[216,217]
T2D	n = 52	Inulin 10 g/day	Placebo	8 weeks	↓ LPS *	[217]
T2D	n = 29	GOS 5.5 g/day	Placebo	12 weeks	↑ bacterial diversity and richness **	[255]
T2D	n = 52	GOS 10 g/day	Placebo	4 weeks	↑ *Bifidobacteriaceae* *, ↓ *Peptostreptococcaceae, Ruminococcaceae, Lachnospiraceae, Porphyromonadaceae, Erysipelotrichaceea* **	[58]
Prediabetes	n = 44	GOS 15 g/day	Placebo	12 weeks	↑ *Bifidobacterium* *	[256]
T2D	n = 25	ITFs 16 g/day	Placebo	6 weeks	↑ *Bifidobacterium*, SCFAs *	[254]
T2D	n = 192	RS, OBG + diet	Placebo Diet	12 weeks	↑ *Roseburia faecis, Anaerostipes hadrus*, ↓ HbA_{1c} *	[257]
NASH	n = 14	ITF 8 g/day ITF 16 g/day	Placebo	12 weeks 24 weeks	↑ *Bifidobacterium*, ↓ *Clostridium* clusters XI and I, steatosis *	[258]
NAFLD	n = 19	ITF 16 g/day	Placebo	12 weeks	↑ *Bifidobacterium* *	[259]

* Statistically significant between groups ($p < 0.05$); ** Statistically significant from baseline ($p < 0.05$); "↓", decreased; "↑", increased. Abbreviations: GOS, galactooligosaccharides; HbA_{1c}, glycosylated hemoglobin; ITFs, inulin-type fructans; LPS, lipopolysaccharide; RS, resistant starch; OBG, oat beta-glucan; SCFAs, short-chain fatty acids.

Pedersen et al. (2016) conducted a RCT investigating the relationship among intestinal permeability, glucose control, and intestinal bacteria in men with well-controlled T2D (n = 29). Compared to a placebo, supplementation with a mixture of GOS (5.5 g/day for 12 weeks) had no significant effects on glucose tolerance or bacterial populations. Nevertheless, prebiotic-treated patients displayed a significant increase in microbial diversity and richness indices after the intervention. In addition, an inverse relationship between changes in *Veillonellaceae* and changes in both glucose response and IL-6 levels was reported. The authors argued that the lack of significant shifts in GM composition could be attributed to metformin use and high variability in T2D characteristics among the study participants [255].

Another RCT was performed by Gonai et al. (2017) involving 52 patients with T2D who were given either 10 g/day of GOS syrup (n = 27) or 10 g/day of a placebo (n = 25) for 1 month. The baseline assessment revealed that compared to healthy controls (n = 25), *Veillonellaceae* was significantly more abundant in the T2D group and was positively correlated with BMI, FBG, HbA_{1c}, TGs, and LBP. It was proposed that *Veillonellaceae* might play a role in the onset of glucose intolerance. In contrast, the abundance of *Bifidobacteriaceae, Clostridiales, Incertae sedis XIV*, and *Peptostreptococcaceae* were significantly lower in patients with T2D. Moreover, T2D patients also exhibited significantly lower microbial diversity compared to controls. However, while LPS were not detected in any study participant, LBP was significantly higher in patients with T2D and was also correlated with FBG and HbA_{1c} levels. No significant differences regarding IL-6, IL-10, and TNF-α were observed between T2D patients and healthy controls. Results showed that GOS supplementation led to a significant restoration of *Bifidobacteriaceae* abundance in patients with T2D but had no significant effect on LPB or glucose tolerance. Also, the levels of *Peptostreptococcaceae, Ruminococcaceae, Lachnospiraceae, Porphyromonadaceae*, and *Erysipelotrichaceae* significantly decreased compared to baseline after GOS intake. Both inflammatory and anti-inflammatory markers remained unchanged [58].

In 2017, Canfora et al. investigated the effect of supplementation with GOS (15 g/day for 12 weeks) versus a placebo on the GM composition and metabolic parameters of 44 individuals with excess weight and prediabetes. GOS supplementation led to a fivefold increase in the abundance of *Bifidobacterium* species. However, microbial richness and diversity were not significantly affected by prebiotic intake compared to the placebo group. In addition, no significant differences between the two groups were reported regarding the levels of fecal or plasma SCFAs or concentrations of incretins, gut hormones, insulin sensitivity, anthropometric indices, LBP, or other inflammatory markers (IL-6, IL-8, TNF-α) [256].

Birkeland et al. (2020) reported in a crossover RCT that 6-week supplementation with ITFs (16 g/day) led to a significant increase in bifidobacteria (*B. adolescentis*) and SCFAs in the feces of patients with T2D (n = 25) compared to a placebo. No effects on butyric acid or overall microbial diversity were observed [254].

A 2022 SRMA conducted by Ojo et al. revealed that, in patients with T2D, prebiotic supplementation led to a significant reduction in HbA_{1c} levels compared to the controls. Prebiotic intake was also associated with an increase in the relative abundance of beneficial bacteria, including *Bifidobacterium* and *Akkermansia*, although this increase was not statistically significant compared to the control group. Metformin, on the other hand, decreased *Bifidobacterium* but increased *Lactobacillus* and *Akkermansia*; however, these changes were not significantly different compared to those in the control groups. Neither prebiotics nor oral antidiabetic medication exerted significant effects on BMI, FBG, or PBG compared to the controls [252].

Finally, in a 2023 12-week double-blind placebo-controlled RCT, 192 participants with T2D were assigned to receive either a prebiotic fiber-rich supplement (n = 95), a placebo fiber-absent supplement (n = 48), or dietary advice alone (n = 49). All study participants were asked to follow nutritional recommendations. The fiber-based supplement featured a mixture of resistant starch (RS) and oat beta-glucan, which may attenuate postprandial glycemic response. Pivotal bacterial species involved in RS degradation to enhance butyrate-producing species include *Ruminococcus bromii* and *Bifidobacterium* ssp. (primary degraders) and *Clostridia* clusters IV and XIVa (secondary degraders). The results showed no significant changes in microbial composition (alpha diversity) at the end of the study in either group. Compared to the diet-managed patients, the relative abundance of RS primary degraders increased in the prebiotic-treated patients, but not significantly. Instead, there was a significant increase in the relative abundance of secondary degraders, specifically butyrate-producing bacteria (*Roseburia faecis* and *Anaerostipes hadrus*) after prebiotic intake. Also, HbA_{1c} levels and BW were significantly reduced after supplementation in the prebiotic-treated group versus the placebo group. Since FBG levels showed no significant changes either within or between groups after 12 weeks, and weight loss was rather modest, the authors suggested that glycemic control was improved, probably due to attenuation of PBG and other factors [257].

Only two studies specifically investigated the effects of prebiotic supplementation on GM in patients with NAFLD/NASH (Table 14). In a 2019 pilot clinical trial, Bomhof et al. demonstrated that the administration of oligofructose (8 g/day for 12 weeks followed by 16 g/day for 24 weeks, n = 8) compared to a placebo (n = 6) led to improved liver steatosis and an improved overall NAS score, independently of weight loss, in patients with NASH. However, no changes in liver enzyme levels (ALT, ALP, GGT) or glycemic indices were observed after the intervention. IL-6 and TNF-α concentrations decreased after prebiotic consumption, but not significantly compared to the placebo group. Oligofructose has also been shown to enhance *Bifidobacterium* and decrease microorganisms within *Clostridium* clusters XI and I. While the beneficial bifidogenic effect is well-documented, the implications of reduced bacteria from *Clostridium* clusters XI and I in NASH are not clear [258].

Reshef et al. (2024) investigated the effect of prebiotic supplementation on liver function, fecal GM, metabolism, and inflammation in patients with NAFLD and MS. All study participants were advised to follow a weight-maintenance diet. Patients supplemented with 16 g of ITFs/day for 12 weeks (n = 8) exhibited a significant increase in *Bifidobacterium* compared to placebo recipients (n = 11). However, no other significant changes were observed regarding hepatic (liver enzymes—ALT, AST, GGT—or HFC), metabolic (FBG, HbA_{1c}, HOMA-IR, insulin, TC, TGs, LDL-c, HDL-c), or inflammatory markers (CRP) between the two groups. Notably, patients' weight did not fluctuate throughout the course of the study. The authors concluded that prebiotics, in the absence of weight loss, may not alleviate NAFLD-related outcomes [259].

Safety. There are no safety-related concerns regarding the intake of ITFs and GOS [260,261]. ITFs are well tolerated in dosages up to 20 g/day [260], while the recommended dose for GOS ranges from 8 to 15 g/day. Higher intakes may lead to gastrointestinal discomfort, flatulence, diarrhea, or cramping [261].

Summary. So far, prebiotics possess great potential as an approach to ameliorate metabolic dysfunction in T2D and MASLD via GM modulation. However, although evidence regarding their beneficial health effects is accumulating, there is still insufficient clinical data, and the results of available studies are less conclusive.

6. Conclusions

NBCs have sparked significant interest in recent decades, with evidence highlighting their role in improving glycemic control, lipid profile, and liver function by providing powerful antioxidant and anti-inflammatory benefits. Our findings show that certain NBCs, particularly BBR, CRM, soluble fibers, and omega-3 fatty acids, have substantial evidence regarding their efficacy and safety in the management of T2D and MASLD. The ability of NBCs to counteract metabolic dysfunction positions them as a promising adjunct therapy to conventional treatment, as well as candidates for new drug development. Future well-designed investigations are needed to deepen our understanding of NBCs' specific action mechanisms, determine optimal dosage and intervention duration, and optimize their therapeutic potential in T2D and MASLD.

Author Contributions: Conceptualization, D.C. and A.F.C.; methodology, D.C. and L.G.; writing—original draft preparation, D.C., A.F.C. and R.B.; writing—review and editing, R.B., L.G., D.M. and L.F.; supervision, D.M. and L.F. All authors have read and agreed to the published version of the manuscript.

Funding: This research received no external funding.

Conflicts of Interest: The authors declare no conflicts of interest.

References

1. Ruze, R.; Liu, T.; Zou, X.; Song, J.; Chen, Y.; Xu, R.; Yin, X.; Xu, Q. Obesity and type 2 diabetes mellitus: Connections in epidemiology, pathogenesis, and treatments. *Front. Endocrinol.* **2023**, *21*, 1161521. [CrossRef]
2. Younossi, Z.M.; Golabi, P.; Paik, J.M.; Henry, A.; Van Dongen, C.; Henry, L. The global epidemiology of nonalcoholic fatty liver disease (NAFLD) and nonalcoholic steatohepatitis (NASH): A systematic review. *Hepatology* **2023**, *77*, 1335–1347. [CrossRef] [PubMed]
3. DeFronzo, R.A.; Ferrannini, E.; Groop, L.; Henry, R.R.; Herman, W.H.; Holst, J.J.; Hu, F.B.; Roland Kahn, C.; Raz, I.; Shulman, I.G.; et al. Type 2 diabetes mellitus. *Nat. Rev. Dis. Primers* **2015**, *23*, 15019. [CrossRef] [PubMed]
4. Einarson, T.R.; Ludwig, C.; Panton, U.H. Prevalence of cardiovascular disease in type 2 diabetes: A systematic literature review of scientific evidence from across the world in 2007–2017. *Cardiovasc. Diabetol.* **2018**, *17*, 83. [CrossRef]
5. Low Wang, C.C.; Hess, C.N.; Hiatt, W.R.; Goldfine, A.B. Clinical Update: Cardiovascular Disease in Diabetes Mellitus. *Circulation* **2016**, *133*, 2459–2502. [CrossRef]
6. Samy, A.M.; Kandeil, M.A.; Sabry, D.; Abdel-Ghany, A.A.; Mahmoud, M.O. From NAFLD to NASH: Understanding the spectrum of non-alcoholic liver diseases and their consequences. *Heliyon* **2024**, *10*, e30387. [CrossRef] [PubMed]
7. Targher, G.; Corey, K.E.; Byrne, C.D.; Roden, M. The complex link between NAFLD and type 2 diabetes mellitus—Mechanisms and treatments. *Nat. Rev. Gastroenterol. Hepatol.* **2021**, *18*, 599–612. [CrossRef]

8. Targher, G.; Lonardo, A.; Byrne, C.D. Nonalcoholic fatty liver disease and chronic vascular complications of diabetes mellitus. *Nat. Rev. Endocrinol.* **2018**, *14*, 99–114. [CrossRef] [PubMed]
9. Barton Duell, P.; Welty, F.K.; Miller, M.; Hammond, G.; Ahmad, Z.; Cohen, D.E.; Horton, J.D.; Pressman, G.S.; Toth, P.P. Nonalcoholic Fatty Liver Disease and Cardiovascular Risk: A Scientific Statement From the American Heart Association. *Arterioscler. Thromb. Vasc. Biol.* **2022**, *42*, E168–E185. [CrossRef]
10. Mellemkjær, A.; Kjær, M.B.; Haldrup, D.; Grønbæk, H.; Thomsen, K.L. Management of cardiovascular risk in patients with metabolic dysfunction-associated steatotic liver disease. *Eur. J. Intern. Med.* **2024**, *122*, 28–34. [CrossRef]
11. Crudele, L.; Gadaleta, R.M.; Cariello, M.; Moschetta, A. Gut microbiota in the pathogenesis and therapeutic approaches of diabetes. *eBioMedicine* **2023**, *97*, 104821. [CrossRef] [PubMed]
12. Fianchi, F.; Liguori, A.; Gasbarrini, A.; Grieco, A.; Miele, L. Nonalcoholic Fatty Liver Disease (NAFLD) as Model of Gut–Liver Axis Interaction: From Pathophysiology to Potential Target of Treatment for Personalized Therapy. *Int. J. Mol. Sci.* **2021**, *22*, 6485. [CrossRef]
13. Stefan, N.; Yki-Järvinen, H.; Neuschwander-Tetri, B.A. Metabolic dysfunction-associated steatotic liver disease: Heterogeneous pathomechanisms and effectiveness of metabolism-based treatment. *Lancet Diabetes Endocrinol.* **2024**, *13*, 134–148. [CrossRef]
14. Rinella, M.E.; Lazarus, J.V.; Ratziu, V.; Francque, S.M.; Sanyal, A.J.; Kanwal, F.; Romero, D.; Abdelmalek, M.F.; Anstee, Q.M.; Arab, J.P.; et al. NAFLD Nomenclature consensus group. A multisociety Delphi consensus statement on new fatty liver disease nomenclature. *Hepatology* **2023**, *78*, 1966–1986. [CrossRef]
15. Shang, Y.; Grip, E.T.; Modica, A.; Skröder, H.; Ström, O.; Ntanios, F.; Gudbjörnsdottir, S.; Hagström, H. Metabolic Syndrome Traits Increase the Risk of Major Adverse Liver Outcomes in Type 2 Diabetes. *Diabetes Care* **2024**, *47*, 978–985. [CrossRef]
16. Zhou, Y.Y.; Zhou, X.D.; Wu, S.J.; Hu, X.Q.; Tang, B.; Poucke, S.V.; Pan, X.Y.; Wu, W.J.; Gu, X.M.; Fu, S.W.; et al. Synergistic increase in cardiovascular risk in diabetes mellitus with nonalcoholic fatty liver disease: A meta-analysis. *Eur. J. Gastroenterol. Hepatol.* **2018**, *30*, 631–636. [CrossRef] [PubMed]
17. Ferguson, D.; Finck, B.N. Emerging therapeutic approaches for the treatment of NAFLD and type 2 diabetes mellitus. *Nat. Rev. Endocrinol.* **2021**, *17*, 484–495. [CrossRef] [PubMed]
18. Shahzad, N.; Alzahrani, A.R.; Aziz Ibrahim, I.A.; Shahid, I.; Alanazi, I.M.; Falemban, A.H.; Imam, M.T.; Mohsin, N.; Azlina, M.F.N.; Arulselvan, P. Therapeutic strategy of biological macromolecules based natural bioactive compounds of diabetes mellitus and future perspectives: A systematic review. *Heliyon* **2024**, *10*, e24207. [CrossRef] [PubMed]
19. Stahel, P.; Xiao, C.; Hegele, R.A.; Lewis, G.F. The Atherogenic Dyslipidemia Complex and Novel Approaches to Cardiovascular Disease Prevention in Diabetes. *Can. J. Cardiol.* **2018**, *34*, 595–604. [CrossRef] [PubMed]
20. Leiter, L.A.; Lundman, P.; da Silva, P.M.; Drexel, H.; Jünger, C.; Gitt, A.K. Persistent lipid abnormalities in statin-treated patients with diabetes mellitus in Europe and Canada: Results of the Dyslipidaemia International Study. *Diabet. Med.* **2011**, *28*, 1343–1351. [CrossRef]
21. Katzmann, J.L.; Stürzebecher, P.E.; Kruppert, S.; Laufs, U. LDL cholesterol target attainment in cardiovascular high- and very-high-risk patients with statin intolerance: A simulation study. *Sci. Rep.* **2024**, *14*, 474. [CrossRef] [PubMed]
22. Fappa, E.; Yannakoulia, M.; Pitsavos, C.; Skoumas, I.; Valourdou, S.; Stefanadis, C. Lifestyle intervention in the management of metabolic syndrome: Could we improve adherence issues? *Nutrition* **2008**, *24*, 286–291. [CrossRef] [PubMed]
23. Grundy, S.M. Drug therapy of the metabolic syndrome: Minimizing the emerging crisis in polypharmacy. *Nat. Rev. Drug Discov.* **2006**, *5*, 295–309. [CrossRef]
24. Chew, N.W.S.; Ng, C.H.; Tan, D.J.H.; Kong, G.; Lin, C.; Chin, Y.H.; Lim, W.H.; Huang, D.Q.; Quek, J.; Fu, C.E.; et al. The global burden of metabolic disease: Data from 2000 to 2019. *Cell Metab.* **2023**, *35*, 414–428.e3. [CrossRef]
25. Eslam, M.; Valenti, L.; Romeo, S. Genetics and epigenetics of NAFLD and NASH: Clinical impact. *J. Hepatol.* **2018**, *68*, 268–279. [CrossRef]
26. DeFronzo, R.A. Insulin resistance, lipotoxicity, type 2 diabetes and atherosclerosis: The missing links. The Claude Bernard Lecture 2009. *Diabetologia* **2010**, *53*, 1270–1287. [CrossRef]
27. Godoy-Matos, A.F.; Silva Júnior, W.S.; Valerio, C.M. NAFLD as a continuum: From obesity to metabolic syndrome and diabetes. *Diabetol. Metab. Syndr.* **2020**, *12*, 60. [CrossRef] [PubMed]
28. Bellavite, P.; Fazio, S.; Affuso, F. A Descriptive Review of the Action Mechanisms of Berberine, Quercetin and Silymarin on Insulin Resistance/Hyperinsulinemia and Cardiovascular Prevention. *Molecules* **2023**, *28*, 4491. [CrossRef] [PubMed]
29. Fazakerley, D.J.; Krycer, J.R.; Kearney, A.L.; Hocking, S.L.; James, D.E. Muscle and adipose tissue insulin resistance: Malady without mechanism? *J. Lipid Res.* **2019**, *60*, 1720–1732. [CrossRef] [PubMed]
30. Petersen, M.C.; Shulman, G.I. Mechanisms of Insulin Action and Insulin Resistance. *Physiol. Rev.* **2018**, *98*, 2133–2223. [CrossRef]
31. Mota, M.; Banini, B.A.; Cazanave, S.C.; Sanyal, A.J. Molecular mechanisms of lipotoxicity and glucotoxicity in nonalcoholic fatty liver disease. *Metabolism* **2016**, *65*, 1049–1061. [CrossRef] [PubMed]
32. Stumvoll, M.; Goldstein, B.J.; Van Haeften, T.W. Type 2 diabetes: Principles of pathogenesis and therapy. *Lancet* **2005**, *365*, 1333–1346. [CrossRef] [PubMed]

33. Merz, K.E.; Thurmond, D.C. Role of Skeletal Muscle in Insulin Resistance and Glucose Uptake. *Compr. Physiol.* **2020**, *10*, 785–809. [CrossRef] [PubMed]
34. da Silva Rosa, S.C.; Nayak, N.; Caymo, A.M.; Gordon, J.W. Mechanisms of muscle insulin resistance and the cross-talk with liver and adipose tissue. *Physiol. Rep.* **2020**, *8*, e14607. [CrossRef] [PubMed]
35. Heni, M. The insulin resistant brain: Impact on whole-body metabolism and body fat distribution. *Diabetologia* **2024**, *67*, 1181–1191. [CrossRef] [PubMed]
36. Klein, S.; Gastaldelli, A.; Yki-Järvinen, H.; Scherer, P.E. Why does obesity cause diabetes? *Cell Metab.* **2022**, *34*, 11–20. [CrossRef]
37. Nogueira, J.P.; Cusi, K. Role of insulin resistance in the development of nonalcoholic fatty liver disease in people with type 2 diabetes: From bench to patient care. *Diabetes Spectr.* **2024**, *37*, 20–28. [CrossRef]
38. Esler, W.P.; Cohen, D.E. Pharmacologic inhibition of lipogenesis for the treatment of NAFLD. *J. Hepatol.* **2024**, *80*, 362–377. [CrossRef]
39. Gallego-Durán, R.; Albillos, A.; Ampuero, J.; Arechederra, M.; Bañares, R.; Blas-García, A.; Berná, G.; Caparrós, E.; Delgado, T.C.; Falcón-Pérez, J.M.; et al. Metabolic-associated fatty liver disease: From simple steatosis toward liver cirrhosis and potential complications. Proceedings of the Third Translational Hepatology Meeting, organized by the Spanish Association for the Study of the Liver (AEEH). *Gastroenterol. Hepatol.* **2022**, *45*, 724–734. [CrossRef]
40. Ola, M.S. Reduced Tyrosine and Serine-632 Phosphorylation of Insulin Receptor Substrate-1 in the Gastrocnemius Muscle of Obese Zucker Rat. *Curr. Issues Mol. Biol.* **2022**, *44*, 6015–6027. [CrossRef]
41. Li, M.; Chi, X.; Wang, Y.; Setrerrahmane, S.; Xie, W.; Xu, H. Trends in insulin resistance: Insights into mechanisms and therapeutic strategy. *Signal Transduct. Target. Ther.* **2022**, *7*, 216. [CrossRef] [PubMed]
42. Lira, F.S.; Rosa, J.C.; Pimentel, G.D.; Seelaender, M.; Damaso, A.R.; Oyama, L.M.; do Nascimento, C.O. Both adiponectin and interleukin-10 inhibit LPS-induced activation of the NF-κB pathway in 3T3-L1 adipocytes. *Cytokine* **2012**, *57*, 98–106. [CrossRef] [PubMed]
43. Engin, A. Adiponectin-Resistance in Obesity. *Adv. Exp. Med. Biol.* **2017**, *960*, 415–441. [CrossRef] [PubMed]
44. Hotamisligil, G.S. Inflammation and metabolic disorders. *Nature* **2006**, *444*, 860–867. [CrossRef]
45. Sykiotis, G.P.; Papavassiliou, A.G. Serine Phosphorylation of Insulin Receptor Substrate-1: A Novel Target for the Reversal of Insulin Resistance. *Mol. Endocrinol.* **2001**, *15*, 1864–1869. [CrossRef] [PubMed]
46. Rohm, T.V.; Meier, D.T.; Olefsky, J.M.; Donath, M.Y. Inflammation in obesity, diabetes, and related disorders. *Immunity* **2022**, *55*, 31–55. [CrossRef]
47. Goldberg, R.B. Cytokine and cytokine-like inflammation markers, endothelial dysfunction, and imbalanced coagulation in development of diabetes and its complications. *J. Clin. Endocrinol. Metab.* **2009**, *94*, 3171–3182. [CrossRef]
48. Yaribeygi, H.; Sathyapalan, T.; Atkin, S.L.; Sahebkar, A. Molecular Mechanisms Linking Oxidative Stress and Diabetes Mellitus. *Oxid. Med. Cell. Longev.* **2020**, *9*, 8609213. [CrossRef]
49. Wang, J.; Jiang, Y.; Jin, L.; Qian, C.; Zuo, W.; Lin, J.; Xie, L.; Jin, B.; Zhao, Y.; Huang, L.; et al. Alantolactone attenuates high-fat diet-induced inflammation and oxidative stress in non-alcoholic fatty liver disease. *Nutr. Diabetes* **2024**, *14*, 41. [CrossRef]
50. Volpe, C.M.O.; Villar-Delfino, P.H.; dos Anjos, P.M.F.; Nogueira-Machado, J.A. Cellular death, reactive oxygen species (ROS) and diabetic complications. *Cell Death Dis.* **2018**, *9*, 119. [CrossRef]
51. Poitout, V.; Robertson, P. Minireview: Secondary β-Cell Failure in Type 2 Diabetes—A Convergence of Glucotoxicity and Lipotoxicity. *Endocrinology* **2002**, *143*, 339–342. [CrossRef] [PubMed]
52. Lee, H.M.; Kim, J.J.; Kim, H.J.; Shong, M.; Ku, B.J.; Jo, E.K. Upregulated NLRP3 inflammasome activation in patients with type 2 diabetes. *Diabetes* **2013**, *62*, 194–204. [CrossRef]
53. Dixit, V.D. Nlrp3 Inflammasome Activation in Type 2 Diabetes: Is It Clinically Relevant? *Diabetes* **2013**, *62*, 22–24. [CrossRef] [PubMed]
54. Menini, S.; Iacobini, C.; Vitale, M.; Pugliese, G. The Inflammasome in Chronic Complications of Diabetes and Related Metabolic Disorders. *Cells* **2020**, *9*, 1812. [CrossRef]
55. Anand, S.; Mande, S.S. Host-microbiome interactions: Gut-Liver axis and its connection with other organs. *NPJ Biofilms Microbiomes* **2022**, *8*, 89. [CrossRef] [PubMed]
56. Nawrot, M.; Peschard, S.; Lestavel, S.; Staels, B. Intestine-liver crosstalk in type 2 diabetes and non-alcoholic fatty liver disease. *Metabolism* **2021**, *123*, 154844. [CrossRef] [PubMed]
57. Martín-Mateos, R.; Albillos, A. The Role of the Gut-Liver Axis in Metabolic Dysfunction-Associated Fatty Liver Disease. *Front. Immunol.* **2021**, *12*, 660179. [CrossRef] [PubMed]
58. Gonai, M.; Shigehisa, A.; Kigawa, I.; Kurasaki, K.; Chonan, O.; Matsuki, T.; Yoshida, Y.; Aida, M.; Hamano, C.; Terauchi, Y. Galacto-oligosaccharides ameliorate dysbiotic Bifidobacteriaceae decline in Japanese patients with type 2 diabetes. *Benef. Microbes* **2017**, *8*, 705–716. [CrossRef]
59. Lee, G.; You, H.J.; Bajaj, J.S.; Joo, S.K.; Yu, J.; Park, S.; Kang, H.; Park, J.H.; Kim, J.H.; Lee, D.H.; et al. Distinct signatures of gut microbiome and metabolites associated with significant fibrosis in non-obese NAFLD. *Nat. Commun.* **2020**, *11*, 4982. [CrossRef]

60. Abouelkheir, M.; Taher, I.; Eladl, A.S.R.; Shabaan, D.A.; Soliman, M.F.M.; Taha, A.E. Detection and Quantification of Some Ethanol-Producing Bacterial Strains in the Gut of Mouse Model of Non-Alcoholic Fatty Liver Disease: Role of Metformin. *Pharmaceuticals* **2023**, *16*, 658. [CrossRef]
61. Sharma, B.R.; Jaiswal, S.; Ravindra, P.V. Modulation of gut microbiota by bioactive compounds for prevention and management of type 2 diabetes. *Biomed. Pharmacother.* **2022**, *152*, 113148. [CrossRef]
62. Dixit, V.; Joseph Kamal, S.W.; Bajrang Chole, P.; Dayal, D.; Chaubey, K.K.; Pal, A.K.; Xavier, J.; Manjunath, B.T.; Bachheti, R.K. Functional Foods: Exploring the Health Benefits of Bioactive Compounds from Plant and Animal Sources. *J. Food Qual.* **2023**, *2023*, 5546753. [CrossRef]
63. Noce, A.; Di Lauro, M.; Di Daniele, F.; Pietroboni Zaitseva, A.; Marrone, G.; Borboni, P.; Di Daniele, N. Natural Bioactive Compounds Useful in Clinical Management of Metabolic Syndrome. *Nutrients* **2021**, *13*, 630. [CrossRef] [PubMed]
64. Figueiredo, P.S.; Inada, A.C.; Fernandes, M.R.; Arakaki, D.G.; De Cássia Freitas, K.; De Cássia Avellaneda Guimarães, R.; do Nascimento, V.A.; Hiane, P.A. An overview of novel dietary supplements and food ingredients in patients with metabolic syndrome and non-alcoholic fatty liver disease. *Molecules* **2018**, *23*, 877. [CrossRef] [PubMed]
65. Guo, J.; Chen, H.; Zhang, X.; Lou, W.; Zhang, P.; Qiu, Y.; Zhang, C.; Wang, Y.; Liu, W.J. The Effect of Berberine on Metabolic Profiles in Type 2 Diabetic Patients: A Systematic Review and Meta-Analysis of Randomized Controlled Trials. *Oxid. Med. Cell. Longev.* **2021**, *2021*, 2074610. [CrossRef] [PubMed]
66. Shrivastava, S.; Sharma, A.; Saxena, N.; Bhamra, R.; Kumar, S. Addressing the preventive and therapeutic perspective of berberine against diabetes. *Heliyon* **2023**, *9*, e21233. [CrossRef] [PubMed]
67. Xie, W.; Su, F.; Wang, G.; Peng, Z.; Xu, Y.; Zhang, Y.; Xu, Y.; Zhang, Y.; Xu, N.; Hou, C.; et al. Glucose-lowering effect of berberine on type 2 diabetes: A systematic review and meta-analysis. *Front. Pharmacol.* **2022**, *16*, 1015045. [CrossRef]
68. Yin, J.; Xing, H.; Ye, J. Efficacy of berberine in patients with type 2 diabetes mellitus. *Metabolism* **2008**, *57*, 712–717. [CrossRef]
69. Zhang, H.; Wei, J.; Xue, R.; Wu, J.D.; Zhao, W.; Wang, Z.Z.; Zhou, Z.X.; Song, D.Q.; Wang, Y.M.; Pan, H.N.; et al. Berberine lowers blood glucose in type 2 diabetes mellitus patients through increasing insulin receptor expression. *Metabolism* **2010**, *59*, 285–292. [CrossRef] [PubMed]
70. Gu, Y.; Zhang, Y.; Shi, X.; Li, X.; Hong, J.; Chen, J.; Gu, W.; Lu, X.; Xu, G.; Ning, G. Effect of traditional Chinese medicine berberine on type 2 diabetes based on comprehensive metabonomics. *Talanta* **2010**, *81*, 766–772. [CrossRef] [PubMed]
71. Di Pierro, F.; Putignano, P.; Montesi, L.; Moscatiello, S.; Marchesini Reggiani, G.; Villanova, N. Preliminary study about the possible glycemic clinical advantage in using a fixed combination of *Berberis aristata* and *Silybum marianum* standardized extracts versus only *Berberis aristata* in patients with type 2 diabetes. *Clin. Pharmacol.* **2013**, *19*, 167–174. [CrossRef] [PubMed]
72. Di Pierro, F.; Bellone, I.; Rapacioli, G.; Putignano, P. Clinical role of a fixed combination of standardized *Berberis aristata* and *Silybum marianum* extracts in diabetic and hypercholesterolemic patients intolerant to statins. *Diabetes Metab. Syndr. Obes.* **2015**, *8*, 89–96. [CrossRef]
73. Dai, P.; Wang, J.; Lin, L.; Zhang, Y.; Wang, Z. Renoprotective effects of berberine as adjuvant therapy for hypertensive patients with type 2 diabetes mellitus: Evaluation via biochemical markers and color Doppler ultrasonography. *Exp. Ther. Med.* **2015**, *10*, 869–876. [CrossRef]
74. Yan, H.M.; Xia, M.F.; Wang, Y.; Chang, X.X.; Yao, X.Z.; Rao, S.X.; Zeng, M.S.; Tu, Y.F.; Feng, R.; Jia, W.P.; et al. Efficacy of Berberine in Patients with Non-Alcoholic Fatty Liver Disease. *PLoS ONE* **2015**, *10*, e0134172. [CrossRef] [PubMed]
75. Chang, X.; Wang, Z.; Zhang, J.; Yan, H.; Bian, H.; Xia, M.; Lin, H.; Jiang, J.; Gao, X. Lipid profiling of the therapeutic effects of berberine in patients with nonalcoholic fatty liver disease. *J. Transl. Med.* **2016**, *14*, 266. [CrossRef] [PubMed]
76. Harrison, S.A.; Gunn, N.; Neff, G.W.; Kohli, A.; Liu, L.; Flyer, A.; Goldkind, L.; di Bisceglie, A.M. A phase 2, proof of concept, randomised controlled trial of berberine ursodeoxycholate in patients with presumed non-alcoholic steatohepatitis and type 2 diabetes. *Nat. Commun.* **2021**, *12*, 5503. [CrossRef]
77. Koperska, A.; Moszak, M.; Seraszek-Jaros, A.; Bogdanski, P.; Szulinska, M. Does berberine impact anthropometric, hepatic, and metabolic parameters in patients with metabolic dysfunction-associated fatty liver disease? Randomized, double-blind placebo-controlled trial. *J. Physiol. Pharmacol.* **2024**, *75*, 291–302. [CrossRef]
78. Kong, W.J.; Wei, J.; Zuo, Z.Y.; Wang, Y.M.; Song, D.Q.; You, X.F.; Zhao, L.X.; Pan, H.N.; Jiang, J.D. Combination of simvastatin with berberine improves the lipid-lowering efficacy. *Metabolism* **2008**, *57*, 1029–1037. [CrossRef] [PubMed]
79. Schmidt, A.F.; Carter, J.P.L.; Pearce, L.S.; Wilkins, J.T.; Overington, J.P.; Hingorani, A.D.; Casas, J.P. PCSK9 monoclonal antibodies for the primary and secondary prevention of cardiovascular disease. *Cochrane Database Syst. Rev.* **2020**, *2020*, CD011748. [CrossRef]
80. He, N.Y.; Li, Q.; Wu, C.Y.; Ren, Z.; Gao, Y.; Pan, L.H.; Wang, M.M.; Wen, H.Y.; Jiang, Z.S.; Tang, Z.H.; et al. Lowering serum lipids via PCSK9-targeting drugs: Current advances and future perspectives. *Acta Pharmacol. Sin.* **2017**, *38*, 301–311. [CrossRef] [PubMed]
81. Nie, Q.; Li, M.; Huang, C.; Yuan, Y.; Liang, Q.; Ma, X.; Qiu, T.; Li, J. The clinical efficacy and safety of berberine in the treatment of non-alcoholic fatty liver disease: A meta-analysis and systematic review. *J. Transl. Med.* **2024**, *22*, 225. [CrossRef] [PubMed]

82. Pivari, F.; Mingione, A.; Brasacchio, C.; Soldati, L. Curcumin and Type 2 Diabetes Mellitus: Prevention and Treatment. *Nutrients* **2019**, *11*, 1837. [CrossRef]
83. Panahi, Y.; Khalili, N.; Sahebi, E.; Namazi, S.; Reiner, Ž.; Majeed, M.; Sahebkar, A. Curcuminoids modify lipid profile in type 2 diabetes mellitus: A randomized controlled trial. *Complement. Ther. Med.* **2017**, *33*, 1–5. [CrossRef]
84. Asghari, K.M.; Saleh, P.; Salekzamani, Y.; Dolatkhah, N.; Aghamohammadzadeh, N.; Hashemian, M. The effect of curcumin and high-content eicosapentaenoic acid supplementations in type 2 diabetes mellitus patients: A double-blinded randomized clinical trial. *Nutr. Diabetes* **2024**, *14*, 14. [CrossRef]
85. Na, L.X.; Li, Y.; Pan, H.Z.; Zhou, X.L.; Sun, D.J.; Meng, M.; Li, X.X.; Sun, C.H. Curcuminoids exert glucose-lowering effect in type 2 diabetes by decreasing serum free fatty acids: A double-blind, placebo-controlled trial. *Mol. Nutr. Food Res.* **2013**, *57*, 1569–1577. [CrossRef] [PubMed]
86. Rahimi, H.R.; Hooshang Mohammadpour, A.; Dastani, M.; Jaafari, M.R.; Abnous, K.; Mobarhan, M.G.; Oskuee, R.K. The effect of nano-curcumin on HbA1c, fasting blood glucose, and lipid profile in diabetic subjects: A randomized clinical trial. *Avicenna J. Phytomed.* **2016**, *6*, 567–577.
87. Yaikwawong, M.; Jansarikit, L.; Jirawatnotai, S.; Chuengsamarn, S. Curcumin extract improves beta cell functions in obese patients with type 2 diabetes: A randomized controlled trial. *Nutr. J.* **2024**, *23*, 119. [CrossRef] [PubMed]
88. Yaikwawong, M.; Jansarikit, L.; Jirawatnotai, S.; Chuengsamarn, S. The Effect of Curcumin on Reducing Atherogenic Risks in Obese Patients with Type 2 Diabetes: A Randomized Controlled Trial. *Nutrients* **2024**, *16*, 2441. [CrossRef]
89. Rahmani, S.; Asgary, S.; Askari, G.; Keshvari, M.; Hatamipour, M.; Feizi, A.; Sahebkar, A. Treatment of Non-alcoholic Fatty Liver Disease with Curcumin: A Randomized Placebo-controlled Trial. *Phytother. Res.* **2016**, *30*, 1540–1548. [CrossRef] [PubMed]
90. Saadati, S.; Sadeghi, A.; Mansour, A.; Yari, Z.; Poustchi, H.; Hedayati, M.; Hatami, B.; Hekmatdoost, A. Curcumin and inflammation in non-alcoholic fatty liver disease: A randomized, placebo controlled clinical trial. *BMC Gastroenterol.* **2019**, *19*, 133. [CrossRef] [PubMed]
91. Naseri, K.; Saadati, S.; Yari, Z.; Askari, B.; Mafi, D.; Hoseinian, P.; Asbaghi, O.; Hekmatdoost, A.; de Courten, B. Curcumin Offers No Additional Benefit to Lifestyle Intervention on Cardiometabolic Status in Patients with Non-Alcoholic Fatty Liver Disease. *Nutrients* **2022**, *14*, 3224. [CrossRef] [PubMed]
92. Sharifi, S.; Bagherniya, M.; Khoram, Z.; Ebrahimi Varzaneh, A.; Atkin, S.L.; Jamialahmadi, T.; Sahebkar, A.; Askari, G. Efficacy of curcumin plus piperine co-supplementation in moderate-to-high hepatic steatosis: A double-blind, randomized, placebo-controlled clinical trial. *Phytother. Res.* **2023**, *37*, 2217–2229. [CrossRef]
93. Pathomwichaiwat, T.; Jinatongthai, P.; Prommasut, N.; Ampornwong, K.; Rattanavipanon, W.; Nathisuwan, S.; Thakkinstian, A. Effects of turmeric (*Curcuma longa*) supplementation on glucose metabolism in diabetes mellitus and metabolic syndrome: An umbrella review and updated meta-analysis. *PLoS ONE* **2023**, *18*, e0288997. [CrossRef] [PubMed]
94. Molani-Gol, R.; Dehghani, A.; Rafraf, M. Effects of curcumin/turmeric supplementation on the liver enzymes, lipid profiles, glycemic index, and anthropometric indices in non-alcoholic fatty liver patients: An umbrella meta-analysis. *Phytother. Res.* **2024**, *38*, 539–555. [CrossRef]
95. Servida, S.; Panzeri, E.; Tomaino, L.; Marfia, G.; Garzia, E.; Appiani, G.C.; Moroncini, G.; De Gennaro Colonna, V.; La Vecchia, C.; Vigna, L. Overview of Curcumin and Piperine Effects on Glucose Metabolism: The Case of an Insulinoma Patient's Loss of Consciousness. *Int. J. Mol. Sci.* **2023**, *24*, 6621. [CrossRef] [PubMed]
96. Gu, W.; Geng, J.; Zhao, H.; Li, X.; Song, G. Effects of Resveratrol on Metabolic Indicators in Patients with Type 2 Diabetes: A Systematic Review and Meta-Analysis. *Int. J. Clin. Pract.* **2022**, *2022*, 9734738. [CrossRef] [PubMed]
97. Bhatt, J.K.; Thomas, S.; Nanjan, M.J. Resveratrol supplementation improves glycemic control in type 2 diabetes mellitus. *Nutr. Res.* **2012**, *32*, 537–541. [CrossRef] [PubMed]
98. Thazhath, S.S.; Wu, T.; Bound, M.J.; Checklin, H.L.; Standfield, S.; Jones, K.L.; Horowitz, M.; Rayner, C.K. Administration of resveratrol for 5 wk has no effect on glucagon-like peptide 1 secretion, gastric emptying, or glycemic control in type 2 diabetes: A randomized controlled trial. *Am. J. Clin. Nutr.* **2016**, *103*, 66–70. [CrossRef]
99. Timmers, S.; de Ligt, M.; Phielix, E.; van de Weijer, T.; Hansen, J.; Moonen-Kornips, E.; Schaart, G.; Kunz, I.; Hesselink, M.K.C.; Schrauven-Hinderling, V.B. Resveratrol as Add-on Therapy in Subjects With Well-Controlled Type 2 Diabetes: A Randomized Controlled Trial. *Diabetes Care* **2016**, *39*, 2211–2217. [CrossRef] [PubMed]
100. Bo, S.; Ponzo, V.; Ciccone, G.; Evangelista, A.; Saba, F.; Goitre, I.; Procopio, M.; Pagano, G.F.; Cassader, M.; Gambino, R. Six months of resveratrol supplementation has no measurable effect in type 2 diabetic patients. A randomized, double blind, placebo-controlled trial. *Pharmacol. Res.* **2016**, *111*, 896–905. [CrossRef] [PubMed]
101. Hoseini, A.; Namazi, G.; Farrokhian, A.; Reiner, Ž.; Aghadavod, E.; Bahmani, F.; Asemi, Z. The effects of resveratrol on metabolic status in patients with type 2 diabetes mellitus and coronary heart disease. *Food Funct.* **2019**, *10*, 6042–6051. [CrossRef]
102. Mahjabeen, W.; Khan, D.A.; Mirza, S.A. Role of resveratrol supplementation in regulation of glucose hemostasis, inflammation and oxidative stress in patients with diabetes mellitus type 2: A randomized, placebo-controlled trial. *Complement. Ther. Med.* **2022**, *66*, 102819. [CrossRef]

103. Chachay, V.S.; Macdonald, G.A.; Martin, J.H.; Whitehead, J.P.; O'Moore–Sullivan, T.M.; Lee, P.; Franklin, M.; Klein, K.; Taylor, P.J.; Ferguson, M.; et al. Resveratrol Does Not Benefit Patients With Nonalcoholic Fatty Liver Disease. *Clin. Gastroenterol. Hepatol.* **2014**, *12*, 2092–2103.e6. [CrossRef]
104. Faghihzadeh, F.; Adibi, P.; Hekmatdoost, A. The effects of resveratrol supplementation on cardiovascular risk factors in patients with non-alcoholic fatty liver disease: A randomised, double-blind, placebo-controlled study. *Br. J. Nutr.* **2015**, *114*, 796–803. [CrossRef] [PubMed]
105. Chen, S.; Zhao, X.; Ran, L.; Wan, J.; Wang, X.; Qin, Y.; Shu, F.; Gao, Y.; Yuan, L.; Zhang, Q.; et al. Resveratrol improves insulin resistance, glucose and lipid metabolism in patients with non-alcoholic fatty liver disease: A randomized controlled trial. *Dig. Liver Dis.* **2015**, *47*, 226–232. [CrossRef] [PubMed]
106. Heebøll, S.; Kreuzfeldt, M.; Hamilton-Dutoit, S.; Kjær Poulsen, M.; Stødkilde-Jørgensen, H.; Møller, H.J.; Jessesn, N.; Thorsen, K.; Hellberg, Y.K.; Pedersen, S.B.; et al. Placebo-controlled, randomised clinical trial: High-dose resveratrol treatment for non-alcoholic fatty liver disease. *Scand. J. Gastroenterol.* **2016**, *51*, 456–464. [CrossRef] [PubMed]
107. Rafiee, S.; Mohammadi, H.; Ghavami, A.; Sadeghi, E.; Safari, Z.; Askari, G. Efficacy of resveratrol supplementation in patients with nonalcoholic fatty liver disease: A systematic review and meta-analysis of clinical trials. *Complement. Ther. Clin. Pract.* **2021**, *42*, 101281. [CrossRef]
108. Zeraattalab-Motlagh, S.; Jayedi, A.; Shab-Bidar, S. The effects of resveratrol supplementation in patients with type 2 diabetes, metabolic syndrome, and nonalcoholic fatty liver disease: An umbrella review of meta-analyses of randomized controlled trials. *Am. J. Clin. Nutr.* **2021**, *114*, 1675–1685. [CrossRef]
109. Shaito, A.; Posadino, A.M.; Younes, N.; Hasan, H.; Halabi, S.; Alhababi, D.; Al-Mohannadi, A.; Abdel-Rahman, W.M.; Eid, A.H.; Nasrallah, G.N.; et al. Potential Adverse Effects of Resveratrol: A Literature Review. *Int. J. Mol. Sci.* **2020**, *21*, 2084. [CrossRef] [PubMed]
110. Khoo, H.E.; Azlan, A.; Tang, S.T.; Lim, S.M. Anthocyanidins and anthocyanins: Colored pigments as food, pharmaceutical ingredients, and the potential health benefits. *Food Nutr. Res.* **2017**, *61*, 1361779. [CrossRef] [PubMed]
111. Mao, T.; Akshit, F.N.U.; Mohan, M.S. Effects of anthocyanin supplementation in diet on glycemic and related cardiovascular biomarkers in patients with type 2 diabetes: A systematic review and meta-analysis of randomized controlled trials. *Front. Nutr.* **2023**, *10*, 1199815. [CrossRef] [PubMed]
112. Kianbakht, S.; Abasi, B.; Dabaghian, F.H. Anti-hyperglycemic effect of Vaccinium arctostaphylos in type 2 diabetic patients: A randomized controlled trial. *Forsch. Komplementmed.* **2013**, *20*, 17–22. [CrossRef] [PubMed]
113. Li, D.; Zhang, Y.; Liu, Y.; Sun, R.; Xia, M. Purified Anthocyanin Supplementation Reduces Dyslipidemia, Enhances Antioxidant Capacity, and Prevents Insulin Resistance in Diabetic Patients. *J. Nutr.* **2015**, *145*, 742–748. [CrossRef]
114. Yang, L.; Ling, W.; Qiu, Y.; Liu, Y.; Wang, L.; Yang, J.; Wang, C.; Ma, J. Anthocyanins increase serum adiponectin in newly diagnosed diabetes but not in prediabetes: A randomized controlled trial. *Nutr. Metab.* **2020**, *17*, 78. [CrossRef] [PubMed]
115. Stote, K.S.; Wilson, M.M.; Hallenbeck, D.; Thomas, K.; Rourke, J.M.; Sweeney, M.I.; Gottschall-Pass, K.T.; Gosmanov, A.R. Effect of Blueberry Consumption on Cardiometabolic Health Parameters in Men with Type 2 Diabetes: An 8-Week, Double-Blind, Randomized, Placebo-Controlled Trial. *Curr. Dev. Nutr.* **2020**, *4*, nzaa030. [CrossRef] [PubMed]
116. Chan, S.W.; Chu, T.T.W.; Choi, S.W.; Benzie, I.F.F.; Tomlinson, B. Impact of short-term bilberry supplementation on glycemic control, cardiovascular disease risk factors, and antioxidant status in Chinese patients with type 2 diabetes. *Phytother. Res.* **2021**, *35*, 3236–3245. [CrossRef] [PubMed]
117. Nikbakht, E.; Singh, I.; Vider, J.; Williams, L.T.; Vugic, L.; Gaiz, A.; Kundur, A.R.; Colson, N. Potential of anthocyanin as an anti-inflammatory agent: A human clinical trial on type 2 diabetic, diabetic at-risk and healthy adults. *Inflamm. Res.* **2021**, *70*, 275–284. [CrossRef] [PubMed]
118. Chang, H.C.; Peng, C.H.; Yeh, D.M.; Kao, E.S.; Wang, C.J. Hibiscus sabdariffa extract inhibits obesity and fat accumulation, and improves liver steatosis in humans. *Food Funct.* **2014**, *5*, 734. [CrossRef]
119. Zhang, P.W.; Chen, F.X.; Li, D.; Ling, W.H.; Guo, H.H. A CONSORT-Compliant, Randomized, Double-Blind, Placebo-Controlled Pilot Trial of Purified Anthocyanin in Patients with Nonalcoholic Fatty Liver Disease. *Medicine* **2015**, *94*, e758. [CrossRef]
120. Sangsefidi, Z.S.; Yarhosseini, F.; Hosseinzadeh, M.; Ranjbar, A.; Akhondi-Meybodi, M.; Fallahzadeh, H.; Mozaffari-Khosravi, H. The effect of (*Cornus mas* L.) fruit extract on liver function among patients with nonalcoholic fatty liver: A double-blind randomized clinical trial. *Phytother. Res.* **2021**, *35*, 5259–5268. [CrossRef]
121. Bayram, H.M.; Iliaz, R.; Gunes, F.E. Effects of *Cornus mas* L. on anthropometric and biochemical parameters among metabolic associated fatty liver disease patients: Randomized clinical trial. *J. Ethnopharmacol.* **2024**, *318*, 117068. [CrossRef]
122. Khan, N.N.; Zurayyir, E.J.; Almuslem, M.Y.; Alshamrani, R.; Alamri, R.A.; Sulaimani, G.H.T.; Sulimani, M.H.T.; Albalawi, M.S.F.; Alqahani, R.M.A.; Alanazi, E.M.; et al. Anthocyanins as Adjuvant Treatment for Non-alcoholic Fatty Liver Disease: A Systematic Review and Meta-Analysis. *Cureus* **2024**, *16*, e63445. [CrossRef]
123. Frumuzachi, O.; Kieserling, H.; Rohn, S.; Mocan, A.; Crișan, G. The Impact of Cornelian Cherry (*Cornus mas* L.) on Cardiometabolic Risk Factors: A Meta-Analysis of Randomised Controlled Trials. *Nutrients* **2024**, *16*, 2173. [CrossRef] [PubMed]

124. Gonçalves, A.C.; Nunes, A.R.; Falcão, A.; Alves, G.; Silva, L.R. Dietary Effects of Anthocyanins in Human Health: A Comprehensive Review. *Pharmaceuticals* **2021**, *14*, 690. [CrossRef] [PubMed]
125. Liu, C.Y.; Huang, C.J.; Huang, L.H.; Chen, I.J.; Chiu, J.P.; Hsu, C.H. Effects of Green Tea Extract on Insulin Resistance and Glucagon-Like Peptide 1 in Patients with Type 2 Diabetes and Lipid Abnormalities: A Randomized, Double-Blinded, and Placebo-Controlled Trial. *PLoS ONE* **2014**, *9*, e91163. [CrossRef] [PubMed]
126. Mozaffari-Khosravi, H.; Ahadi, Z.; Fallah, T.M. The Effect of Green Tea versus Sour Tea on Insulin Resistance, Lipids Profiles and Oxidative Stress in Patients with Type 2 Diabetes Mellitus: A Randomized Clinical Trial. *Iran. J. Med. Sci.* **2014**, *39*, 424–432. [PubMed]
127. Nagao, T.; Meguro, S.; Hase, T.; Otsuka, K.; Komikado, M.; Tokimitsu, I.; Yamamoto, T.; Yamamoto, K. A Catechin-rich Beverage Improves Obesity and Blood Glucose Control in Patients with Type 2 Diabetes. *Obesity* **2009**, *17*, 310–317. [CrossRef]
128. Hsu, C.H.; Liao, Y.L.; Lin, S.C.; Tsai, T.H.; Huang, C.J.; Chou, P. Does supplementation with green tea extract improve insulin resistance in obese type 2 diabetics? A randomized, double-blind, and placebo-controlled clinical trial. *Altern. Med. Rev.* **2011**, *16*, 157–163.
129. Mousavi, A.; Vafa, M.; Neyestani, T.; Khamseh, M.; Hoseini, F. The effects of green tea consumption on metabolic and anthropometric indices in patients with Type 2 diabetes. *J. Res. Med. Sci.* **2013**, *18*, 1080–1086. [PubMed]
130. Bazyar, H.; Hosseini, S.A.; Saradar, S.; Mombaini, D.; Allivand, M.; Labibzadeh, M.; Alipour, M. Effects of epigallocatechin-3-gallate of *Camellia sinensis* leaves on blood pressure, lipid profile, atherogenic index of plasma and some inflammatory and antioxidant markers in type 2 diabetes mellitus patients: A clinical trial. *J. Complement. Integr. Med.* **2020**, *18*, 405–411. [CrossRef]
131. Yazdanpanah, Z.; Salehi-Abargouei, A.; Mozaffari, Z.; Hemayati, R. The effect of green tea (*Camellia sinensis*) on lipid profiles and renal function in people with type 2 diabetes and nephropathy: A randomized controlled clinical trial. *Front. Nutr.* **2023**, *10*, 1253275. [CrossRef] [PubMed]
132. Asbaghi, O.; Fouladvand, F.; Gonzalez, M.J.; Ashtary-Larky, D.; Choghakhori, R.; Abbasnezhad, A. Effect of green tea on glycemic control in patients with type 2 diabetes mellitus: A systematic review and meta-analysis. *Diabetes Metab. Syndr.* **2021**, *15*, 23–31. [CrossRef] [PubMed]
133. Sakata, R.; Nakamura, T.; Torimura, T.; Ueno, T.; Sata, M. Green tea with high-density catechins improves liver function and fat infiltration in non-alcoholic fatty liver disease (NAFLD) patients: A double-blind placebo-controlled study. *Int. J. Mol. Med.* **2013**, *32*, 989–994. [CrossRef] [PubMed]
134. Pezeshki, A.; Safi, S.; Feizi, A.; Askari, G.; Karami, F. The effect of green tea extract supplementation on liver enzymes in patients with nonalcoholic fatty liver disease. *Int. J. Prev. Med.* **2016**, *1*, 28. [CrossRef]
135. Tabatabaee, S.M.; Alavian, S.M.; Ghalichi, L.; Miryounesi, S.M.; Mousavizadeh, K.; Jazayeri, S.; Vafa, M.R. Green Tea in Non-Alcoholic Fatty Liver Disease: A Double Blind Randomized Clinical Trial. *Hepat. Mon.* **2017**, *17*, 949746. [CrossRef]
136. Hussain, M.; Rehman, H.U.; Akhtar, L. Therapeutic benefits of green tea extract on various parameters in non-alcoholic fatty liver disease patients. *Pak. J. Med. Sci.* **2017**, *33*, 931–936. [CrossRef]
137. Mahmoodi, M.; Hosseini, R.; Kazemi, A.; Ofori-Asenso, R.; Mazidi, M.; Mazloomi, S.M. Effects of green tea or green tea catechin on liver enzymes in healthy individuals and people with nonalcoholic fatty liver disease: A systematic review and meta-analysis of randomized clinical trials. *Phytother. Res.* **2020**, *34*, 1587–1598. [CrossRef] [PubMed]
138. Isomura, T.; Suzuki, S.; Origasa, H.; Hosono, A.; Suzuki, M.; Sawada, T.; Terao, S.; Muto, Y.; Koga, T. Liver-related safety assessment of green tea extracts in humans: A systematic review of randomized controlled trials. *Eur. J. Clin. Nutr.* **2016**, *70*, 1340. [CrossRef] [PubMed]
139. Younes, M.; Aggett, P.; Aguilar, F.; Crebelli, R.; Dusemund, B.; Filipič, M.; Frutos, M.J.; Galtier, P.; Gott, D.; Gundert-Remy, U.; et al. Scientific opinion on the safety of green tea catechins. *EFSA J.* **2018**, *16*, e05239. [CrossRef]
140. Ebrahimi-Mameghani, M.; Asghari-Jafarabadi, M.; Rezazadeh, K. TCF7L2-rs7903146 polymorphism modulates the effect of artichoke leaf extract supplementation on insulin resistance in metabolic syndrome: A randomized, double-blind, placebo-controlled trial. *J. Integr. Med.* **2018**, *16*, 329–334. [CrossRef] [PubMed]
141. Osama, H.; Hamed, E.O.; Mahmoud, M.A.; Abdelrahim, M.E.A. The Effect of Hesperidin and Diosmin Individually or in Combination on Metabolic Profile and Neuropathy among Diabetic Patients with Metabolic Syndrome: A Randomized Controlled Trial. *J. Diet. Suppl.* **2023**, *20*, 749–762. [CrossRef] [PubMed]
142. Inoue, T.; Yoshida, K.; Sasaki, E.; Aizawa, K.; Kamioka, H. Effect of Lycopene Intake on the Fasting Blood Glucose Level: A Systematic Review with Meta-Analysis. *Nutrients* **2022**, *15*, 122. [CrossRef] [PubMed]
143. Panahi, Y.; Kianpour, P.; Mohtashami, R.; Atkin, S.L.; Butler, A.E.; Jafari, R.; Badeli, R.; Sahebkar, A. Efficacy of artichoke leaf extract in non-alcoholic fatty liver disease: A pilot double-blind randomized controlled trial. *Phytother. Res.* **2018**, *32*, 1382–1387. [CrossRef] [PubMed]
144. Al-Aubaidy, H.A.; Dayan, A.; Deseo, M.A.; Itsiopoulos, C.; Jamil, D.; Hadi, N.R.; Thomas, C.J. Twelve-Week Mediterranean Diet Intervention Increases Citrus Bioflavonoid Levels and Reduces Inflammation in People with Type 2 Diabetes Mellitus. *Nutrients* **2021**, *13*, 1133. [CrossRef]

145. Fallah Huseini, H.; Kianbakht, S.; Heshmat, R. Cynara scolymus L. in Treatment of Hypercholesterolemic Type 2 Diabetic Patients: A Randomized Double-Blind Placebo-Controlled Clinical Trial. *J. Med. Plants* **2012**, *11*, 58–65.
146. Upritchard, J.E.; Sutherland, W.H.; Mann, J.I. Effect of supplementation with tomato juice, vitamin E, and vitamin C on LDL oxidation and products of inflammatory activity in type 2 diabetes. *Diabetes Care* **2000**, *23*, 733–738. [CrossRef] [PubMed]
147. Homayouni, F.; Haidari, F.; Hedayati, M.; Zakerkish, M.; Ahmadi, K. Blood pressure lowering and anti-inflammatory effects of hesperidin in type 2 diabetes; a randomized double-blind controlled clinical trial. *Phytother. Res.* **2018**, *32*, 1073–1079. [CrossRef] [PubMed]
148. Yari, Z.; Movahedian, M.; Imani, H.; Alavian, S.M.; Hedayati, M.; Hekmatdoost, A. The effect of hesperidin supplementation on metabolic profiles in patients with metabolic syndrome: A randomized, double-blind, placebo-controlled clinical trial. *Eur. J. Nutr.* **2020**, *59*, 2569–2577. [CrossRef] [PubMed]
149. Rangboo, V.; Noroozi, M.; Zavoshy, R.; Rezadoost, S.A.; Mohammadpoorasl, A. The Effect of Artichoke Leaf Extract on Alanine Aminotransferase and Aspartate Aminotransferase in the Patients with Nonalcoholic Steatohepatitis. *Int. J. Hepatol.* **2016**, *2016*, 4030476. [CrossRef]
150. Musolino, V.; Gliozzi, M.; Bombardelli, E.; Nucera, S.; Carresi, C.; Maiuolo, J.; Mollace, R.; Paone, S.; Bosco, F.; Scarano, F.; et al. The synergistic effect of Citrus bergamia and Cynara cardunculus extracts on vascular inflammation and oxidative stress in non-alcoholic fatty liver disease. *J. Tradit. Complement. Med.* **2020**, *10*, 268–274. [CrossRef]
151. Cheraghpour, M.; Imani, H.; Ommi, S.; Alavian, S.M.; Karimi-Shahrbabak, E.; Hedayati, M.; Yari, Z.; Hekmatdoost, A. Hesperidin improves hepatic steatosis, hepatic enzymes, and metabolic and inflammatory parameters in patients with nonalcoholic fatty liver disease: A randomized, placebo-controlled, double-blind clinical trial. *Phytother. Res.* **2019**, *33*, 2118–2125. [CrossRef]
152. Yari, Z.; Cheraghpour, M.; Alavian, S.M.; Hedayati, M.; Eini-Zinab, H.; Hekmatdoost, A. The efficacy of flaxseed and hesperidin on non-alcoholic fatty liver disease: An open-labeled randomized controlled trial. *Eur. J. Clin. Nutr.* **2021**, *75*, 99–111. [CrossRef] [PubMed]
153. Shams-Rad, S.; Mohammadi, M.; Ramezani-Jolfaie, N.; Zarei, S.; Mohsenpour, M.; Salehi-Abargouei, A. Hesperidin supplementation has no effect on blood glucose control: A systematic review and meta-analysis of randomized controlled clinical trials. *Br. J. Clin. Pharmacol.* **2020**, *86*, 13–22. [CrossRef] [PubMed]
154. Mirarchi, A.; Mare, R.; Musolino, V.; Nucera, S.; Mollace, V.; Pujia, A.; Montalcini, T.; Romeo, S.; Maurotti, S. Bergamot Polyphenol Extract Reduces Hepatocyte Neutral Fat by Increasing Beta-Oxidation. *Nutrients* **2022**, *14*, 3434. [CrossRef]
155. Moradi, S.; Shokri-Mashhadi, N.; Saraf-Bank, S.; Mohammadi, H.; Zobeiri, M.; Clark, C.C.T.; Rouhani, M.H. The effects of Cynara scolymus L. supplementation on liver enzymes: A systematic review and meta-analysis. *Int. J. Clin. Pract.* **2021**, *75*, e14726. [CrossRef]
156. Salem, M.B.; Affes, H.; Ksouda, K.; Dhouibi, R.; Sahnoun, Z.; Hammami, S.; Zeghal, K.M. Pharmacological Studies of Artichoke Leaf Extract and Their Health Benefits. *Plant Foods Hum. Nutr.* **2015**, *70*, 441–453. [CrossRef] [PubMed]
157. Tufail, T.; Bader, U.l.; Ain, H.; Noreen, S.; Ikram, A.; Arshad, M.T.; Abdullahi, M.A. Nutritional Benefits of Lycopene and Beta-Carotene: A Comprehensive Overview. *Food Sci. Nutr.* **2024**, *12*, 8715–8741. [CrossRef] [PubMed]
158. Tayal, R.; Munjal, K.; Gauttam, V.K.; Popli, P.; Khurana, L.; Neeraj, C. Potential role of hesperidin in lifestyle disorders: A scoping review. *S. Afr. J. Bot.* **2023**, *161*, 542–554. [CrossRef]
159. Hadi, A.; Pourmasoumi, M.; Mohammadi, H.; Symonds, M.; Miraghajani, M. The effects of silymarin supplementation on metabolic status and oxidative stress in patients with type 2 diabetes mellitus: A systematic review and meta-analysis of clinical trials. *Complement. Ther. Med.* **2018**, *41*, 311–319. [CrossRef] [PubMed]
160. Abenavoli, L.; Izzo, A.A.; Milić, N.; Cicala, C.; Santini, A.; Capasso, R. Milk thistle (*Silybum marianum*): A concise overview on its chemistry, pharmacological, and nutraceutical uses in liver diseases. *Phytother. Res.* **2018**, *32*, 2202–2213. [CrossRef]
161. Huseini, H.F.; Larijani, B.; Heshmat, R.; Fakhrzadeh, H.; Radjabipour, B.; Toliat, T.; Raza, M. The efficacy of *Silybum marianum* (L.) Gaertn. (silymarin) in the treatment of type II diabetes: A randomized, double-blind, placebo-controlled, clinical trial. *Phytother. Res.* **2006**, *20*, 1036–1039. [CrossRef]
162. Ebrahimpour Koujan, S.; Gargari, B.P.; Mobasseri, M.; Valizadeh, H.; Asghari-Jafarabadi, M. Effects of *Silybum marianum* (L.) Gaertn. (silymarin) extract supplementation on antioxidant status and hs-CRP in patients with type 2 diabetes mellitus: A randomized, triple-blind, placebo-controlled clinical trial. *Phytomedicine* **2015**, *22*, 290–296. [CrossRef] [PubMed]
163. Ebrahimpour-Koujan, S.; Gargari, B.P.; Mobasseri, M.; Valizadeh, H.; Asghari-Jafarabadi, M. Lower glycemic indices and lipid profile among type 2 diabetes mellitus patients who received novel dose of *Silybum marianum* (L.) Gaertn. (silymarin) extract supplement: A triple-blinded randomized controlled clinical trial. *Phytomedicine* **2018**, *15*, 39–44. [CrossRef]
164. Ghalandari, K.; Shabani, M.; Khajehlandi, A.; Mohammadi, A. Effect of aerobic training with silymarin consumption on glycemic indices and liver enzymes in men with type 2 diabetes. *Arch. Physiol. Biochem.* **2023**, *129*, 76–81. [CrossRef]
165. Ferdowsi, S.; Shidfar, F.; Heidari, I.; Kashi, M.; Sohouli, M.H.; Sarrafi Zadeh, S. Effect of silymarin on lipid profile and glycemic control in patients with type 2 diabetes mellitus. *Phytother. Res.* **2024**, *38*, 4667–4674. [CrossRef] [PubMed]

166. Aller, R.; Izaola, O.; Gómez, S.; Tafur, C.; González, G.; Berroa, E.; Mora, N.; González, J.M.; de Luis, D.A. Effect of silymarin plus vitamin E in patients with non-alcoholic fatty liver disease.A randomized clinical pilot study. *Eur. Rev. Med. Pharmacol. Sci.* **2015**, *19*, 3118–3124. [PubMed]
167. Anushiravani, A.; Haddadi, N.; Pourfarmanbar, M.; Mohammadkarimi, V. Treatment options for nonalcoholic fatty liver disease: A double-blinded randomized placebo-controlled trial. *Eur. J. Gastroenterol. Hepatol.* **2019**, *31*, 613–617. [CrossRef]
168. Wah Kheong, C.; Nik Mustapha, N.R.; Mahadeva, S. A Randomized Trial of Silymarin for the Treatment of Nonalcoholic Steatohepatitis. *Clin. Gastroenterol. Hepatol.* **2017**, *15*, 1940–1949.e8. [CrossRef]
169. Jin, Y.; Wang, X.; Chen, K.; Chen, Y.; Zhou, L.; Zeng, Y.; Zhou, Y.; Pan, Z.; Wang, D.; Li, Z.; et al. Silymarin decreases liver stiffness associated with gut microbiota in patients with metabolic dysfunction-associated steatotic liver disease: A randomized, double-blind, placebo-controlled trial. *Lipids Health Dis.* **2024**, *23*, 239. [CrossRef] [PubMed]
170. de Avelar, C.R.; Pereira, E.M.; de Farias Costa, P.R.; de Jesus, R.P.; de Oliveira, L.P.M. Effect of silymarin on biochemical indicators in patients with liver disease: Systematic review with meta-analysis. *World J. Gastroenterol.* **2017**, *23*, 5004. [CrossRef]
171. Voroneanu, L.; Nistor, I.; Dumea, R.; Apetrii, M.; Covic, A. Silymarin in Type 2 Diabetes Mellitus: A Systematic Review and Meta-Analysis of Randomized Controlled Trials. *J. Diabetes Res.* **2016**, *2016*, 5147468. [CrossRef]
172. Costello, R.B.; Dwyer, J.T.; Saldanha, L.; Bailey, R.L.; Merkel, J.; Wambogo, E. Do Cinnamon Supplements Have a Role in Glycemic Control in Type 2 Diabetes? A Narrative Review. *J. Acad. Nutr. Diet.* **2016**, *116*, 1794–1802. [CrossRef] [PubMed]
173. Gruenwald, J.; Freder, J.; Armbruester, N. Cinnamon and health. *Crit. Rev. Food Sci. Nutr.* **2010**, *50*, 822–834. [CrossRef] [PubMed]
174. Khan, A.; Safdar, M.; Ali Khan, M.M.; Khattak, K.N.; Anderson, R.A. Cinnamon Improves Glucose and Lipids of People with Type 2 Diabetes. *Diabetes Care* **2003**, *26*, 3215–3218. [CrossRef] [PubMed]
175. Akilen, R.; Tsiami, A.; Devendra, D.; Robinson, N. Glycated haemoglobin and blood pressure-lowering effect of cinnamon in multi-ethnic Type 2 diabetic patients in the UK: A randomized, placebo-controlled, double-blind clinical trial. *Diabet. Med.* **2010**, *27*, 1159–1167. [CrossRef]
176. Lu, T.; Sheng, H.; Wu, J.; Cheng, Y.; Zhu, J.; Chen, Y. Cinnamon extract improves fasting blood glucose and glycosylated hemoglobin level in Chinese patients with type 2 diabetes. *Nutr. Res.* **2012**, *32*, 408–412. [CrossRef] [PubMed]
177. Vafa, M.; Mohammadi, F.; Shidfar, F.; Sormaghi, M.S.; Heidari, I.; Golestan, B.; Amiri, F. Effects of Cinnamon Consumption on Glycemic Status, Lipid Profile and Body Composition in Type 2 Diabetic Patients. *Int. J. Prev. Med.* **2012**, *3*, 531–536. [PubMed]
178. Zare, R.; Nadjarzadeh, A.; Zarshenas, M.M.; Shams, M.; Heydari, M. Efficacy of cinnamon in patients with type II diabetes mellitus: A randomized controlled clinical trial. *Clin. Nutr.* **2019**, *38*, 549–556. [CrossRef]
179. Davari, M.; Hashemi, R.; Mirmiran, P.; Hedayati, M.; Sahranavard, S.; Bahreini, S.; Tavakoly, R.; Talaei, B. Effects of cinnamon supplementation on expression of systemic inflammation factors, NF-kB and Sirtuin-1 (SIRT1) in type 2 diabetes: A randomized, double blind, and controlled clinical trial. *Nutr. J.* **2020**, *19*, 1. [CrossRef]
180. Askari, F.; Rashidkhani, B.; Hekmatdoost, A. Cinnamon may have therapeutic benefits on lipid profile, liver enzymes, insulin resistance, and high-sensitivity C-reactive protein in nonalcoholic fatty liver disease patients. *Nutr. Res.* **2014**, *34*, 143–148. [CrossRef]
181. Santos, H.O.; da Silva, G.A.R. To what extent does cinnamon administration improve the glycemic and lipid profiles? *Clin. Nutr. ESPEN* **2018**, *27*, 1–9. [CrossRef] [PubMed]
182. de Moura, S.L.; Gomes, B.G.R.; Guilarducci, M.J.; Coelho, O.G.L.; Guimarães, N.S.; Gomes, J.M.G. Effects of cinnamon supplementation on metabolic biomarkers in individuals with type 2 diabetes: A systematic review and meta-analysis. *Nutr. Rev.* **2025**, *83*, 249–279. [CrossRef] [PubMed]
183. Gu, D.T.; Tung, T.H.; Jiesisibieke, Z.L.; Chien, C.W.; Liu, W.Y. Safety of Cinnamon: An Umbrella Review of Meta-Analyses and Systematic Reviews of Randomized Clinical Trials. *Front. Pharmacol.* **2022**, *18*, 790901. [CrossRef]
184. Vajdi, M.; Noshadi, N.; Bonyadian, A.; Golpour-Hamedani, S.; Alipour, B.; Pourteymour Fard Tabrizi, F.; Abbasalizad-Farhangi, M.; Askari, G. Therapeutic effect of fenugreek supplementation on type 2 diabetes mellitus: A systematic review and meta-analysis of clinical trials. *Heliyon* **2024**, *10*, e36649. [CrossRef] [PubMed]
185. Gupta, A.; Gupta, R.; Lal, B. Effect of Trigonella foenum-graecum (fenugreek) seeds on glycaemic control and insulin resistance in type 2 diabetes mellitus: A double-blind placebo-controlled study. *J. Assoc. Physicians India* **2001**, *49*, 1057–1061.
186. Lu, F.-r.; Shen, L.; Qin, Y.; Gao, L.; Li, H.; Dai, Y. Clinical observation on trigonella foenum-graecum L. total saponins in combination with sulfonylureas in the treatment of type 2 diabetes mellitus. *Chin. J. Integr. Med.* **2008**, *14*, 56–60. [CrossRef]
187. Rafraf, M.; Malekiyan, M.; Asghari-Jafarabadi, M.; Aliasgarzadeh, A. Effect of Fenugreek Seeds on Serum Metabolic Factors and Adiponectin Levels in Type 2 Diabetic Patients. *Int. J. Vitam. Nutr. Res.* **2014**, *84*, 0196–0205. [CrossRef] [PubMed]
188. Najdi, R.A.; Hagras, M.M.; Kamel, F.O.; Magadmi, R.M. A randomized controlled clinical trial evaluating the effect of Trigonella foenum-graecum (fenugreek) versus glibenclamide in patients with diabetes. *Afr. Health Sci.* **2019**, *19*, 1594. [CrossRef]
189. Geberemeskel, G.A.; Debebe, Y.G.; Nguse, N.A. Antidiabetic Effect of Fenugreek Seed Powder Solution (*Trigonella foenum-graecum* L.) on Hyperlipidemia in Diabetic Patients. *J. Diabetes Res.* **2019**, *2019*, 8507453. [CrossRef] [PubMed]

190. Hadi, A.; Arab, A.; Hajianfar, H.; Talaei, B.; Miraghajani, M.; Babajafari, S.; Marx, W.; Tavakoly, R. The effect of fenugreek seed supplementation on serum irisin levels, blood pressure, and liver and kidney function in patients with type 2 diabetes mellitus: A parallel randomized clinical trial. *Complement. Ther. Med.* **2020**, *49*, 102315. [CrossRef]
191. Chehregosha, F.; Maghsoumi-Norouzabad, L.; Mobasseri, M.; Fakhr, L.; Tarighat-Esfanjani, A. The effect of Fenugreek seed dry extract supplement on glycemic indices, lipid profile, and prooxidant-antioxidant balance in patients with type 2 diabetes: A double-blind randomized clinical trial. *J. Cardiovasc. Thorac. Res.* **2024**, *16*, 184–193. [CrossRef]
192. Babaei, A.; Taghavi, S.; Mohammadi, A.; Mahdiyar, M.; Iranpour, P.; Ejtehadi, F.; Mohagheghzadeh, A. Comparison of the efficacy of oral fenugreek seeds hydroalcoholic extract versus placebo in nonalcoholic fatty liver disease; a randomized, triple-blind controlled pilot clinical trial. *Indian. J. Pharmacol.* **2020**, *52*, 86–93. [CrossRef] [PubMed]
193. Aryaeian, N.; Sedehi, S.K.; Arablou, T. Polyphenols and their effects on diabetes management: A review. *Med. J. Islam. Repub. Iran.* **2017**, *31*, 134. [CrossRef]
194. Mahluji, S.; Attari, V.E.; Mobasseri, M.; Payahoo, L.; Ostadrahimi, A.; Golzari, S.E. Effects of ginger (*Zingiber officinale*) on plasma glucose level, HbA1c and insulin sensitivity in type 2 diabetic patients. *Int. J. Food Sci. Nutr.* **2013**, *64*, 682–686. [CrossRef] [PubMed]
195. Rafie, R.; Hosseini, S.A.; Hajiani, E.; Saki Malehi, A.; Mard, S.A. Effect of Ginger Powder Supplementation in Patients with Non-Alcoholic Fatty Liver Disease: A Randomized Clinical Trial. *Clin. Exp. Gastroenterol.* **2020**, *13*, 35–45. [CrossRef] [PubMed]
196. Mozaffari-Khosravi, H.; Talaei, B.; Jalali, B.A.; Najarzadeh, A.; Mozayan, M.R. The effect of ginger powder supplementation on insulin resistance and glycemic indices in patients with type 2 diabetes: A randomized, double-blind, placebo-controlled trial. *Complement. Ther. Med.* **2014**, *22*, 9–16. [CrossRef] [PubMed]
197. Arablou, T.; Aryaeian, N.; Valizadeh, M.; Sharifi, F.; Hosseini, A.; Djalali, M. The effect of ginger consumption on glycemic status, lipid profile and some inflammatory markers in patients with type 2 diabetes mellitus. *Int. J. Food Sci. Nutr.* **2014**, *65*, 515–520. [CrossRef]
198. Shidfar, F.; Rajab, A.; Rahideh, T.; Khandouzi, N.; Hosseini, S.; Shidfar, S. The effect of ginger (*Zingiber officinale*) on glycemic markers in patients with type 2 diabetes. *J. Complement. Integr. Med.* **2015**, *12*, 165–170. [CrossRef] [PubMed]
199. Makhdoomi Arzati, M.; Mohammadzadeh Honarvar, N.; Saedisomeolia, A.; Anvari, S.; Effatpanah, M.; Makhdoomi Arzati, R.; Yekaninejad, M.S.; Hashemi, R.; Djalali, M. The Effects of Ginger on Fasting Blood Sugar, Hemoglobin A1c, and Lipid Profiles in Patients with Type 2 Diabetes. *Int. J. Endocrinol. Metab.* **2017**, *15*, e57927. [CrossRef]
200. Carvalho, G.C.N.; Lira-Neto, J.C.G.; Araújo, M.F.M.; Freitas, R.W.J.; Zanetti, M.L.; Damasceno, M.M.C. Effectiveness of ginger in reducing metabolic levels in people with diabetes: A randomized clinical trial. *Rev. Lat. Am. Enferm.* **2020**, *28*, e3369. [CrossRef] [PubMed]
201. Ebrahimzadeh, A.; Ebrahimzadeh, A.; Mirghazanfari, S.M.; Hazrati, E.; Hadi, S.; Milajerdi, A. The effect of ginger supplementation on metabolic profiles in patients with type 2 diabetes mellitus: A systematic review and meta-analysis of randomized controlled trials. *Complement. Ther. Med.* **2022**, *65*, 102802. [CrossRef]
202. Rahimlou, M.; Yari, Z.; Hekmatdoost, A.; Alavian, S.M.; Keshavarz, S.A. Ginger Supplementation in Nonalcoholic Fatty Liver Disease: A Randomized, Double-Blind, Placebo-Controlled Pilot Study. *Hepat. Mon.* **2016**, *16*, e34897. [CrossRef] [PubMed]
203. Ghoreishi, P.S.; Shams, M.; Nimrouzi, M.; Zarshenas, M.M.; Lankarani, K.B.; Fallahzadeh Abarghooei, E.; Talebzadeh, M.; Hashempur, M.H. The Effects of Ginger (Zingiber Officinale Roscoe) on Non-Alcoholic Fatty Liver Disease in Patients with Type 2 Diabetes Mellitus: A Randomized Double-Blinded Placebo-Controlled Clinical Trial. *J. Diet. Suppl.* **2024**, *21*, 294–312. [CrossRef]
204. Huang, F.Y.; Deng, T.; Meng, L.X.; Ma, X.L. Dietary ginger as a traditional therapy for blood sugar control in patients with type 2 diabetes mellitus: A systematic review and meta-analysis. *Medicine* **2019**, *98*, e15054. [CrossRef] [PubMed]
205. Jovanovski, E.; Khayyat, R.; Zurbau, A.; Komishon, A.; Mazhar, N.; Sievenpiper, J.L.; Blanco Mejia, S.; Ho, H.V.T.; Li, D.; Jenkins, A.L.; et al. Should Viscous Fiber Supplements Be Considered in Diabetes Control? Results From a Systematic Review and Meta-analysis of Randomized Controlled Trials. *Diabetes Care* **2019**, *42*, 755–766. [CrossRef] [PubMed]
206. Li, J.; Chen, R.; Chen, Y.; Zhu, D.; Wu, Z.; Chen, F.; Huang, X.; Khan, B.A.; Al Hennawi, H.E.; Albazee, E.; et al. The effect of guar gum consumption on the lipid profile in type 2 diabetes mellitus: A systematic review and meta-analysis of randomized controlled trials. *Crit. Rev. Food Sci. Nutr.* **2023**, *63*, 2886–2895. [CrossRef]
207. Liu, F.; Prabhakar, M.; Ju, J.; Long, H.; Zhou, H.W. Effect of inulin-type fructans on blood lipid profile and glucose level: A systematic review and meta-analysis of randomized controlled trials. *Eur. J. Clin. Nutr.* **2017**, *71*, 9–20. [CrossRef]
208. Stachowska, E.; Portincasa, P.; Jamioł-Milc, D.; Maciejewska-Markiewicz, D.; Skonieczna-Żydecka, K. The Relationship between Prebiotic Supplementation and Anthropometric and Biochemical Parameters in Patients with NAFLD—A Systematic Review and Meta-Analysis of Randomized Controlled Trials. *Nutrients* **2020**, *12*, 3460. [CrossRef]
209. Slavin, J. Fiber and Prebiotics: Mechanisms and Health Benefits. *Nutrients* **2013**, *5*, 1417–1435. [CrossRef]
210. Sartore, G.; Reitano, R.; Barison, A.; Magnanini, P.; Cosma, C.; Burlina, S.; Manzato, E.; Fedele, D.; Lapolla, A. The effects of psyllium on lipoproteins in type II diabetic patients. *Eur. J. Clin. Nutr.* **2009**, *63*, 1269–1271. [CrossRef]

211. Feinglos, M.N.; Gibb, R.D.; Ramsey, D.L.; Surwit, R.S.; McRorie, J.W. Psyllium improves glycemic control in patients with type-2 diabetes mellitus. *Bioact. Carbohydr. Diet. Fibre* **2013**, *1*, 156–161. [CrossRef]
212. Gibb, R.D.; McRorie, J.W.; Russell, D.A.; Hasselblad, V.; D'Alessio, D.A. Psyllium fiber improves glycemic control proportional to loss of glycemic control: A meta-analysis of data in euglycemic subjects, patients at risk of type 2 diabetes mellitus, and patients being treated for type 2 diabetes mellitus. *Am. J. Clin. Nutr.* **2015**, *102*, 1604–1614. [CrossRef]
213. Abutair, A.S.; Naser, I.A.; Hamed, A.T. The Effect of Soluble Fiber Supplementation on Metabolic Syndrome Profile among Newly Diagnosed Type 2 Diabetes Patients. *Clin. Nutr. Res.* **2018**, *7*, 31. [CrossRef] [PubMed]
214. Kamalpour, M.; Ghalandari, H.; Nasrollahzadeh, J. Short-Term Supplementation of a Moderate Carbohydrate Diet with Psyllium Reduces Fasting Plasma Insulin and Tumor Necrosis Factor-α in Patients with Type 2 Diabetes Mellitus. *J. Diet. Suppl.* **2018**, *15*, 507–515. [CrossRef]
215. Pourghassem Gargari, B.; Dehghan, P.; Aliasgharzadeh, A.; Asghari Jafar-Abadi, M. Effects of High-Performance Inulin Supplementation on Glycemic Control and Antioxidant Status in Women with Type 2 Diabetes. *Diabetes Metab. J.* **2013**, *37*, 140. [CrossRef]
216. Dehghan, P.; Gargari, B.P.; Jafar-Abadi, M.A.; Aliasgharzadeh, A. Inulin controls inflammation and metabolic endotoxemia in women with type 2 diabetes mellitus: A randomized-controlled clinical trial. *Int. J. Food Sci. Nutr.* **2014**, *65*, 117–123. [CrossRef] [PubMed]
217. Dehghan, P.; Pourghassem Gargari, B.; Asghari Jafar-Abadi, M. Oligofructose-enriched inulin improves some inflammatory markers and metabolic endotoxemia in women with type 2 diabetes mellitus: A randomized controlled clinical trial. *Nutrition* **2014**, *30*, 418–423. [CrossRef] [PubMed]
218. Farhangi, M.A.; Javid, A.Z.; Dehghan, P. The effect of enriched chicory inulin on liver enzymes, calcium homeostasis and hematological parameters in patients with type 2 diabetes mellitus: A randomized placebo-controlled trial. *Prim. Care Diabetes* **2016**, *10*, 265–271. [CrossRef]
219. Dall'Alba, V.; Silva, F.M.; Antonio, J.P.; Steemburgo, T.; Royer, C.P.; Almeida, J.C.; Gross, J.L.; Azevedo, M.J. Improvement of the metabolic syndrome profile by soluble fibre—Guar gum—In patients with type 2 diabetes: A randomized clinical trial. *Br. J. Nutr.* **2013**, *110*, 1601–1610. [CrossRef]
220. Watson, L.E.; Phillips, L.K.; Wu, T.; Bound, M.J.; Checklin, H.L.; Grivell, J.; Jones, K.L.; Clifton, P.M.; Horowitz, M.; Rayner, C.K. A whey/guar "preload" improves postprandial glycaemia and glycated haemoglobin levels in type 2 diabetes: A 12-week, single-blind, randomized, placebo-controlled trial. *Diabetes Obes. Metab.* **2019**, *21*, 930–938. [CrossRef]
221. Daubioul, C.A.; Horsmans, Y.; Lambert, P.; Danse, E.; Delzenne, N.M. Effects of oligofructose on glucose and lipid metabolism in patients with nonalcoholic steatohepatitis: Results of a pilot study. *Eur. J. Clin. Nutr.* **2005**, *59*, 723–726. [CrossRef]
222. Akbarzadeh, M.; Nourian, M.; Askari, G.; Maracy, M.R. The effect of psyllium on anthropometric measurements and liver enzymes in overweight or obese adults with nonalcoholic fatty liver disease (NAFLD). *Isfahan Med. Sch.* **2015**, *33*, 1771–1783.
223. Akbarian, S.A.; Asgary, S.; Feizi, A.; Iraj, B.; Askari, G. Comparative study on the effect of Plantago psyllium and Ocimum basilicum seeds on anthropometric measures in nonalcoholic fatty liver patients. *Int. J. Prev. Med.* **2016**, *7*, 114. [CrossRef]
224. Gholami, Z.; Clark, C.C.T.; Paknahad, Z. The effect of psyllium on fasting blood sugar, HbA1c, HOMA IR, and insulin control: A GRADE-assessed systematic review and meta-analysis of randomized controlled trials. *BMC Endocr. Disord.* **2024**, *24*, 82. [CrossRef] [PubMed]
225. Wang, L.; Yang, H.; Huang, H.; Zhang, C.; Zuo, H.X.; Xu, P.; Niu, Y.M.; Wu, S.S. Inulin-type fructans supplementation improves glycemic control for the prediabetes and type 2 diabetes populations: Results from a GRADE-assessed systematic review and dose–response meta-analysis of 33 randomized controlled trials. *J. Transl. Med.* **2019**, *17*, 410. [CrossRef] [PubMed]
226. Javad Alaeian, M.; Pourreza, S.; Yousefi, M.; Golalipour, E.; Setayesh, L.; Zeinali Khosroshahi, M.; Bagheri, R.; Ashtary-Larky, D.; Wong, A.; Zamani, M.; et al. The effects of guar gum supplementation on glycemic control, body mass and blood pressure in adults: A GRADE-assessed systematic review and meta-analysis of randomized clinical trials. *Diabetes Res. Clin. Pract.* **2023**, *199*, 110604. [CrossRef] [PubMed]
227. Jenko Pražnikar, Z.; Mohorko, N.; Gmajner, D.; Kenig, S.; Petelin, A. Effects of Four Different Dietary Fibre Supplements on Weight Loss and Lipid and Glucose Serum Profiles during Energy Restriction in Patients with Traits of Metabolic Syndrome: A Comparative, Randomized, Placebo-Controlled Study. *Foods* **2023**, *12*, 2122. [CrossRef] [PubMed]
228. Delpino, F.M.; Figueiredo, L.M.; da Silva, B.G.C.; da Silva, T.G.; Mintem, G.C.; Bielemann, R.M.; Gigante, D.P. Omega-3 supplementation and diabetes: A systematic review and meta-analysis. *Crit. Rev. Food Sci. Nutr.* **2022**, *62*, 4435–4448. [CrossRef] [PubMed]
229. Crochemore, I.C.C.; Souza, A.F.P.; De Souza, A.C.F.; Rosado, E.L. Ω-3 polyunsaturated fatty acid supplementation does not influence body composition, insulin resistance, and lipemia in women with type 2 diabetes and obesity. *Nutr. Clin. Pract.* **2012**, *27*, 553–560. [CrossRef]
230. Spooner, M.H.; Jump, D.B. Omega-3 fatty acids and nonalcoholic fatty liver disease in adults and children. *Curr. Opin. Clin. Nutr. Metab. Care* **2019**, *22*, 103–110. [CrossRef] [PubMed]

231. Hartweg, J.; Farmer, A.J.; Holman, R.R.; Neil, A. Potential impact of omega-3 treatment on cardiovascular disease in type 2 diabetes. *Curr. Opin. Lipidol.* **2009**, *20*, 30–38. [CrossRef]
232. Malekshahi Moghadam, A.; Saedisomeolia, A.; Djalali, M.; Djazayery, A.; Pooya, S.; Sojoudi, F. Efficacy of omega-3 fatty acid supplementation on serum levels of tumour necrosis factor-alpha, C-reactive protein and interleukin-2 in type 2 diabetes mellitus patients. *Singap. Med. J.* **2012**, *53*, 615–619.
233. Zheng, J.; Lin, M.; Fang, L.; Yu, Y.; Yuan, L.; Jin, Y.; Feng, J.; Wang, L.; Yang, H.; Chen, W.; et al. Effects of *n*-3 fatty acid supplements on glycemic traits in Chinese type 2 diabetic patients: A double-blind randomized controlled trial. *Mol. Nutr. Food Res.* **2016**, *60*, 2176–2184. [CrossRef]
234. Wang, F.; Wang, Y.; Zhu, Y.; Liu, X.; Xia, H.; Yang, X.; Sun, G. Treatment for 6 months with fish oil-derived n-3 polyunsaturated fatty acids has neutral effects on glycemic control but improves dyslipidemia in type 2 diabetic patients with abdominal obesity: A randomized, double-blind, placebo-controlled trial. *Eur. J. Nutr.* **2017**, *56*, 2415–2422. [CrossRef] [PubMed]
235. Jacobo-Cejudo, M.G.; Valdés-Ramos, R.; Guadarrama-López, A.L.; Pardo-Morales, R.V.; Martínez-Carrillo, B.E.; Harbige, L.S. Effect of n-3 Polyunsaturated Fatty Acid Supplementation on Metabolic and Inflammatory Biomarkers in Type 2 Diabetes Mellitus Patients. *Nutrients* **2017**, *9*, 573. [CrossRef]
236. Werida, R.H.; Ramzy, A.; Ebrahim, Y.N.; Helmy, M.W. Effect of coadministration of omega-3 fatty acids with glimepiride on glycemic control, lipid profile, irisin, and sirtuin-1 in type 2 diabetes mellitus patients: A randomized controlled trial. *BMC Endocr. Disord.* **2023**, *23*, 259. [CrossRef] [PubMed]
237. Spadaro, L.; Magliocco, O.; Spampinato, D.; Piro, S.; Oliveri, C.; Alagona, C.; Papa, G.; Rabuazzo, A.M.; Purrello, F. Effects of n-3 polyunsaturated fatty acids in subjects with nonalcoholic fatty liver disease. *Dig. Liver Dis.* **2008**, *40*, 194–199. [CrossRef] [PubMed]
238. Qin, Y.; Zhou, Y.; Chen, S.H.; Zhao, X.L.; Ran, L.; Zeng, X.L.; Wu, Y.; Chen, J.L.; Kang, C.; Shu, F.R.; et al. Fish Oil Supplements Lower Serum Lipids and Glucose in Correlation with a Reduction in Plasma Fibroblast Growth Factor 21 and Prostaglandin E2 in Nonalcoholic Fatty Liver Disease Associated with Hyperlipidemia: A Randomized Clinical Trial. *PLoS ONE* **2015**, *10*, e0133496. [CrossRef] [PubMed]
239. Sanyal, A.J.; Abdelmalek, M.F.; Suzuki, A.; Cummings, O.W.; Chojkier, M.; EPE-A Study Group. No significant effects of ethyl-eicosapentanoic acid on histologic features of nonalcoholic steatohepatitis in a phase 2 trial. *Gastroenterology* **2014**, *147*, 377–384.e1. [CrossRef]
240. Dasarathy, S.; Dasarathy, J.; Khiyami, A.; Yerian, L.; Hawkins, C.; Sargent, R.; McCullough, A.J. Double-blind Randomized Placebo-controlled Clinical Trial of Omega 3 Fatty Acids for the Treatment of Diabetic Patients with Nonalcoholic Steatohepatitis. *J. Clin. Gastroenterol.* **2015**, *49*, 137–144. [CrossRef] [PubMed]
241. Šmíd, V.; Dvořák, K.; Šedivý, P.; Kosek, V.; Leníček, M.; Dezortová, M.; Hajšlová, J.; Hájek, M.; Vítek, L.; Bechyňská, K.; et al. Effect of Omega-3 Polyunsaturated Fatty Acids on Lipid Metabolism in Patients with Metabolic Syndrome and NAFLD. *Hepatol. Commun.* **2022**, *6*, 1336–1349. [CrossRef] [PubMed]
242. O'Mahoney, L.L.; Matu, J.; Price, O.J.; Birch, K.M.; Ajjan, R.A.; Farrar, D.; Tapp, R.; West, D.J.; Deighton, K.; Campbell, M.D. Omega-3 polyunsaturated fatty acids favourably modulate cardiometabolic biomarkers in type 2 diabetes: A meta-analysis and meta-regression of randomized controlled trials. *Cardiovasc. Diabetol.* **2018**, *17*, 98. [CrossRef] [PubMed]
243. Parker, H.M.; Johnson, N.A.; Burdon, C.A.; Cohn, J.S.; O'Connor, H.T.; George, J. Omega-3 supplementation and non-alcoholic fatty liver disease: A systematic review and meta-analysis. *J. Hepatol.* **2012**, *56*, 944–951. [CrossRef]
244. He, X.X.; Wu, X.L.; Chen, R.P.; Chen, C.; Liu, X.G.; Wu, B.J.; Huang, Z.M. Effectiveness of Omega-3 Polyunsaturated Fatty Acids in Non-Alcoholic Fatty Liver Disease: A Meta-Analysis of Randomized Controlled Trials. *PLoS ONE* **2016**, *11*, e0162368. [CrossRef]
245. Li, Y.; Chen, D. The optimal dose of omega-3 supplementation for non-alcoholic fatty liver disease. *J. Hepatol.* **2012**, *57*, 468–469. [CrossRef]
246. Gurung, M.; Li, Z.; You, H.; Rodrigues, R.; Jump, D.B.; Morgun, A.; Shulzhenko, N. Role of gut microbiota in type 2 diabetes pathophysiology. *eBioMedicine* **2020**, *51*, 102590. [CrossRef]
247. Aron-Wisnewsky, J.; Vigliotti, C.; Witjes, J.; Le, P.; Holleboom, A.G.; Verheij, J.; Nieuwdorp, M.; Clément, K. Gut microbiota and human NAFLD: Disentangling microbial signatures from metabolic disorders. *Nat. Rev. Gastroenterol. Hepatol.* **2020**, *17*(5), 279–297. [CrossRef] [PubMed]
248. Hrncir, T.; Hrncirova, L.; Kverka, M.; Hromadka, R.; Machova, V.; Trckova, E.; Kostovcikova, K.; Kralickova, P.; Krejsek, J.; Tlaskalova-Hogenova, H. Gut Microbiota and NAFLD: Pathogenetic Mechanisms, Microbiota Signatures, and Therapeutic Interventions. *Microorganisms* **2021**, *9*, 957. [CrossRef]
249. Barchetta, I.; Cimini, F.A.; Sentinelli, F.; Chiappetta, C.; Di Cristofano, C.; Silecchia, G.; Leonetti, F.; Baroni, M.G.; Cavallo, M.G. Reduced Lipopolysaccharide-Binding Protein (LBP) Levels Are Associated with Non-Alcoholic Fatty Liver Disease (NAFLD) and Adipose Inflammation in Human Obesity. *Int. J. Mol. Sci.* **2023**, *24*, 17174. [CrossRef]

250. Moreno-Navarrete, J.M.; Ortega, F.; Serino, M.; Luche, E.; Waget, A.; Pardo, G.; Salvador, J.; Ricart, W.; Frühbeck, G.; Burcelin, R.; et al. Circulating lipopolysaccharide-binding protein (LBP) as a marker of obesity-related insulin resistance. *Int. J. Obes.* **2012**, *36*, 1442–1449. [CrossRef] [PubMed]
251. Kitabatake, H.; Tanaka, N.; Fujimori, N.; Komatsu, M.; Okubo, A.; Kakegawa, K.; Kimura, T.; Sugiura, A.; Yamazaki, T.; Shibata, S.; et al. Association between endotoxemia and histological features of nonalcoholic fatty liver disease. *World J. Gastroenterol.* **2017**, *23*, 712–722. [CrossRef] [PubMed]
252. Ojo, O.; Wang, X.; Ojo, O.O.; Brooke, J.; Jiang, Y.; Dong, Q.; Thompson, T. The Effect of Prebiotics and Oral Anti-Diabetic Agents on Gut Microbiome in Patients with Type 2 Diabetes: A Systematic Review and Network Meta-Analysis of Randomised Controlled Trials. *Nutrients* **2022**, *14*, 5139. [CrossRef] [PubMed]
253. Robertson, M.D. Prebiotics and type 2 diabetes: Targeting the gut microbiota for improved glycaemic control? *Pract. Diabetes* **2020**, *37*, 133–137. [CrossRef]
254. Birkeland, E.; Gharagozlian, S.; Birkeland, K.I.; Valeur, J.; Måge, I.; Rud, I.; Aas, A.M. Prebiotic effect of inulin-type fructans on faecal microbiota and short-chain fatty acids in type 2 diabetes: A randomised controlled trial. *Eur. J. Nutr.* **2020**, *59*, 3325–3338. [CrossRef] [PubMed]
255. Pedersen, C.; Gallagher, E.; Horton, F.; Ellis, R.J.; Ijaz, U.Z.; Wu, H.; Jaiyeola, E.; Diribe, O.; Duparc, T.; Cani, P.; et al. Host–microbiome interactions in human type 2 diabetes following prebiotic fibre (galacto-oligosaccharide) intake. *Br. J. Nutr.* **2016**, *116*, 1869–1877. [CrossRef]
256. Canfora, E.E.; van der Beek, C.M.; Hermes, G.D.A.; Goossens, G.H.; Jocken, J.W.E.; Holst, J.J.; van Eijk, H.M.; Venema, K.; Smidt, H.; Zoetendal, E.G.; et al. Supplementation of Diet with Galacto-oligosaccharides Increases Bifidobacteria, but Not Insulin Sensitivity, in Obese Prediabetic Individuals. *Gastroenterology* **2017**, *153*, 87–97.e3. [CrossRef]
257. Frias, J.P.; Lee, M.L.; Carter, M.M.; Ebel, E.R.; Lai, R.; Rikse, L.; Washington, M.E.; Sonnenburg, J.L.; Damman, C.J. A microbiome-targeting fibre-enriched nutritional formula is well tolerated and improves quality of life and haemoglobin A1c in type 2 diabetes: A double-blind, randomized, placebo-controlled trial. *Diabetes Obes. Metab.* **2023**, *25*, 1203–1212. [CrossRef] [PubMed]
258. Bomhof, M.R.; Parnell, J.A.; Ramay, H.R.; Crotty, P.; Rioux, K.P.; Probert, C.S.; Jayakumar, S.; Raman, M.; Reimer, R.A. Histological improvement of non-alcoholic steatohepatitis with a prebiotic: A pilot clinical trial. *Eur. J. Nutr.* **2019**, *58*, 1735–1745. [CrossRef]
259. Reshef, N.; Gophna, U.; Reshef, L.; Konikoff, F.; Gabay, G.; Zornitzki, T.; Knobler, H.; Maor, Y. Prebiotic Treatment in Patients with Nonalcoholic Fatty Liver Disease (NAFLD)—A Randomized Pilot Trial. *Nutrients* **2024**, *16*, 1571. [CrossRef]
260. Schaafsma, G.; Slavin, J.L. Significance of Inulin Fructans in the Human Diet. *Compr. Rev. Food Sci. Food Saf.* **2015**, *14*, 37–47. [CrossRef]
261. Macfarlane, G.T.; Steed, H.; Macfarlane, S. Bacterial metabolism and health-related effects of galacto-oligosaccharides and other prebiotics. *J. Appl. Microbiol.* **2008**, *104*, 305–344. [CrossRef]

pharmaceuticals

MDPI

Review

Medicinal Plant Extracts against Cardiometabolic Risk Factors Associated with Obesity: Molecular Mechanisms and Therapeutic Targets

Jorge Gutiérrez-Cuevas [1,*], Daniel López-Cifuentes [1,2], Ana Sandoval-Rodriguez [1], Jesús García-Bañuelos [1] and Juan Armendariz-Borunda [1,3]

1 Department of Molecular Biology and Genomics, Institute for Molecular Biology in Medicine and Gene Therapy, University Center of Health Sciences, University of Guadalajara, Guadalajara 44340, Jalisco, Mexico; daniel.2cifuentes@gmail.com (D.L.-C.); anasol44@hotmail.com (A.S.-R.); armdbo@gmail.com (J.A.-B.)
2 Doctorate in Sciences in Molecular Biology in Medicine, University Center of Health Sciences, University of Guadalajara, Guadalajara 44340, Jalisco, Mexico
3 Escuela de Medicina y Ciencias de la Salud (EMCS), Tecnologico de Monterrey, Campus Guadalajara, Zapopan 45201, Jalisco, Mexico
* Correspondence: gutierrezcj05@gmail.com; Tel.: +52-331-062-2083

Abstract: Obesity has increasingly become a worldwide epidemic, as demonstrated by epidemiological and clinical studies. Obesity may lead to the development of a broad spectrum of cardiovascular diseases (CVDs), such as coronary heart disease, hypertension, heart failure, cerebrovascular disease, atrial fibrillation, ventricular arrhythmias, and sudden cardiac death. In addition to hypertension, there are other cardiometabolic risk factors (CRFs) such as visceral adiposity, dyslipidemia, insulin resistance, diabetes, elevated levels of fibrinogen and C-reactive protein, and others, all of which increase the risk of CVD events. The mechanisms involved between obesity and CVD mainly include insulin resistance, oxidative stress, inflammation, and adipokine dysregulation, which cause maladaptive structural and functional alterations of the heart, particularly left-ventricular remodeling and diastolic dysfunction. Natural products of plants provide a diversity of nutrients and different bioactive compounds, including phenolics, flavonoids, terpenoids, carotenoids, anthocyanins, vitamins, minerals, fibers, and others, which possess a wide range of biological activities including antihypertensive, antilipidemic, antidiabetic, and other activities, thus conferring cardiometabolic benefits. In this review, we discuss the main therapeutic interventions using extracts from herbs and plants in preclinical and clinical trials with protective properties targeting CRFs. Molecular mechanisms and therapeutic targets of herb and plant extracts for the prevention and treatment of CRFs are also reviewed.

Keywords: obesity; cardiometabolic risk factors; herbs; plants; extracts; molecular mechanisms; therapeutic targets

1. Introduction

Obesity is a worldwide public health problem and is a chronic non-transmissible disease whose incidence has been dramatically increasing around the world. This chronic metabolic disease affects distinct age, ethnic and social classes, and has a tremendous impact on the economy and quality of life. Obesity and being overweight are the fifth main causes of deaths globally [1,2]. According to the World Health Organization (WHO), overweight people are defined as having a body mass index (BMI) > 25, while people with a BMI > 30 are considered obese [1]. The pathophysiology of obesity implicates a combination of genetic/epigenetic, nutritional, and environmental factors that promote a chronic positive energy balance and expansion of body fat mass, specially of white adipose tissue (WAT) in visceral fat depots [1,2]. In obese people, WAT plays a key role in secreting lipolysis or lipid synthesis hormones, including inflammatory cytokines that regulate lipid metabolism, and promotes a low-grade chronic inflammation that has the potential to activate insulin resistance and endothelial dysfunction [1,3–5]. An excessive accumulation of fat in WAT, in addition to obesity, can also cause metabolic disorders such as dyslipidemia, adipocyte dysfunction, metabolic syndrome, hypertension, type 2 diabetes (T2D), metabolic dysfunction-associated steatotic liver disease (MASLD), cardiovascular disease, and even certain cancers [1,6,7]. In obese people, it is presently accepted that oxidative stress is induced by obesity-related diseases such as hyperglycemia, insulin resistance, diabetes, dyslipidemia, atherosclerosis, and inflammation [1,4,8]. Furthermore, adipose tissue inflammation and oxidative stress cause a dysregulation of adipokine secretion, with a reduction in adiponectin and an increase in the secretion of resistin, leptin, and pro-inflammatory adipokines and cytokines, which contribute to cardiovascular stiffness, impaired vascular relaxation, and finally, cardiac diastolic dysfunction [3]. In addition, the cardiac phenotype in obesity includes concentric left-ventricular hypertrophy (LVH), myocardial fibrosis, microvascular dysfunction, arrhythmia, heart failure (HF)—particularly HF with preserved ejection fraction (HFpEF)—atrial fibrillation (AF), cardiac remodeling, myocardial infarction, and left-ventricular systolic dysfunction, causing deterioration in myocardial function and HF [3,9].

The complex interaction between several cardiometabolic dysfunctions and pathological processes plays an essential role in the pathogenesis of obesity, which is associated with the morbidity and mortality of diabetes and cardiovascular disease [1,4,8,10]. Moreover, cardiovascular diseases are closely associated with high cholesterol, obesity, smoking, diabetes, and a lack of physical activity. Therefore, a convenient lifestyle accompanied by healthy nutrition, a reduction in energy-dense food consumption, physical activity and activities that reduce oxidative stress are the most common therapeutic strategies to reduce cardiometabolic risk factors closely linked to obesity, such as hypertension, dyslipidemia, insulin resistance, diabetes, elevated levels of fibrinogen and C-reactive protein (CRP), including low-grade chronic inflammation (Figure 1) [1,11].

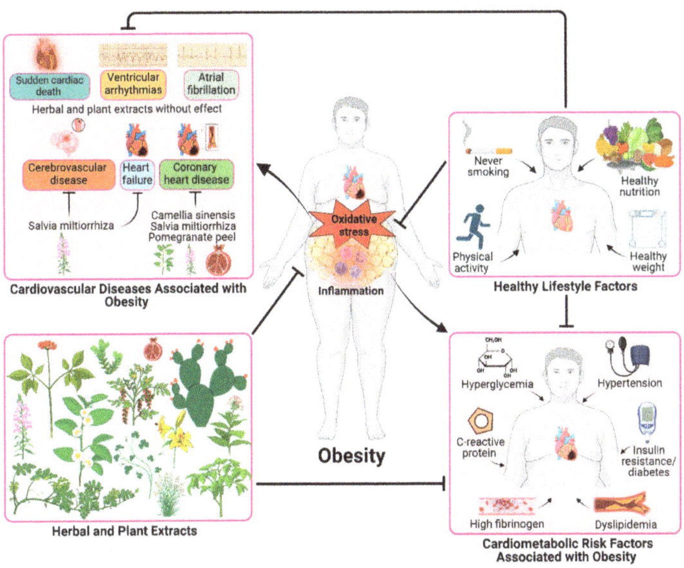

Figure 1. Overview of obesity. Obesity is associated with the development of cardiometabolic risk factors and cardiovascular diseases. However, healthy lifestyle and intake of plant extracts such as those described in this review (21 natural extracts), which have antioxidant and anti-inflammatory properties, can prevent these pathological conditions.

Several antiobesity medications approved by the United States (US) Food and Drug Administration (FDA) exist, which include liraglutide (Saxenda), naltrexone-bupropion (Contrave), orlistat (Xenical), phentermine-topiramate (Qsymia), semaglutide (Wegovy), setmelanotide (IMCIVREE), and tirzepatide (Mounjaro) [12,13]; however, the use of these drugs remains controversial, as they are associated with a number of adverse side effects and weight regain when the medication is stopped [12,13]. Therefore, the WHO (Committee, 1980) recommended the use of indigenous medicinal plants to treat obesity because of their easy availability, low costs, and relatively fewer side effects. Moreover, herbs and plants contain an unlimited source of phytochemicals, macronutrients, micronutrients, and antioxidants such as polyphenols, which are known to prevent diseases associated with oxidative stress such as obesity and its related complications.

In this review article, we discussed the beneficial properties of several herbs and plant extracts (21 natural extracts), as well as their active components against obesity, cardiometabolic risk factors, and associated pathophysiological processes to treat and prevent different cardiovascular diseases in preclinical and clinical trials, considering their molecular mechanisms underlying for their medicinal uses.

2. Phytochemical Constituents and Pharmacological Activities of Herbs and Plants with Cardiovascular Protective Effects

2.1. *Allium sativum, Family Alliaceae*

Garlic is one of the most well-known herbal medicines in the world and has been used as a spice or medicinal herb for many centuries. The major bioactive compounds of bulbs include sulfur compounds such as alliin, allicin, ajoene, vinyldithiins, diallyl disulfide, allyl methanethiosulfinate, diallyltrisulfide, dimethylmonotohexasulfide, and S-allylcysteine [14]. Garlic administered either in liquid form or capsules has different antioxidant, antidiabetic, antihypertensive, antiatherosclerotic, anti-inflammation, endothelial-protecting, lipid-lowering, plasma fibrinogen-lowering, platelet aggregation-inhibiting, fibrinolytic activity-increasing, and other cardiovascular-protective effects [14–16]. In addition, aged garlic extract (AGE) has been used in previous human trials and has been shown to be safe [17].

2.2. *Andrographis paniculata (Burm. F.) Wall. Ex Nees (Family: Acanthaceae)*

Andrographis paniculata (Burm.f.) Nees is considered a potent plant medicinal in most parts of Asia for the treatment of endocrine disorders, inflammation, and hypertension. Based on phytochemical tests, flavonoids, alkaloids, tannins, triterpenoids, and polyphenols have been isolated from *Andrographis paniculata* [18]. In addition, andrographolide is a natural diterpenoid lactone extracted from *Andrographis paniculata* (Burm.f.) Nees, and scientific studies revealed that andrographolide is the main phytoconstituent for its medicinal properties, such as antineoplasm antibacterial, anti-inflammatory, antimalaria, antithrombotic, hepato-protective, antihypertensive, antidiabetic, antioxidant, antiapoptosis, antifibrosis, and cardioprotection activities [19].

2.3. *Aronia melanocarpa (Michx.) Elliott. (Family: Rosaceae)*

Black chokeberry, *Aronia melanocarpa* (Michx.) Elliot is a deciduous shrub native to eastern North America, and *Aronia melanocarpa* (chokeberry) contains a rich source of biologically active polyphenols such as anthocyanins, proanthocyanidins, and phenolic acid, which have strong antioxidant effects and cardioprotective benefits [20,21]. Other bioactive compounds have been identified to be present in the fruits and other parts of the plant, such as neochlorogenic and chlorogenic acids, cyanidin-3-galactoside, cyanidin-3-arabinoside, and (-)-epicatechin [21,22]. *Aronia melanocarpa* or black chokeberry has been found in multiple clinical trials to combat hyperglycemia-induced oxidative stress, blood pressure (BP), cholesterol and the macrovascular complications of diabetes, including cardiovascular disease [21,22]. The berries of *Aronia melanocarpa* also possess therapeutic benefits such as gastroprotective, hepatoprotective, antiproliferative, and anti-inflammatory activities [22].

2.4. *Camellia sinensis (Family: Theaceae)*

Green tea derived from *Camellia sinensis* leaves is one of the most popular beverages consumed worldwide. The plant is native to East Asia, possibly originating in southern China, including border areas of Myanmar and India [23]. Green tea extract (GTE) contains several bioactive components, including polyphenols, catechins, theobromine, caffeine, and flavonoids. The major catechins in green tea are (-)-epigallocatechin-3-gallate (EGCG), (-)-epigallocatechin (EGC), (-)-epicatechin-3-gallate (ECG), (-)-epicatechin (EC), and (þ)-catechin (C). Among them, EGCG represents approximately 50–70% of the total catechins from green tea leaves and is primarily responsible for the beneficial effect of green tea [23,24]. The polyphenolic compounds in green tea possess antioxidant properties preventing oxidative stress-caused diseases such as cancer, cardiovascular (e.g., stroke, coronary heart disease, and coronary atherosclerosis) and neurodegenerative diseases. In addition, green tea has beneficial effects on cardiovascular risk factors such as hypertension, lipid disorders, diabetes, endothelial dysfunction, and inflammation. Other beneficial effects include antibacterial, antiviral, antimicrobial, antiobesity, antiangiogenic, and antimetabolic syndrome activities [23,24].

2.5. *Caralluma fimbriata (Family: Apocynaceae)*

Caralluma fimbriata, an edible succulent and wild medicinal plant growing in dry places, is found throughout Asia (Afghanistan, India, Iran, Pakistan, and Sri Lanka), Africa, Arabian Peninsula, Canary Islands, and Southeast Europe. The key phytochemical constituents of the herb are pregnane glycosides, flavone glycosides, megastigmane glycosides, and saponins, including bitter principles, triterpenoids, and other flavonoids [25]. Pregnane glycosides, particularly rich in this plant, are known to suppress hunger and increase endurance. In addition, extracts of *Caralluma fimbriata* have hypoglycaemic, antioxidant, antiadipogenic, antihypertensive properties [25–27]. The herb is also used to treat pain, fever, inflammation, and is commonly consumed by ethnic populations of Central India to manage obesity. Bioactive compounds derived from *Caralluma fimbriata* such as flavonoids, saponins, alkaloids, tannins/gallic-tannins, and trigonelline have antioxidant effects. Meanwhile, the compounds flavonoids, saponins, tannins/gallic-tannins, phytosterol, terpenoids, anthraquinones, pregnane glycosides, and trigonelline are responsible for anti-inflammatory properties of *Caralluma fimbriata.* Alkaloids and quercetin found in *Caralluma fimbriata* have antiadipogenic effects. Phytochemicals such as diterpenes, phytosterol, flavonoids, and quercetin have been reported to have antihyperlipidemic effects. Flavonoids modulate blood pressure through the restoration of endothelial function or by affecting nitric oxide levels [25].

2.6. *Cinnamomum zeylanicum (Ceylon cinnamon), Family: Lauraceae*

Ceylon cinnamon is scientifically known as *Cinnamomum zeylanicum* Blume. Cinnamon is native to Sri Lanka and is one of the most important spices used daily by people around the world. The most important compounds of cinnamon are cinnamaldehyde and trans-cinnamaldehyde, which also are found in the essential oil, and both contribute to fragrance and to the various biological activities observed with cinnamon. In addition, this plant contains a variety of resinous compounds, such as cinnamate, cinnamic acid, and numerous essential oils [28]. Cinnamon has many health benefits, including anti-inflammatory, antioxidant, blood-glucose regulation, insulin sensitivity improvement, antidiabetic, lipid-lowering, antimicrobial, anticancer, and anticardiovascular properties; cinnamon has also been reported to have benefits against neurological disorders, such as Parkinson's and Alzheimer's diseases [28–30].

2.7. *Citrullus colocynthis (Family: Cucurbitacea)*

Citrullus colocynthis (L.) Schrad is widely distributed in desert areas around the world, including Sudan, Morocco, Arabian Desert, Jordan, Tunisia, Iran, India, and Pakistan. *Citrullus colocynthis* contains several compounds, mainly cucurbitacins and others such as alkaloids, flavonoids, coumarins, steroids, and phenolic acids [31]. Parts of this plant have been used in traditional medicine, and are widely used to treat constipation, mastitis, joint pain, diabetes, hypertension, inflammation, leukemia, epilepsy, asthma, bronchitis, jaundice, leprosy, rheumatism, common cold, cough, toothache, wounds, and bacterial infection [31–33]. Moreover, in diabetic and nondiabetic animal models, aqueous extracts of *Citrullus colocynthis* have hypoglycemic, antidiabetic, hypolipidemic, and antihyperlipidemic effects, including antiplatelet and profibrinolytic activity [31,33,34]. Antioxidant effects of *Citrullus colocynthis* leaf and root extracts have been described; these effects were reported with triterpenoids spinasterol and 22,23-dihydrospinasterol from leaves of *Citrullus colocynthis* [35]. Other compounds, such as their polyphenols, and flavonoids, remove free radicals and thus have a protective effect [33]. Aqueous extracts from roots and stems of the plant and from fruits and seeds displayed anti-inflammatory activities at different doses without inducing acute toxicity [36]. Saponins and catechic tannins from *Citrullus colocynthis* seed extract are bioactive components that contribute to hypolipidemic activity [37]. However, some side effects caused by *Citrullus colocynthis* have been reported, such as nausea, vomiting, colic, diarrhea, hematochezia, and nephrosis [38].

2.8. *Cacao (Theobroma cacao L.), Family: Malvaceae*

Theobroma cacao is native to the jungles of South America and then extended to Mexico. Cocoa beans are the seeds, which are used mainly to produce chocolate, cocoa, and fat. Cocoa is one of the richest sources of polyphenols (about 6–8% by dry weight), which include mainly flavonoids, flavanols, flavanones, isoflavones, and nonflavonoids, as well as catechins, anthocyanidins/anthocyanins, flavonol glycosides, and procynanidins [39]. Polyphenols are beneficial on blood pressure, insulin resistance, lipid profile, endothelial dysfunction, and oxidative stress, thus contributing to the prevention of cardiometabolic disorders. Flavanols in cocoa are found as (-)-epicatechin, (+)-catechin, and procyanidins. (-)-epicatechin has the capacity to modulate lipid metabolism (e.g., hypocholesterolemic effect). Black chocolate is considered one of the major sources of antioxidants, and the compounds theobromine, caffeine, (-)-epicatechin, catechins, and oligomeric procyanidins in cocoa have strong antioxidative activities [39–42]. Dry cocoa powder can contain approximately 200 mg of caffeine per cup, and caffeine progressively reduces body fat mass and body fat in rats fed an HFD [43]. Several therapeutic effects have been attributed to cocoa-derived polyphenols, such as the improvement of lipid peroxidation, insulin resistance, lipid profile, endothelial dysfunction, postprandial systolic blood pressure (SBP), oxidative stress, and inflammation, including lipid metabolism, and glucose metabolism [39,41,42]. Cocoa and its products play an important role in the prevention and treatment of CVDs, including the inhibition of platelet activation and aggregation [44].

2.9. *Corni Fructus (Cornus officinalis Sieb. et Zucc.), Family: Cornaceae*

Cornus officinalis Siebold et Zuccarini, usually known as Corni Fructus, is a herb and food plant in East Asia used in traditional Chinese medicine. Several chemical constituents have been identified in Corni Fructus, which are terpenoids, flavonoids, tannins, polysaccharides, phenylpropanoids, sterols, carboxylic acids, furans, saponins, phenolic acid (gallic acid and tannic acid), loganin, and mineral substances. In addition, other phytochemicals are reported in Corni Fructus extracts, such as morroniside, 1,6-α-glucans, loganin, ursolic acid, oleanolic acid, cornuside, polymeric proanthocyanidins, 1,2,3-tri-O-galloyl-beta-D-glucose, 1,2,3,6-tetra-O-galloyl-beta-D-glucose, among others [45,46]. The components in Corni Fructus, such as iridoid glycoside, morroniside, loganin, and polyphenols, exhibit protective effects against hyperglycemia, oxidative stress, and cancer. In vivo and in vitro experimental studies indicate that Corni Fructus has several biological activities, including hypoglycemic, antioxidant, anti-inflammatory, antineoplastic, antimicrobial, anticancer, antiapoptosis, anti-inflammation, antiosteoporosis, immunoregulation, neuroprotective, hepatoprotective, nephroprotective, and cardiovascular protection [45–48]. However, clinical studies are still needed to confirm the reported pharmacological activities.

On the other hand, Corni Fructus has been frequently used for the treatment of asthenia diseases, liver, and kidney diseases, including reproductive system diseases since ancient times. Moreover, it is commonly used for the treatment of several conditions such as diabetes, frequent urination, impotence, and collapse with profuse sweating [45,46].

2.10. *Cydonia oblonga Miller (Family: Rosaceae)*

Cydonia oblonga Miller (COM) is a plant known by various names, including quince, aiva, bier, and marmelo. The fruit of COM contains various polyphenolic compounds, organic acids, ionone glycosides, and tetracyclic sesterterpenes, including chlorogenic acid, cryptochlorogenic acid, neochlorogenic acid, isochlorogenic acid, quercetin 3-rutinoside, quercetin 3-galactoside, quercetin 3-glucoside, kaempferol 3-glucoside, kaempferol 3-glycoside, and kaempferol 3-rutinoside. In the pulp, leaves, peel, seeds, and complete fruits of COM, several citric, ascorbic, malic, oxalic, quinic, fumaric, and shikimic acids have been discovered [49,50]. The fruit of COM is commonly used in the Mediterranean region to prevent or treat obesity. In addition, the fruit of COM has been used for the treatment of hypertension, diabetes, cancer, cardiovascular diseases, respiratory disorders, hemolysis, and ulcers [49,51–53]. Several studies have reported the beneficial effects of COM extracts, such as antioxidant, anti-inflammatory, antiallergic, antidepressant, and antistress, including positive effects on cardiovascular-associated factors such as BP, glucose metabolism, lipid profile, liver dysfunction, and thrombosis [49,52,53]. Moreover, the plant's seeds have been used to treat diarrhea, dysentery, constipation, cough, sore throat, and bronchitis [49].

2.11. *Ginkgo biloba (Family: Ginkgoaceae)*

For centuries, the herb *Ginkgo biloba* has been used in traditional Chinese medicine to treat various medical conditions. The extracts of *Ginkgo biloba* (EGb) leaves have a wide variety of bioactive compounds, such as flavonoid heterosides (between 22% and 27%), represented by flavonol glycosides (kaempferol, quercetin, myricetin, apigenin, isorhamnetin, luteolin, and tamarixetin), diterpenes, sesquiterpenes, between 5% and 7% of terpene trilactones (ginkgolide A, ginkgolide B, ginkgolide C, ginkgolide J, ginkgolide M, ginkgolide K, ginkgolide L, and bilobalide), 2.8–3.4% corresponding to ginkgolides A, B, and C, and 2.6–3.2% consisting of bilobalide, phenolic acids, polysaccharides, steroids, and a content of less than 5 mg/kg of ginkgolic acids, of which flavonoids and terpene lactones are usually considered to be responsible for the pharmacological activity associated with this plant [54,55]. For instance, ginkgolide B is a potent anti-inflammatory agent and inhibits the platelet-activating factor, and the flavonols of *Ginkgo biloba* have cardioprotective, antioxidant, antibacterial, and neuroprotective properties. Current pharmacological studies have shown that flavonoids from *Ginkgo biloba* have prominent cardioprotective activities, such as regulating blood lipids, lowering blood sugar, inhibiting cardiomyocyte apoptosis, dilating blood vessels, antagonizing platelet-activating factor, and preventing myocardial ischemic injury and vascular rupture [54–57]. It is important to note that many types of preparations based on *Ginkgo biloba* extract have been developed for the treatment of cardiovascular diseases. *Ginkgo biloba* is also used for the prevention and treatment of hypertension, atherosclerosis, peripheral arterial disease, peripheral venous disease, Raynaud's phenomenon, and erectile dysfunction. The plant has also been used for diseases such as cognitive decline, dementia, and tinnitus [54,56,58,59].

2.12. *Coffea (Genus Coffea)*, Family: *Rubiaceae*

Coffee is widely consumed in the world and has a variety of phytochemicals. The main coffee polyphenols include the glycosylated derivate forms of the polyphenol and chlorogenic acids (CGAs), such as esters of caffeic acid and quinic acid. Green coffee is raw coffee beans that have not been roasted, and it is rich in bioactive phytochemical compounds, mainly CGAs, caffeine, and soluble fiber (mostly galactomannans and arabinogalactan) [60,61]. Green coffee bean extract (GCBE) has antioxidant properties and neutralizes reactive oxygen species. In addition, studies have found that the CGA from GCBE regulates vasoreactivity and glucose metabolism, including properties such as anticancer, anti-inflammatory, antilipidemic, antihypertensive, and antidiabetic effects [62–64]. Concerning hypolipidemic effects, GCBE and its CGA reduce triglyceride (TG) and total cholesterol (TC) levels; however, the effects on high- and low-density lipoprotein cholesterol (LDL-C) levels are inconsistent. Some studies have reported an increase in serum high-density lipoprotein cholesterol (HDL-C) after GCBE intake, while others have reported non-significant results [65].

2.13. *Hibiscus sabdariffa* (Roselle), Family: *Malvaceae*

Hibiscus sabdariffa Linn is commonly known as roselle, which probably originated in West Africa and grows in tropical and subtropical regions. Roselle contains several bioactive compounds that have medicinal properties, such as phenolic acids (protocatechuic, chlorogenic caffeic acid, and gallic acids), flavonoids (quercetin-3-glucoside, methyl epigallocatechin, myricetin, quercetin, rutin, and kaempferol), anthocyanins (delphinidin-3-sambubioside and cyanidin-3-sambubioside), and organic acids (hibiscus acid, citric acid, hydroxycitric acid, malic acid, and tartaric acid), which are responsible for many biological activities [66,67]. This plant is commonly used as a traditional drink material and folk medicine against hypertension, pyrexia, liver disease, fever, inflammation, kidney and urinary bladder stones, and obesity. Roselle, mainly its calyx, has phytochemicals with various health benefits, such as antihyperglycemic, antihyperlipidemic, antihypertensive, antioxidative, anti-inflammatory, and antifibrosis effects [66–69]. Roselle water extracts also show anticancer, antibacterial, nephro- and hepato-protective, renal/diuretic effect, anticholesterol, and antidiabetic effects among others; this might be related to the inhibition of α-glucosidase and α-amylase, inhibition of angiotensin-converting enzymes (ACE), including the direct vasorelaxant effect or calcium channel modulation [66,67,70,71]. Additionally, *Hibiscus sabdariffa* relaxes other smooth muscles, including the intestine, uterus, and bladder [67].

2.14. *Ilex paraguariensis A.St.-Hil.* (Mate), Family: *Aquifoliaceae*

Ilex paraguariensis, commonly known as yerba mate, is one of the most widely consumed plants in subtropical regions of South America (Brazil, Paraguay, Uruguay, and Argentina). This tree or shrub contains polyphenols derived from caffeoyl, manly monocaffeoyl quinic isomers (3-O-caffeoyl quinic or neochlorogenic acid, 5-O-caffeoyl quinic or chlorogenic acid and 4-O-caffeoyl quinic or cryptochlorogenic acid), caffeic acid, and dicaffeoyl quinic isomers (3,4-dicaffeoylquinic acid, 3,5-dicaffeoylquinic acid, and 4,5-dicaffeoylquinic acid), methylxanthines (caffeine, theophylline, and theobromine), flavonoids (quercetin, kaempferol, and rutin), tannins, and numerous triterpenic saponins that are derived from ursolic acid and are named metesaponins [72,73]. Yerba mate exhibits various biological activities such as antioxidant, anti-inflammatory, antiobesity, anticancer, immunomodulatory, improvement in glycemic and lipid metabolism, reversion of insulin resistance, inhibition of glycation and atherosclerosis, thermogenic and vasodilatation effects, a protective effect against induced DNA damage, and reduction in cardiovascular risk [72–77]. Moreover, yerba mate facilitates recovery from physical and mental fatigue, reduces the feeling of hunger, and works as a diuretic; an aqueous extract of this medicinal plant protects the myocardium against ischemia-reperfusion injury and decreases oxidative damage, which can be attributed to the potent antioxidant properties of the extract [72,78].

2.15. *Moringa oleifera Lam., Family: Moringaceae*

Moringa oleifera Lam. is native to the sub-Himalayan northern parts of India and commonly cultivated throughout tropical and sub-tropical countries. *Moringa* leaves are rich in many nutritious and bioactive compounds, including carotenoids, polyphenols, glucosinolates [the most abundant of them is 4-O-(α-l-rhamnopyranosyl-oxy)-benzylglucosinolate or also named glucomoringin], tannins, among others. Polyphenolic compounds are represented by flavonoids (mostly quercetin and kaempferol in their 3′-O-glycoside forms) and phenolic acids such as gallic, chlorogenic, which is an ester of dihydrocinnamic acid (caffeic acid), ellagic, quinic, and ferulic acids [79,80]. The following compounds have hypotensive properties, such as sothiocyanates, thiocyanates, and nitriles, which are formed by enzymatic hydrolysis of the glucosinolates; niaziminin, also a hypotensive, is a mustard oil glycoside isolated along with other glycosides (niazinin and niazimicin) from ethanolic extracts of *Moringa oleifera* leaves. The flavonol quercetin is a potent antioxidant and is found at concentrations as high as 100 mg/100 g of dried *Moringa oleifera* leaves [79,80]. The bioactive compounds of *Moringa oleifera* are accountable for many medicinal properties such as cholesterol-lowering, antiobesity, antihyperlipidemic, antidiabetic, antihypertensive, neuroprotective, antiasthmatic, antitumor, anti-inflammatory, antioxidant, antipyretic, antiepileptic, antiulcer, antispasmodic, diuretic, hepatoprotective, antiviral, antimicrobial, antifungal, and cardioprotective activity, as well as protection against signs of aging, typhoid fever, malaria, diarrhea, and dysentery [79–84].

2.16. *Nigella sativa, Family: Ranunculaceae*

This medicinal plant is popularly known as black seed or black cumin and is mainly distributed in North Africa, the Middle East, Europe, and Asia. The major phytochemical constituent of the seeds from *Nigella sativa* is thymoquinone (particularly the essential oil), but they also include phytosterols (β-sitosterol and stigmasterol), alkaloids (e.g., nigellamines), saponins, dithymoquinone, nigellin, terpenes and terpenoids (such as thymoquinone and its derivatives), tocopherols, polyphenols (such as quercitrin and kaempferol), and miscellaneous components [85,86]. These bioactive components of the seeds are responsible for the pleiotropic pharmacological properties, such as antioxidant, anti-inflammatory, antihypertensive, antihepatotoxic, anticancer, hypoglycemic, antimicrobial, antifungal, antinephrotoxic, antihepatotoxic, lipid-lowering properties, and immunostimulating activities. The seeds of *Nigella sativa* are also used for the treatment of cardiovascular diseases, respiratory diseases (asthma and bronchitis), cough, headache, rheumatic disorders, fever, influenza, obesity, epilepsy, back pain, and gastrointestinal disorders (indigestion and diarrhea) as well as in cases of amenorrhea, dysmenorrhea, and skin infections [85–87].

2.17. *Opuntia ficus Indica, Family: Cactaceae*

The species of genus *Opuntia* (approximately 200) grow extensively in desert or semi-desert regions in Mexico, the United States, and Mediterranean countries, among other countries. This plant is native to Mexico and is known there as nopal, prickly-pear cactus in the Southern United States, and Indian fig cactus in Europe. Cladodes of *Opuntia ficus-indica* provide dietary fiber and bioactive compounds such as carotenoids (lutein, β-carotene, and β-cryptoxanthin), flavonoids (isorhamnetin-3-O-glucoside, kaempferol, quercetin, isoquercetin, nicotiflorin, and rutin), and phenolic compounds (coumaric callic acid, and 3,4-dihydroxybenzoic 4-hydroxybenzoic, and ferulic acid). Moreover, cladodes are rich in pectin, mucilage, minerals, malic acid, vitamins, and antioxidants. Meanwhile, prickly-pear fruits contain bioactive compounds such as pigments (betaxanthins, betacyanins, and betalains) and flavonoids (kaempferol, quercetin, and isorhamnetin) [88,89]. *Opuntia ficus-indica* has actions against atherosclerotic cardiovascular diseases, diabetes, obesity, hypertension, asthma, burns, edema, and indigestion, as well as other pharmacological effects including antioxidant, neuroprotective, anti-inflammatory, antihypercholesterolemic, antiulcer, antimicrobial, antiviral potential, wound-healing, skin-protective, hepatoprotective, anticancer, human infertility, and chemopreventive effects. Moreover, *Opuntia ficus-indica* has effects on the bone health, kidneys, and gastrointestinal tract, including gastroprotective, sedative, analgesic, anxiolytic, cognitive, and memory effects [88–92].

2.18. *Platycodon grandiflorus, Family: Campanulaceae*

Platycodon grandiflorus, a common Chinese herb, is mainly distributed in Northeast Asia, including China, the Korean Peninsula, Japan, and Siberia, where it has been used for decades as a traditional medicinal herb. A phytochemical investigation revealed that *Platycodon grandiflorus* contains at least 100 compounds, including steroidal saponins, flavonoids, polyacetylenes, sterols (e.g., stigmasterol), phenolic acids, and other bioactive compounds, among which, saponins are considered the main active compounds [93,94]. Triterpenoid saponins such as platycodin A, C, D and polygalacin D, which contain sterol components including stigmasterol, have various effects such as improving blood glucose and cholesterol metabolism, anticancer and anti-inflammatory effects, and relieving atopic dermatitis. Platycodin A, platycodin C, deapioplatycodin D, and 16-oxo-platycodin D have antiobesity effects. Platycodin D is the main phytochemical in *Platycodon grandiflorus* extract, which has shown antioxidant, anti-inflammation, antiadipogeneic, antiobesity, antifibrosis, and antitumor properties. Furthermore, platycodin D inhibits pancreatic lipase activity [93,94] and inhibits the adipogenesis of 3T3-L1 cells by upregulating Kruppel like factor 2 (KLF2) and subsequent downregulation of peroxisome proliferator-activated receptor gamma (PPARγ) [95]. Platycodin D improves obesity in db/db mice by an AMPK-associated decrease in adipogenic (PPARγ and CCAAT/enhancer-binding protein alpha, C/EBPα) and increase in thermogenesis markers (UCP1 and PGC1α) [96]. Moreover, total saponins of *Platycodon grandiflorus* reduce the levels of blood glucose, serum cholesterol, TG, and LDL-C, increase serum HDL-C, and improve liver function, thereby reducing T2D in rats [94]. In summary, *Platycodon grandiflorus* exhibit pharmacological activities, such as antidiabetic, antibacterial, antiapoptosis, hypocholesterolemic, hypoglycemic, immune enhancement, and liver protection effects, improve insulin resistance and the lipid profile, decrease BP, alleviate atopic dermatitis, as well as relieving cough and asthma activities, apophlegmatic, antitussive, and cardiovascular system activities [93,94,97–100]. *Platycodon grandiflorus* has also been reported to be used for the treatments of chest congestion, chest distress, diphtheria, dyspnea, mastitis, measles, dermatitis, dysentery, suppuration, chronic rhinitis, chronic tonsillitis, bronchitis, asthma, pulmonary abscesses, pulmonary tuberculosis, faucitis, bronchial asthma, and other conditions [93,94].

2.19. *Punica granatum L., Family: Lythraceae*

Punica granatum Linn., commonly known as pomegranate, is a small shrub with tasty fruit native to the Middle East, growing in subtropical and temperate regions and having a variety of planting distributions around the world. More than 60 bioactive components have been identified in pomegranate, which are categorized as phenols, flavonoids, triterpenes, alkaloids, sterols, vitamins, and unsaturated fatty acids. In addition, pomegranates are rich in polyphenolic antioxidants, such as tannins, anthocyanin, and flavonoids; these active components are the most abundant in pomegranates. The main compounds isolated from pomegranate flowers are polyphenols, flavonoids, terpenoids, and triterpenoids, such as leanolic acid and ursolic acid. The pomegranate fruit includes hydrolyzable tannins like gallotannins and ellagitannins, as well as ellagic acid and its derivatives, gallic acid, anthocyanins, proanthocyanidins, flavonoids, sterols, lignans, terpenes, and terpenoids. Pomegranate peel is abundant in a variety of phenolics, ellagitannins, proanthocyanidins, microelements, and flavonoids, including kaempferol-3-O-glucoside. *Punica granatum* bark is rich in tannins, proanthocyanidins, anthocyanins, and terpenoids. Pomegranate juice is rich in antioxidants, such as polyphenols, flavonoids, ellagitannins, tannins, and anthocyanins [101–103]. In vivo and in vitro studies have shown that extracts of different pomegranate fractions (peels, flowers, seeds, and juice) improve lipid metabolism in diseases such as atherosclerosis, metabolic dysfunction-associated steatotic liver disease (MASLD), metabolic syndrome, and type 2 diabetes, including a wide range of diseases, such as inflammation, Alzheimer's disease, ulcers, diarrhea, erectile dysfunction, obesity, cancer, brain ischaemia, fibrosis, and fungal and microbial infections. Pomegranate flowers are used for the treatment of cardiovascular disorders, diabetes, obesity, and some microbial infections (Salmonella entteriditis and Kentucky). Pomegranate seeds are used to treat heart diseases, diabetes, cancer, obesity, urinary disorders, and to prevent miscarriage and to improve male fertility. Additionally, pomegranate seeds have antimicrobial and antioxidant properties. Pomegranate peel extracts are traditionally used to treat diarrhea and ulcers. Other pharmaceutical properties reported in pomegranate peels include antiproliferative, anti-inflammatory, antioxidant, and anticancerous effects. *Punica granatum* bark has been used traditionally for the treatment of inflammation, diarrhea, malaria, nose bleeding, sore throat, ulcer, and hoarseness. Pomegranate juice has important biological actions, including antioxidant activity and cardiovascular protection. Moreover, the consumption of pomegranate can relieve dental infections and menopausal symptoms, as well as improve the intestinal microbiota, thus preventing obesity and diabetes [101–106].

2.20. *Salvia miltiorrhiza Bunge, Family: Lamiaceae*

Salvia miltiorrhiza Bunge, commonly called danshen, is a perennial herb used in traditional Chinese medicine. *Salvia miltiorrhiza* contains more than 100 compounds, including salvianolic acid A/B/C/D/E/F/G, lithospermic acid, danshensu, caffeic acid, and rosmarinic acid, tanshinone I/IIA/IIB/V/VI, tanshindiol A, cryptotanshinone, dihydrotanshinone I, miltirone, dehydro miltirone, and isotanshinone, among others. The bioactive compounds in *Salvia miltiorrhiza* extract are classified into two major groups, water-soluble phenolics (salvianolic acid and comfrey acid) and liposoluble tanshinones (diterpenoids), which are responsible for the main pharmacological properties of *Salvia miltiorrhiza* [107,108]. Tanshinone IIA and salvianolate have various cardiovascular and pharmacological effects, including antioxidative, anti-inflammatory, endothelial protective, anticoagulation, vasodilation, myocardial protective, anticoagulation, vasodilation, and antiatherosclerosis, as well as effects on reducing the proliferation and migration of vascular smooth muscle cells. Additionally, salvianolates are composed of salvianolic acid B, rosmarinic acid, and lithospermic acid, which are widely used in the treatment of coronary heart disease. Meanwhile, tanshinones are more effective in the treatment of cardiovascular diseases and cerebrovascular diseases, including atherosclerosis, myocardial infarction, cardiac hypertrophy, myocardial ischemia-reperfusion (I/R), and chronic heart failure. *Salvia miltiorrhiza* has other effects such as antidiabetic, anti-inflammation, antioxidant, antifibrosis, and antiapoptosis effects. *Salvia miltiorrhiza* is also used to treat malignant tumors, neurological, lung diseases, inflammatory diseases, gynecological diseases, liver diseases, renal diseases, and metabolic disorders such as atherosclerosis, hyperlipidemia, obesity, and other dyslipidemia-related diseases [107–110].

2.21. *Taraxacum officinale L. (Dandelion), Family: Asteraceae*

Taraxacum officinale L., also known as dandelion, a perennial herb and commonly regarded as a weed, is native to Eurasia and grows in America, Africa, New Zealand, and Australia. Dandelion has phenolic acids (chlorogenic acid and chicoric acid), flavonoids (luteolin derivatives and quercetin), and terpenes (sesquiterpene lactones). The leaves contain bitter sesquiterpene lactones (taraxinic acid and triterpenoids such as cycloartenol), while the roots have phenolic acids, inulin, sesquiterpene lactones, triterpenes, sterols (taraxasterol, taraxerol, cycloartenol, beta-sitosterol, and stigmasterol), and the compounds already mentioned, which contribute to their therapeutic properties [111,112]. Dandelion has been used as a phytomedicine for its holeretic, antirheumatic, diuretic, antibacterial, hypolipidemic, hypoglycemic, antithrombotic, anti-inflammatory, antiobesity, antioxidant, and antiplatelet effects, as well its use against cancer and cardiovascular ailments. Moreover, dandelion is used as a remedy for kidney diseases, and liver, kidney, and spleen disorders. Dandelion has high levels of phenolic acids, with antioxidant effects; coumarins with anti-inflammatory, anticancer, antibacterial, and antithrombotic properties; sesquiterpene lactones with anti-inflammatory and antibacterial effects; and triterpenes or phytosterols, which possess antiatherosclerotic effects. Dandelion leaves and flowers contain polyphenols, predominantly hydroxycinnamic acid derivatives, and flavonoids (apigenin and luteolin derivatives), all of which have antioxidant and hypocholesterolemic properties. Dandelion roots are rich in inulin, which has a hypoglycemic, probiotic, and immune-boosting effect; meanwhile, its phytochemicals such as phenolic acids and sesquiterpene lactones are responsible for its antidiabetic properties. In general, bioactive compounds from dandelion roots possess bifidogenic, anti-inflammatory, and antifibrotic activities [111–116].

3. Pathological Processes Involved in Obesity

Overweight and obesity are increasingly common conditions in the world due to the intake of calorie-dense foods and relatively inactive lifestyles, which create long-term imbalances between energy uptake and expenditure, and these conditions promote the deposition of fat mass in the body's WAT, leading to phenotypic changes in this tissue such as adipocyte hypertrophy (cell size increase) and subsequently hyperplasia (cell number increase) [1,3,117]. In obesity, the hypertrophied WAT visceral adipocytes show lipolysis activation, leading to high levels of circulating non-esterified fatty acids (NEFAs) [118]. NEFAs in normal conditions are catabolized by the β-oxidation to provide energy to tissues such as the liver and muscle; however, high concentrations contribute to the development of insulin resistance [119]. Furthermore, hypertrophic visceral adipocytes contribute to elevated circulating triacylglycerol (TAG) levels mainly from de novo lipogenesis, in which fatty acids (FAs) are synthesized from carbohydrates or FAs are provided from chylomicrons and very low-density lipoproteins (VLDL) [120]. Several studies suggest that oxidative stress plays a fundamental role as a factor linking obesity and its related complications. Furthermore, oxidative stress can increase with preadipocyte proliferation, adipocyte differentiation, and the size of mature adipocytes. Nuclear factor erythroid 2-related factor 2 (NRF2) is a key transcription factor that protects against oxidative stress and electrophilic stress. NRF2 is abundantly expressed in WAT. The deficiency of NRF2 leads to imparting adipocyte differentiation in 3T3-L1 cells and human subcutaneous preadipocytes. Meanwhile, its transfection stimulates hormone-induced adipocyte differentiation. Oxidative stress is increased in WAT from obese mice and from human individuals with obesity. NRF2 in response to oxidative stress activates *Srebf1* promoter and induces target gene transcription and subsequent lipogenesis, which promotes lipid accumulation in adipocytes, thus exacerbating the development of obesity [121]. However, the effects of NRF2 are controversial and even contradictory in animal models of diet-induced obesity. mRNA expression and protein levels of *Nrf2* gene were reduced or increased in WAT and liver in obese mouse models with different percentages of fat calories and feeding duration [122]. Obesity per se can also induce systemic oxidative stress through superoxide generation from NADPH oxidases, oxidative phosphorylation, protein kinase C activation (PKC), glyceraldehyde auto-oxidation, and polyol and hexosamine pathways. Additionally, elevated plasma-free FAs promote the generation of superoxide radicals, hyperleptinemia, low antioxidant defense, and low-grade chronic inflammation. Additionally, postprandial reactive oxygen species generation are other factors that also contribute to oxidative stress in obesity. Obesity-associated oxidative stress induces various pathological events, including insulin resistance and diabetes, liver failure, cardiovascular complications, sleep disorders, and asthma, including reproductive, oncological, and rheumatological problems [1,3,123]. Adipose tissue produces several adipokines including cytokines and hormones, which regulate energy homeostasis, glucose and lipid metabolism, and cardiovascular functions [124]. Because obesity is directly associated with low-grade chronic inflammation, the hypertrophy and hyperplasia of adipose tissue leads to the organ's dysfunction and development of a pro-inflammatory microenvironment, and the signaling pathway of NF-κB is activated and increases the expression of interleukin-6 (IL-6), tumor necrosis factor-α (TNF-α), and IL-1β through the TLR4/MyD88 signaling pathway; other molecules increased with excessive adiposity are leptin, IL-8, CRP, PAI-1, haptoglobin, angiotensinogen, inducible nitric oxide synthase, platelet-activating factor (PAF) and chemokines, such as monocyte chemotactic protein 1 (MCP1), which promotes the migration of macrophages into the adipose tissue and induces the release of cytokines. Furthermore, in obese subjects, the levels of interleukin 10 (IL-10) are decreased, which worsens the metabolic profile due to IL-10 inhibiting the synthesis of pro-inflammatory cytokines [3,19,123,125,126]. The activation of NF-κB, TLR4, and mTOR leads to the attenuation of insulin signaling and insulin resistance in several tissues, which contribute to obesity-related complications, including diabetes and atherosclerosis [127,128]. Platelets are key players in thrombotic processes, and various platelet markers have been reported elevated in obese and T2D individuals, including the mean platelet volume, circulating levels of platelet microparticles, oxidation products, platelet-derived soluble P-selectin, and CD40L. Therefore, these markers contribute to an intersection between obesity, inflammation, and thrombotic phenotype [129]. Obesity is an altered health condition with changes in gut microbiota due to the consumption of improper diet, which affects the health status of the host. The gut microbiota plays an important role in energy balance, intestinal integrity, and immunity against invading pathogens. Approximately 100 trillion microbes colonize the human gut, which are represented by microorganisms such as bacteria, archaea, fungi, protozoa, and viruses. The gut microbiota is represented by the phyla Bacteroidetes, Firmicutes, Proteobacteria, Actinobacteria, and Verrucomicrobia, and approximately 90% of the total bacterial species belong to Bacteroidetes and Firmicutes. Obese individuals exhibit reduced proportions of Bacteroidetes and elevated levels of Actinobacteria with no significant differences in Firmicutes; thus, an increased Firmicutes/Bacteroidetes ratio is a biomarker of obesity susceptibility [130,131].

Plant and Herb Extracts with Antiobesity Activity

Previous studies have shown the nutritional and beneficial effects on the metabolism of plant and herb consumption, showing a wide range of bioactive compounds, many of them with different properties for healthy humans. There are several papers in which the use of various medicinal plants and herbs to treat obesity has been investigated. For instance, green tea is associated with beneficial health effects due to its body-fat-reducing and hypocholesterolemic properties [132,133], and green tea aqueous extract (GTAE, 1.1% and 2%) administered in rats fed with a high-fat diet, lowed atherogenic index, reduced body weight gain (only with 2% of GTAE), and prevented visceral fat accumulation [134]. The visceral weight loss and improvement of lipid profile with green tea in rats may be due to increased thermogenesis and fat oxidation [135]. The main phytochemicals in *Caralluma fimbriata* are pregnane glycosides, which are known to suppress hunger and increase endurance. Therefore, pregnane glycosides and diterpenes from *Caralluma fimbriata*, have antiobesity activities [25]. In a diet-induced obesity (DIO) rat model, *Caralluma fimbriata* extract (CFE) showed dose-dependent appetite suppressant, prevented liver weight and fat pad mass, and protected against atherogenesis in rats fed a cafeteria diet [136]. In overweight adults, CFE preserved body weight, decreased waist circumference, and reduced daily caloric intake over a 16-week period in overweight patients compared to a placebo. The mechanism for appetite suppression by CFE includes a reduction in ghrelin synthesis in the stomach and neuropeptide Y in the hypothalamus [26]. Bioactive compounds derived from *cacao*, which are rich in polyphenols (flavonoids), are beneficial against overweight and lipid disorders. In an obesity model induced by a high-fat diet (HFD) and fructose ingestion in rats, cocoa extracts made with outer pod husk and kernel husk decreased weight gain, reduced SBP, and improved lipid profiles [42]. *Ginkgo biloba* extract (GBE), which contains a mixture of polyphenols with antioxidant properties, has several potentially beneficial effects, such as reducing food and energy intake, reducing body adiposity, improving insulin sensitivity, enhancing insulin receptor and AKT phosphorylation, reducing NF-κB p65 phosphorylation in retroperitoneal adipose tissue of obese rats, and reducing weight gain in models of obesity induced by diet and ovariectomy [137–139]. These findings were confirmed in HFD-induced obese male rats; GBE supplementation reduced energy intake and epididymal adipocyte volume [140]. Green coffee beans contain phytochemicals with beneficial effects on cardiometabolic disorders. The 3-caffeoylquinic acid (3-CQA) in green coffee bean extract (GCBE) was evaluated in HFD-induced obese mice, and this extract decreased body weight gain, liver weight and WAT weights, regulating adipogenesis and lipid metabolism-linked genes and proteins in WAT and liver [141]. In addition, in male albino Wistar rats fed with a HFD, and intervened with GCBE when obesity was established, the extract decreased the body and organ weights, and reduced TC, TG, LDL-C, VLDL, glucose, and insulin levels. GCBE also exhibited an increase in adiponectin levels and decreased the expression of RBP4, whereas an increase in GLUT4 expression was observed in the adipose tissue [142]. *Moringa oleifera* leaf extracts (MOLE) possess antiobesity effects in experimental animal models and were tested in HFD-induced obesity in rats. Thirteen metabolites were identified in MOLE, including flavanols, flavones, and phenolic acid. MOLE reduced weight gain and adiposity index, including glucose, insulin and HOMA-IR, and Revised Quantitative Insulin Sensitivity Check Index (R-QUICKI) was significantly increased by MOLE. In visceral fat mass, MOLE significantly reduced the levels of leptin and vaspin; meanwhile, adiponectin, omentin and glucose transporter 4 (GLUT4) expression were increased. MOLE significantly inhibited FAS and HMG-CoA reductase and elevated the mRNA expression of MC4R and PPARα. In obese patients, the administration of *Moringa oleifera* hard gelatin capsules showed a significant reduction in the average BMI, TC and LDL-C [81]. Previous studies have shown that *Ilex paraguariensis* (yerba mate) aqueous extracts inhibited the progression of atherosclerosis and decreased body weight, visceral fat, serum lipids, glucose, leptin, and insulin levels in HFD-fed-rats [143,144]. Treatment with *Ilex paraguariensis* extracts (IPE) in C57BL/6J mice fed a HFD also reduced the accumulation of lipids in adipocytes, body weight gain, and obesity. Additionally, the extract reduced serum cholesterol, serum TG, and glucose levels [76]. These findings were confirmed in another study, in which Yerba mate extract was also evaluated in mice fed with a HFD, and obese mice treated with yerba mate exhibited marked attenuation of weight gain, adiposity, a reduction in epididymal fat pad weight, and restoration of the serum levels of cholesterol, TGs, LDL-C, and glucose [75]. In obese rats primed by early weaning, IPE reversed abdominal obesity, leptin resistance and hypertriglyceridemia [145]. Chlorogenic acid in yerba mate is mainly responsible for these effects [146]. In another study *Ilex paraguariensis* was investigated in Korean subjects with obesity. Individuals with obesity were given oral supplements of Yerba Mate capsules, and this supplementation decreased body fat mass, percentage body fat, and waist–hip ratio, which suggests that Yerba Mate supplementation may be an alternative for treating obese patients [147]. *Platycodon grandiflorus* root extract (PGE) was analyzed in obese Korean adults and revealed a significant decrease in body fat mass and body fat percentage, suggesting antiobesogenic effects in overweight or obese adult humans [148]. Pomegranate extract (PomE) is rich in punicalagins and increases markers related to browning and thermogenesis in human differentiated adipocytes [149]. In addition, in a preclinical study of HFD-induced obesity, PomE increased systemic energy expenditure, thus contributing to a reduction in the low grade of chronic inflammation and insulin resistance associated with obesity [104].

Oxidative stress results from the elevated production of free radicals along with reduced levels of antioxidants and plays an important role in cardiovascular diseases, including atherosclerosis and coronary artery disease [123]. CFE improves HFD-induced cardiac damage through reducing cardiac lipids such as total lipids, TG, TC, and free fatty acids (FFAs). Furthermore, CFE improves the activities of antioxidant enzymes, such as glutathione peroxidase (GPx), glutathione reductase (GR), glutathione peroxidase (GPx), catalase (CAT), superoxide dismutase (SOD), and glutathione-s-transferase (GST) [27]. *Moringa oleifera* leaf extracts (MOLE) were evaluated in HFD-induced obesity and cardiac damage in rats. The activities of antioxidant enzymes were decreased in animals that received an HFD; however, these antioxidant enzymes were significantly, and dose-dependently, enhanced by administration with MOLE [150].

Several diseases associated with obesity, such as dyslipidemia, T2D, and cardiovascular disease, are closely related to low-grade inflammation. In WAT from obese mice, TNF-α, IL-6, leptin, CCR2, CCL2, and PAI-1 genes were upregulated. However, yerba mate extract administration decreased the expression of these genes [75]. In addition, yerba mate extract intake blunted the proinflammatory effects of HFD-induced obesity in rats through the phosphorylation of hypothalamic IKK and NF-κB p65 expression and increasing the protein levels of IκBα, adiponectin receptor-1, and IRS-2 [151]. *Andrographis paniculata* extract (APE) and its bioactive constituent andrographolide are known to possess anti-inflammatory and antiapoptotic effects. APE was analyzed in myocardial tissue from HFD-induced obese mice. The animals fed with HFD developed myocardial inflammation, which potentially contributed to cardiac hypertrophy and myocardial apoptosis, but APE showed significant inhibition of these effects in obese mice [152].

Aronia melanocarpa contains a high content of procyanidins and anthocyanins. It was found that *Aronia melanocarpa* extract significantly inhibits the amidolytic activity of thrombin and plasmin, the latter being the main fibrinolytic enzyme [153]. Moreover, patients with metabolic syndrome showed a significant reduction in the levels of TC, LDL-C, and TG, as well as an improvement in platelet aggregation, clotting, and fibrinolysis after *Aronia melanocarpa* extract supplementation [154]. The effect of *Citrullus colocynthis* was investigated on blood hemostasis in HFD-induced obese rats, and it was found that *Citrullus colocynthis* reversed HFD-induced increases in fibrinogen and von Willebrand factor; thus, *Citrullus colocynthis* has antiplatelets and profibrinolytic properties due to its potent hypoglycaemic and hypolipidaemic effect, its ability to reduced levels of circulatory TNF-α and IL-6, and its ability to lower prothrombotic leptin levels and elevate antithrombic adiponectin levels [34]. *Cydonia oblonga* is traditionally used in Uyghur medicine to prevent cardiovascular diseases. *Cydonia oblonga* extract (COE) was explored on models (mice and rats) and markers of thrombosis. COE dose-dependently prolonged bleeding and the clotting time. In addition, COE reduced pulmonary embolism mortality, dose-dependently increased thrombolysis, and reduced TXB2. Therefore, COE has an antithrombotic effect, probably at least in part related to antithromboxane activity [53]. Garlic also inhibits platelet aggregation, and aged garlic extract (AGE) blocks both the activation and aggregation of human platelets. The mechanism implicated by AGEs in the inhibition of platelet aggregation includes an increase in cAMP levels through inhibition of cAMP phosphodiesterase activity, resulting in reduction in calcium mobilization and, therefore, suppresses the binding of GPIIa/IIIb receptors to fibrinogen [155]. GBE was investigated on experimental cardiac remodeling in rats induced by acute myocardial infarction. The results suggest that GBE may inhibit experimental myocardial remodeling in rats after acute myocardial infarction by reducing the transcription of TGF-β1, MMP-2 and MMP-9 genes and attenuating extracellular matrix deposition by decreasing the levels of proteins such as type I collagen, MMP-2, and MMP-9 [156].

Cardiometabolic parameters were evaluated in $ApoE^{-/-}$ mice fed an atherogenic diet and green coffee extract (GCE). Although GCE did not decrease atherosclerotic lesion progression or plasma lipid levels, it improved metabolic parameters, such as fasting glucose, insulin resistance, serum leptin, urinary catecholamines, and liver TGs. GCE also decreased weight gain, reduced adiposity, lowered inflammatory infiltrate in adipose tissue, and protection against hepatic damage. Furthermore, the number of observed operational taxonomic units (alpha diversity) diminished in $ApoE^{-/-}$ mice with an atherogenic diet, and it was recovered in the GCE-treated $ApoE^{-/-}$ mice [157]. *Hibiscus sabdariffa* extract (HSE) was evaluated in an experimental model of HFD-induced obesity in mice. HSE reduced weight in mice fed an HFD and improved glucose tolerance, insulin sensitivity and normalized LDL-C/HDL-C cholesterol ratio. HSE reduced the expression of different adipokines and pro-inflammatory mediators, and reinforced gut integrity by reducing the Firmicutes/Bacteroidetes ratio [158]. *Salvia miltiorrhiza* extract (SME) was investigated in rats with HFD-induced obesity. SME treatment markedly reduced weight, body fat index, lipid profile, glucose levels, and adipocyte vacuolation. The beneficial effects were accompanied by elevated concentrations of lipid factors such as cAMP, PKA, and HSL in the liver and adipose tissues, enhanced gut integrity, and ameliorated lipid metabolism. Furthermore, *Salvia miltiorrhiza* extract reversed HFD-induced dysbacteriosis by promoting the abundance of Actinobacteriota and Proteobacteria and reducing the growth of Firmicutes and Desulfobacterita [110]. Therefore, the consumption of products derived from the plants and herbs previously analyzed should be considered a new therapeutic strategy in the control of obesity and its associated disorders (Table 1 and Figure 2).

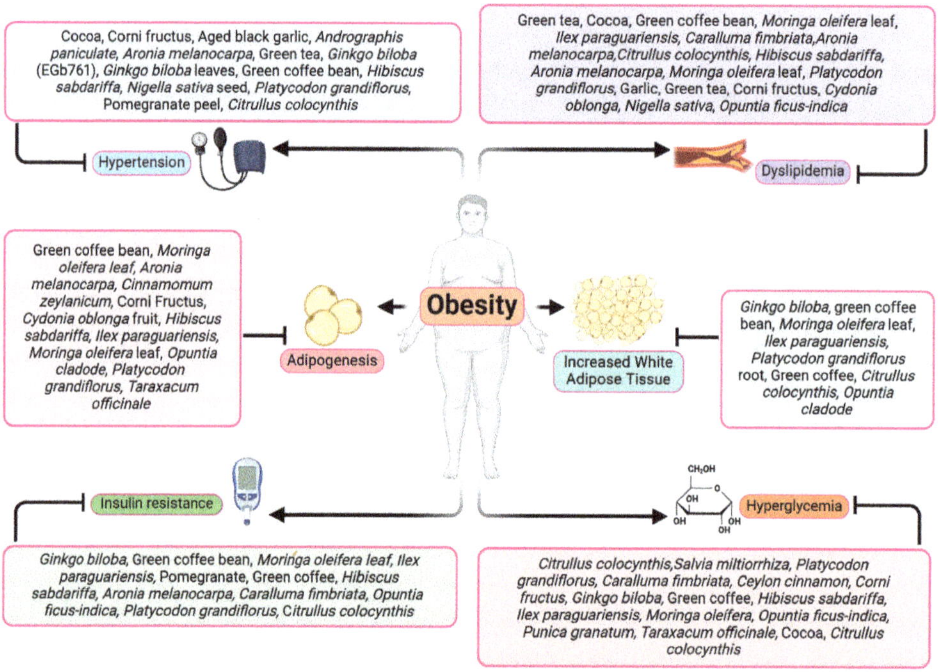

Figure 2. Herb and plant extracts with inhibitory effects on adipogenesis, white adipose tissue accumulation, and cardiometabolic risk factors associated with obesity.

4. Adipogenesis and Obesity

Accumulation and adipocyte differentiation are linked with the development of obesity. In the process of preadipocyte to adipocyte differentiation, several transcription factors participate, the most important being cAMP response element-binding protein (CREB), C/EBPα C/EBPβ, C/EBPδ, and PPARγ, which control adipocyte differentiation. Adipocyte differentiation starts with CREB phosphorylation by PKA and ERK1/ERK2, and at the same time, the activation of C/EBPβ and C/EBPδ occurs, which in turn activate C/EBPα and PPARγ [159]. However, this process is much more complicated because it involves other biological signaling pathways. In addition to adipocyte differentiation, PPARγ plays an important role in lipid storage and glucose homeostasis and is predominantly expressed in adipose tissue [160]. On the other hand, the PI3K/AKT pathway plays a critical role in transmitting insulin action in adipose tissue (increases glucose uptake by the GLUT4 membrane translocation) during the adipogenesis of both WAT and brown adipose tissue (BAT). AKT is essential in inducing PPARγ expression. The activation of PI3K/AKT signaling determines the initiation of adipogenic transformation and adipocyte hyperplasia [161]. AMPK is a serine/threonine kinase that is expressed in several tissues (adipose, skeletal, liver, kidney, and hypothalamus), which regulates lipid/glucose homeostasis, autophagy, mitochondrial biogenesis, protein homeostasis, redox equilibrium, food intake, and insulin signaling. AMPK has a function as a cellular energy sensor. AMPK and adiponectin act in peripheral tissues and the central nervous system by regulating food intake. Consequently, the inhibition of hypothalamic AMPK activity along with an increase in adiponectin levels reduces food intake. In addition, AMPK inhibits de novo synthesis of cholesterol, FAs, and TGs, and activates FAs uptake and β-oxidation. It inhibits and phosphorylates proteins involved in the synthesis of FAs (FAS, ACC1, and SREBP-1c). AMPK inhibits the synthesis of cholesterol (phosphorylates and inhibits HMG-CoA reductase) and, through PGC-1α activation, stimulates mitochondrial biogenesis and β-oxidation. AMPK inhibits adipogenesis via the inhibition of the early mitotic clonal expansion (MCE) phase accompanied with a reduction in early and late adipogenic factors including FAS, SREBP-1c and aP2 [162]. Therefore, the inhibition of differentiation into adipocytes by bioactive compounds from plant and herb extracts is beneficial for the loss of body fat and prevention of obesity (Table 1 and Figure 2).

Adipogenesis as a Possible Target against Obesity

The principal cause of obesity is energy overconsumption and/or insufficient energy expenditure; thereby, excessive food/energy intake leads to the expansion of WAT through de novo adipogenesis with the recruitment of new adipocytes (hyperplasia) and enlargement of existing adipocytes (hypertrophy). Chokeberry extract (*Aronia melanocarpa*) and its active polyphenols (seven antiadipogenic polyphenolic phytochemicals) were investigated in HFD-induced obese mice. Amygdalin and prunasin were shown to inhibit 3T3-L1 adipocyte differentiation by suppressing the expressions of PPARγ, C/EBPα, SREBP-1c, FAS, and aP2. In addition, Chokeberry extract showed in obese mice significant decreases in body weight, serum TG, and LDL-C levels and improved insulin sensitivity [163]. The effects of cinnamon (*Cinnamomum zeylanicum*) extract were examined on the inhibition of adipocyte differentiation in 3T3-L1 fibroblast cells and in male mice fed an HFD. Cinnamon extract inhibited lipid accumulation and increased adiponectin and leptin genes in 3T3-L1 cells. In in vivo experiments, cinnamon extract elevated the expression of lipolysis-related proteins (AMPK, p-ACC, and CPT-1) and decreased the expression of lipid-synthesis-related proteins (SREBP-1c and FAS) in liver tissue [164]. Corni Fructus extract (CFE), which contains Corni Fructus, Dioscoreae Rhizoma, Aurantii Fructus Immaturus, and Platycodonis Radix, was shown to suppress the differentiation of 3T3-L1 adipocytes by reducing the cellular induction of PPARγ, C/EBPα, and lipin-1, including a significant upregulation of AMPK-α phosphorylation. Moreover, CFE in obese mice fed an HFD induced weight loss. Therefore, CFE has a potent antiobesity activity due to the inhibition of adipocyte differentiation and adipogenesis [165]. *Cydonia oblonga* fruit extract (COFE) was tested on adipogenesis in 3T3-L1 preadipocytes. COFE inhibited intracellular TG deposition during adipogenesis. Furthermore, COFE treatment in 3T3-L1 cells induced the upregulation of AMPK-α phosphorylation and downregulation of adipogenic transcription factors (SREBP-1c, PPARγ, and C/EBPα). COFE also reduced the mRNA expression of FAS, ACLY, aP2, and lipoprotein lipase (LPL), including increased HSL and CPT-1 in 3T3-L1 cells [51]. *Hibiscus sabdariffa* extract (HSE) was examined on adipocyte differentiation in 3T3-L1 preadipocytes. HSE significantly inhibited lipid droplet accumulation and attenuated adipogenic transcriptional factors C/EBPα and PPARγ during adipogenesis. HSE also reduced the expression of PI3K/AKT and phosphorylation and expression of MEK1/ERK during adipocyte differentiation. Taken together, HSE inhibits adipocyte differentiation through the regulation of PI3K/AKT and ERK pathways, which play pivotal roles during adipogenesis [166]. *Ilex paraguariensis* extracts (IPE) were investigated in 3T3-L1 adipocytes and HFD-fed obese Sprague Dawley (SD) rats. IPE inhibited intracellular lipid accumulation in 3T3-L1 adipocytes, increased AMPK-α, HSL, CaMKK, LKB1, PKA, C/EBPβ, IRβ, and IRS1(Tyr465), and decreased SREBP-1c, FAS, PPARγ, and IRS1 (Ser1101). Furthermore, an AMPK-α inhibitor abolished the effects exerted by IPE on intracellular lipid accumulation and HSL and FAS expression levels. In animals, IPE inhibited body weight gain and ameliorated serum cholesterol levels, and increased AMPK-α, PKA, ERK1/ERK2 (p44/p42), and UCP1 and reduced those genes of mammalian target of rapamycin, S6 kinase, SREBP-1c, ap2, FAS, Il6, adiponectin, leptin, and FABP4 in obese SD rats [167]. *Moringa oleifera* leaf petroleum ether extract (MOPEE) which has high levels of isoquercitrin, chrysin-7-glucoside, and quercitrin, was studied on lipid accumulation by in vitro and in vivo experiments. MOPEE suppressed adipogenesis in 3T3-L1 adipocytes by downregulating the expression of adipogenesis-associated proteins (PPARγ, C/EBPα and C/EBPβ, and FAS) and upregulating the expression of a lipolysis-associated protein (HSL). MOPEE also significantly increased the phosphorylation of AMPKα and ACC. In HFD-induced obese mice, MOPEE decreased body weight, epididymal, perirenal, and mesenteric fat weight, and fat tissue size, including hepatic fat accumulation. Furthermore, MOPEE also decreased TC, LDL-C, and aspartate transferase (AST). Additionally, MOPEE decreased the expression of adipogenesis-associated proteins (PPARγ and FAS) and upregulated the expression of a lipolysis-associated protein (ATGL) in the liver and epididymal fat tissue. MOPEE also increased the phosphorylation of AMPKα and ACC in the liver and epididymal fat tissue of obese mice. Therefore, MOPEE suppresses fat accumulation by inhibiting adipogenesis and promoting lipolysis [82]. A study explored the antiadipogenic effects of lyophilized *Opuntia* cladode powders (OCP) in an in vitro and an in vivo HFD-induced obesity rat model. Two OCP were tested (O. streptacantha and O. ficus-indica). OCP impaired differentiation in adipocytes (3T3 F442A) and decreased TG content and low glucose uptake, thus suggesting an antiadipogenic effect. In SD rats, OCP slightly reduced body weight gain and liver and abdominal fat weights, improved some metabolic parameters, and augmented TG excretion in the feces [168]. *Platycodon grandiflorus* extract (PGE) was investigated on pre-adipocyte 3T3-L1 differentiation, pancreatic lipase activity, and HFD-induced obese rats. PGE inhibited 3T3-L1 pre-adipocyte differentiation and fat accumulation and reduced pancreatic lipase activity. In SD rats, PGE significantly reduced plasma TC and TG levels, body weight, and subcutaneous adipose tissue weight. PGE also reduced the size of subcutaneous adipocytes [169]. *Taraxacum officinale* (Dandelion) was investigated on adipocyte differentiation and lipogenesis in 3T3-L1 preadipocytes. Leaf and root extracts and a commercial root powder (caffeic and chlorogenic acids as the main phenolic constituents) were used in the study. All extracts tested inhibited adipocyte differentiation and lipid accumulation in 3T3-L1 cells [114]. Therefore, the analyzed herbal and plant extracts play an important role during adipogenesis and lipid metabolism, supporting their therapeutic potential for the prevention and treatment of obesity (Table 1 and Figure 2).

Table 1. Extracts from different herbs and plants with antiobesity properties.

Name of Herbs and Plants and Method of Extraction	Type of Study	Doses and Duration	Outcomes and Side Effects (Humans)
Allium sativum (Garlic) Aged Garlic Extract (15–20% aqueous ethanol). Extract on the market in different brands.	Isolated human platelets stimulated with ADP	1.56 to 25% (*v*/*v*)	Inhibited platelet binding to fibrinogen by 40–70.4%, decreased PAC-1 binding to GPIIb/IIIa by 72%, and increased cAMP levels [155]. Garlic extract may cause breath and body odor, upset stomach, or heartburn.
Andrographis paniculata (ethanolic extract). Extract on the market in different brands.	4-week-old male C57/BL6 mice with HFD (45% kcal from fat)	2 g/kg/day, orally for a week	Attenuated cardiac hypertrophy and apoptosis, decreased ANP and BNP proteins, reduced cardiac collagen accumulation and fibrosis, inhibited COX-2, p-IκBα, and NF-κB proteins, reversed cardiac inflammation and myocardial apoptosis [152]. *Andrographis* can cause diarrhea, vomiting, rash, headache, runny nose, and fatigue.
Aronia melanocarpa (Chokeberry), methanol extract. Extract on the market in different brands.	3T3-L1 adipocytes and 5-week-old male C57BL/6J mice with HFD (60% kcal from fat)	In vitro: 7 polyphenols at 10 µM for 8 days. In vivo: 100 or 200 mg/kg/day, oral-ly for 8 weeks	Inhibited 3T3-L1 adipocyte differentiation, decreased body weight, serum TG, and LDL-C levels; improved insulin sensitivity [163]. Chokeberry extract can cause constipation, diarrhea, or nausea. Taking chokeberry together with drugs that slow blood clotting might increase the risk of bruising and bleeding.
Aronia melanocarpa (Chokeberry) Polyphenol-rich extract (aqueous extract). Extract on the market in different brands.	Human platelets stimulated with ADP	Platelet adhesion assay (range 0.5–100 µg/mL), thrombin activity (0.5–100 mg/mL), Plasmin activity (2.5, 5, 10, 20, 100 µg/mL)	Reduced ADP-activated platelet adhesion, increased overall potential of clotting and lysis, inhibited thrombin and plasmin amidolytic activity [153]. Chokeberry extract can cause constipation, diarrhea, or nausea. Taking chokeberry together with drugs that slow blood clotting might increase the risk of bruising and bleeding.
Aronia melanocarpa (Chokeberry), the extract was purchased from Agropharm SA (Poland).	Patients with metabolic syndrome	100 mg, three times daily for 2 months	Reduced TC, LDL-C, and TG levels, inhibited platelet aggregation (less pronounced after 2 months), decreased potential for coagulation and clot formation, beneficial changes in coagulation and fibrinolysis parameters [154]. No significant adverse effects were recorded [154]. Taking chokeberry together with drugs that slow blood clotting might increase the risk of bruising and bleeding.

Table 1. *Cont.*

Name of Herbs and Plants and Method of Extraction	Type of Study	Doses and Duration	Outcomes and Side Effects (Humans)
Camellia sinensis (Green tea aqueous extract, GTAE). Extract on the market in different brands.	12-week-old male Wistar rats with HFD (50% kcal from fat)	1.1% and 2.0% GTAE for 8 weeks	Reduced body weight gain (5.6% decrease at 2.0% GTAE), prevented visceral fat accumulation (17.8% reduction at 2.0% GTAE), lowered atherogenic index (14.3% reduction at both doses), reduced protein digestion (82.6% and 84.3% at 1.1% and 2.0% GTAE, respectively) [134]. Green tea extracts can cause liver problems, and the symptoms can include yellowing of your skin or the whites of your eyes, stomach pain and nausea.
Caralluma fimbriata (alcohol extract). Extract on the market in different brands.	Male Wistar rats (200–220 g) with cafeteria diet	25, 50, 100 mg/kg/day for 90 days	Inhibited food intake, prevention of body weight, liver weight, and fat pad mass gains, improved serum lipid and leptin profiles, and protection against atherogenesis [136]. No adverse effects were reported [136]. *Caralluma fimbriata* can cause constipation and gas.
Caralluma fimbriata (40% aqueous alcohol). Extract on the market in different brands.	Male Wistar rats (170–190 g) with HFD (60 kcal% from fat)	200 mg/kg/day for 90 days	Attenuated cardiac lipids and oxidative stress, and improved antioxidant enzyme activities [27]. *Caralluma fimbriata* can cause constipation and gas.
Caralluma fimbriata (dry extract concentrate in gelatin capsules). Capsules on the market in different brands.	Double-blind, randomized, placebo-controlled trial	1 g/kg/day for 16 weeks	Reduced waist circumference, calorie intake, maintained body weight, reduced fat mass and BMI, and improved satiety markers [26]. Only 4 of the participants reported rash and minor gastrointestinal symptoms (bloating, loose stools) [26].
Cinnamomum zeylanicum (70% ethylenealcohol). Extract on the market in different brands.	3T3-L1 cells and 7-week-old male C57BL/6J mice with a normal diet with 45% fat	In vitro: 1, 3, 5, 7, 10 µg/mL for 3 days. In vivo: 1% cinnamon extract for 14 weeks	In vitro: Inhibited lipid accumulation, increased adiponectin and leptin gene expression. In vivo: Reduced lipid synthesis, increased lipolysis, decreased VLDL-C, increased HDL-C, and lowered body fat and fatty tissue accumulation [164]. No reported side effects.

Table 1. *Cont.*

Name of Herbs and Plants and Method of Extraction	Type of Study	Doses and Duration	Outcomes and Side Effects (Humans)
Citrullus colocynthis, hydro-alcoholic extract (80/20, *v*/*v*). Extract on the market in different brands.	9-week-old male Sprague Dawley rats with HFD (45% kcal from fat)	50 mg/kg/day, orally for 16 weeks	Enhanced bleeding time and tPA levels, decreased PAI-1 and thromboxane B2, inhibited platelet aggregation, reversed HFD-induced increases in fibrinogen and von Willebrand factor, decreased food intake, pancreatic lipase activity, TNF-a, IL-6, and leptin, and increased adiponectin levels [34]. Colocynth can cause severe irritation of the stomach and intestine lining, bloody diarrhea, bloody urine, kidney damage, and inability to urinate. Also, can cause convulsions, paralysis, and death.
Coffea (Green coffee bean extract, GCBE from KPLC group: Montagne, France).	5-week-old male C57BL/6J mice with HFD (60% Kcal from fat)	Obesity induction for 4 weeks and then with extract (50, 100, 200 mg/kg/day) for 6 weeks	Reduced body weight gain, liver weight, and white adipose tissue weights. Increased adiponectin and reduced leptin. GCBE upregulated mRNA levels of PPARα, ATGL, and HSL, and downregulated adipogenesis-related genes like C/EBPα, SREBP-1c, and PPARγ. GCBE increased pAMPK expression [141]. Consuming large amounts of green coffee might cause headache, anxiety, agitation, and irregular heartbeat.
Coffea Arabica (aqueous extract). Not available as an extract on the market.	Male Wistar rats (160–180 g) with HFD (40% beef tallow)	Obesity induction for 8 weeks and then with extract (200 mg/kg/day) for 8 weeks	Decreased body and organ weights, reduced TC, TG, LDL-C, VLDL-C, glucose, and insulin levels, improved HOMA-IR, increased adiponectin, and reduced adipocyte hypertrophy [142]. Consuming large amounts of green coffee might cause headache, anxiety, agitation, and irregular heartbeat.
Coffea canephora var. robusta beans (hot-water extract). Not available as an extract on the market.	8–12-week-old male ApoE$^{-/-}$ mice with HFD (42% kcal from fat)	At 2 weeks received 220 mg/kg/day for 14 weeks. At 4 weeks received HFD for 12 weeks	Improved fasting glucose, insulin resistance, serum leptin, urinary catecholamines, and liver triglycerides. Reduced weight gain, adiposity, and inflammatory infiltrate in adipose tissue. Recovered operational taxonomic units (alpha diversity) [157]. Consuming large amounts of green coffee might cause headache, anxiety, agitation, and irregular heartbeat.

Table 1. *Cont.*

Name of Herbs and Plants and Method of Extraction	Type of Study	Doses and Duration	Outcomes and Side Effects (Humans)
Combination of Corni Fructus, Dioscoreae Rhizoma, Aurantii Fructus Immaturus, Platycodonis Radix (ethanol extract). Not available on the market.	3T3-L1 adipocytes and 5-week-old male C57BL/6J mice with HFD (60% kcal from fat)	In vitro: 10, 50, 100 µg/mL for 48 h. In vivo: Obesity induction for 4 weeks and then with extract (100 mg/kg/day) for 16 weeks	Inhibited the differentiation of 3T3-L1 adipocytes and expressions of PPARγ, C/EBPα, and lipin-1, increased phosphorylation of AMPK-α, and reduced weight gain in mice [165]. No side effects have been reported.
Cydonia oblonga (30% ethanol). Extract on the market in different brands.	3T3-L1 adipocytes	0–600 µg/mL for 8 days	Inhibited intracellular TG accumulation, induced AMPKα phosphorylation, downregulated adipogenic transcription factors (SREBP-1c, PPARγ, C/EBPα), reduced mRNA expression of FAS, ACL, aP2, LPL, and increased mRNA expression of HSL and CPT-1 [51]. No side effects have been reported.
Cydonia oblonga (aqueous extract). Extract on the market in different brands.	Male ICR mice (18–22 g) and male Wistar rats (300–350 g)	20, 40, 80 mg/kg/day, orally for 14 days	Prolonged bleeding and clotting times reduced pulmonary embolus mortality, increased thrombolysis, shortened ELT, reduced arterial and venous thrombus weights, decreased TXB2 and increased 6-keto-PGF1α levels [53]. No side effects have been reported.
Ginkgo biloba (extract obtained from Huacheng Biotech Inc. China).	2-month-old male Wistar rats with HFD (57.3% from fat)	Obesity induction for 2 months and then with extract (500 mg/kg/day), orally for 2 weeks	Reduced energy intake, epididymal adipocyte volume, and lipid accumulation. It also reduced Plin 1 and Fasn mRNA and FAS protein levels [140]. No side effects were reported [140].
Ginkgo biloba (unspecified extract). Extract on the market in different brands.	Male Sprague Dawley rats (200–250 g) with acute myocardial infarction	100 mg/kg/day, orally for 4 and 8 weeks	Decreased TGF-β1, MMP-2, and MMP-9 mRNA transcription levels, reduced protein levels of type I collagen, MMP-2, and MMP-9, and inhibited myocardial remodeling after AMI [156]. *Ginkgo biloba* can cause stomach upset, headache, dizziness, and allergic skin reactions. *Ginkgo* leaf extract might increase the risk of bruising and bleeding or cause arrhythmia.

Table 1. *Cont.*

Name of Herbs and Plants and Method of Extraction	Type of Study	Doses and Duration	Outcomes and Side Effects (Humans)
Hibiscus sabdariffa (water extract). Extract on the market in different brands.	7–9 weeks old male C57BL/6J mice with HFD (60% kcal from fat)	1, 10, 25 mg/kg/day for 42 days	Inhibited adipogenesis via PI3-K and MAPK pathways, reduced weight gain, improved glucose tolerance and insulin sensitivity, normalized LDL-C/HDL-C ratio, reduced inflammatory state in liver, reinforced gut integrity, and prebiotic effects on gut microbiota [158]. *Hibiscus sabdariffa* can cause stomach upset, gas, and constipation.
Hibiscus sabdariffa (hot-water extract). Extract on the market in different brands.	3T3-L1 adipocytes	2 mg/mL for 5 days	Inhibited adipocyte differentiation through PI3K/AKT and ERK pathways, and decreased lipid droplet accumulation [166]. *Hibiscus sabdariffa* can cause stomach upset, gas, and constipation.
Ilex paraguariensis (Yerba mate), water extract. Extract on the market in different brands.	6-week-old male Swiss strain mice with HFD	Obesity induction for 8 weeks and then with extract (1 mg/kg) for 8 weeks	Attenuation of weight gain, decreased adiposity and epididymal fat-pad weight, restored serum levels of cholesterol, TG, LDL-C, and glucose [75]. Yerba mate can cause insomnia, upset stomach, increased heart rate, and others.
Ilex paraguariensis (Yerba mate), water extract. Available on the market in different brands.	6-week-old male C57BL/6J mice with HFD (60% kcal from fat)	Obesity induction for 6 weeks and then with extract (0.5, 1, or 2 g/kg/day) for 4 weeks	Reduced body weight gain, lower adipose tissue, decreased serum cholesterol, TG, and glucose levels [76]. Yerba mate can cause insomnia, upset stomach, increased heart rate, and others.
Ilex paraguariensis (Yerba mate), 15% etanol extract. Available on the market in different brands.	6-week-old male Sprague Dawley rats with HFD (40% kcal from fat)	Daily supplementation of extract, 0.24% (*w*/*w*) for 60 days	Reduced body weight, visceral fat, blood and Hepatic lipid levels, improved glucose and insulin levels, enhanced AMPK phosphorylation, increased UCP2 and UCP3 expression [144]. Yerba mate can cause insomnia, upset stomach, increased heart rate, and others.
Ilex paraguariensis (Yerba mate), water extract. Available on the market in different brands.	Early weaned Wistar rats	1 g/kg BW/day, gavage for 30 days	Reduced adipose mass (retroperitoneal and epididymal), total body fat, subcutaneous fat, visceral adipocyte area, TG, and hypothalamic NPY content; restored central leptin resistance, hyperphagia, and higher hypothalamic SOCS-3 content [145]. Yerba mate can cause insomnia, upset stomach, increased heart rate, and others.

Table 1. *Cont.*

Name of Herbs and Plants and Method of Extraction	Type of Study	Doses and Duration	Outcomes and Side Effects (Humans)
Ilex paraguariensis (Yerba mate), water extract (capsules). Available on the market in different brands.	A randomized, double-blind, placebo-controlled clinical trial on obese Korean adults	3 g/day for 12 weeks	Decreased body fat mass, percent body fat, and WHR [147]. Yerba Mate supplementation did not cause any adverse side effects [147].
Ilex paraguariensis (Yerba mate), water extract. Available on the market in different brands.	8-week-old male Wistar rats with HFD (45% kcal from lard fat)	100 mg/day in 3rd month of age and 200 mg/day in 4th month of age, daily for 2 months	Reduced hypothalamic IKK phosphorylation and NF-κB p65 expression, increased IκBα and AdipoR1 expression, reduced IL-6 levels, increased IL-10/TNF-α ratio, and reduced low-grade inflammation [151]. Yerba mate can cause insomnia, upset stomach, increased heart rate, and others.
Ilex paraguariensis (Yerba mate), water extract. Available on the market in different brands.	3T3-L1 adipocytes and 8-week-old male Sprague Dawley rats with HFD (507.6 kcal/100 g)	In vitro: 10, 50, 100 μg/mL for 7 days. In vivo: 500 mg/kg/day for 8 weeks	In vitro: Suppressed lipid accumulation, Increased AMPK, HSL, CaMKK, LKB1, PKA, C/EBPβ, Irβ, IRS1 (Tyr465), decreased SREBP-1c, FAS, PPARγ, and IRS1 (Ser1101). In vivo: suppressed body weight gain, improved serum cholesterol levels, increased AMPK, PKA, ERK1/ERK2, UCP1, reduced mTOR, S6K, SREBP-1c, ap2, FAS, IL-6, adiponectin, leptin, and FABP4 [167]. Yerba mate can cause insomnia, upset stomach, increased heart rate, and others.
Moringa oleifera (70% ethanol extract). Extract on the market in different brands.	Male albino rats (100 ± 20 g) with HFD (58% fat) and overweight/obese female patients	In vivo: Obesity induction for 2 months and then with extract (200 and 400 mg/kg/day) for 1 month; patients: gelatine capsules (400 mg/day) for 8 weeks	In rats, reduced final weight, adiposity index, glucose, insulin, and HOMA-IR. Increased R-QUICKI, adiponectin, omentin, GLUT4, and PPARα expression. Reduced leptin and vaspin. Suppressed FAS and HMG-CoA reductase. In patients, reduced BMI, TC, and LDL-C [81]. *Moringa oleifera* is likely safe when the leaves, fruit, and seeds are eaten as food.

Table 1. *Cont.*

Name of Herbs and Plants and Method of Extraction	Type of Study	Doses and Duration	Outcomes and Side Effects (Humans)
Moringa oleifera leaf petroleum ether extract (MOPEE). Extract on the market in different brands.	3T3-L1 adipocytes and 7-week-old male C57BL/6J mice with HFD (60% kcal from fat)	In vitro: 0, 50, 100, 200, and 400 μg/mL for 24 h. In vivo: 0.125, 0.25, 0.5 g/kg/day for 14 weeks	In vitro: Inhibited adipogenesis in a dose-dependent manner. Downregulated PPARγ, C/EBPα, C/EBPβ, FAS. Upregulated HSL, AMPKα, and ACC phosphorylation. In vivo: Decreased body weight, fat pad weight, and hepatic fat accumulation. Reduced TC, LDL-C, and AST levels. Downregulated PPARγ and FAS. Upregulated ATGL, AMPKα, and ACC phosphorylation [82]. *Moringa oleifera* is likely safe when the leaves, fruit, and seeds are eaten as food.
Moringa oleifera (methanol extract from leaves). Extract on the market in different brands.	3-month-old male Wistar rats with HFD	200 and 400 mg/kg/day for 12 weeks	Alleviated serum biochemical abnormalities, balanced antioxidant status, and reestablished normal heart histology [150]. *Moringa oleifera* is likely safe when the leaves, fruit, and seeds are eaten as food.
Opuntia streptacantha and *Opuntia ficus-indica*. *Opuntia* young cladode powders. Not available on the market.	3T3-F442A adipocytes and 6-week-old male Sprague Dawley rats with HFD (60% kcal from fat)	In vitro: 1, 10, 100 μg/mL for 10 days. In vivo: 0.5% *w*/*w* for 8 weeks	In vitro: Impaired adipocyte differentiation and decreased TG, and reduced glucose uptake. In vivo: Slightly reduced body weight gain, liver and abdominal fat weights. Increased TG excretion in feces [168]. *Opuntia ficus-indica* can cause nausea, bloating, mild diarrhea, increased quantity and frequency of stools, and headache.
Platycodon grandiflorus (ethanol extract). Extract on the market in different brands.	Randomized, double-blind, placebo-controlled clinical trial on overweight or moderately obese adults	571 mg, 1142 mg, 2855 mg (in tablets) per day for 12 weeks	Decreased body fat mass and body fat percentage, reduced total abdominal and subcutaneous fat areas, increased muscle mass [148]. Side effects not reported.
Platycodon grandiflorus (water extract). Extract on the market in different brands.	3T3-L1 preadipocytes and 8-week-old male Sprague Dawley rats with HFD (59.8% kcal from fat)	In vitro: various concentrations (10–50 mg/mL). In vivo: 150 mg/kg/day for 7 weeks	Inhibited 3T3-L1 preadipocyte differentiation and fat accumulation. Decreased pancreatic lipase activity. In vivo: Reduced plasma TC) and TG levels, decreased body weight and subcutaneous adipose tissue weight, reduced size of subcutaneous adipocytes, repressed up-regulation of FABP mRNA in subcutaneous adipose tissue [169]. Side effects not reported.

Table 1. *Cont.*

Name of Herbs and Plants and Method of Extraction	Type of Study	Doses and Duration	Outcomes and Side Effects (Humans)
Punica granatum (Pomegranate), ethanol:water 70:30. Extract on the market in different brands.	6-week-old male C57BL/6 mice with HFD (45% of total fat)	0.1 g/kg/3 days per week 0.2 for 12–14 weeks	Increased energy expenditure, reduced chronic inflammation and insulin resistance, promoted browning and thermogenesis in adipose tissue, reduced inflammatory markers, increased the reductive potential [104]. Some people have experienced sensitivity to pomegranate extract such as itching, swelling, runny nose, and difficulty breathing.
Salvia miltiorrhiza (75% etanol extract). Extract on the market in different brands.	8–9-week-old male Sprague Dawley rats with HFD (45% kcal from fat)	0.675, 1.35, 2.70 g/kg/day for 8 weeks	Reduced body weight, body fat index, serum lipid level, hepatic lipid accumulation, and adipocyte vacuolation. Improved gut integrity and lipid metabolism altered gut microbiota composition [110]. *Salvia miltiorrhiza* can cause upset stomach, itching, and reduced appetite.
Taraxacum officinale (95% ethanol extract). Extract on the market in different brands.	Porcine pancreatic lipase and 7-week-old male ICR mice	In vitro: 50–250 µg/mL. In vivo: 400 mg/kg single dose for 240 min	In vitro: inhibited pancreatic lipase activity. In vivo: decreased plasma TG levels and reduced AUC of plasma TG response curve [113]. *Taraxacum officinale* can cause allergic reactions, stomach discomfort, diarrhea, or heartburn in some people.
Taraxacum officinale (leaf and root extracts in ethanol 60%). Extract on the market in different brands.	3T3-L1 adipocytes	300–600 µg/µL for 6 days	Inhibited adipocyte differentiation, reduced lipid and TG accumulation, regulated expression of genes and long non-coding RNAs involved in adipogenesis and lipid metabolism [114]. *Taraxacum officinale* can cause allergic reactions, stomach discomfort, diarrhea, or heartburn in some people.
Theobroma cacao (aqueous extract). Extract on the market in different brands.	Wistar rats (250 ± 20 g) with HFD (45% kcal) and 20% fructose	Obesity induction for 5 weeks and then with 100%, 10%, 1% pellet for 5 weeks	Decreased body weight by 39%, systolic blood pressure by 27%, triglycerides by 55%, TC by 24%, LDL-C by 37%, and TG/HDL-C ratio by 54% [42]. Cocoa can cause allergic skin reactions, migraine headaches, nausea, stomach discomfort, constipation, and gas. Eating large amounts can cause caffeine-related side effects such as nervousness, increased urination, sleeplessness, and a fast heartbeat.

5. Plant and Herb Extracts Targeting Dyslipidemia and Adipokines in Obesity

Obesity-related dyslipidemia is considered as an atherogenic lipoprotein phenotype and one of the major risk factors for ischemic heart disease. The main manifestations of dyslipidemia include elevated plasma concentrations of TC, LDL-C and TGs, and low levels of HDL-C, which are important factors in hypertension and CVD [170]. Visceral obesity promotes insulin resistance in part mediated by high levels of FFAs and adipokines dysregulation. Adipokines such as leptin, resistin, and retinol-binding protein 4 increase insulin resistance, whereas adiponectin with anti-inflammatory and antilipogenic effects increases insulin sensitivity. In addition, in obesity, pro-inflammatory mediators (leptin, resistin, IL-6, and TNF-α) may promote adipose tissue dysregulation and systemic insulin resistance [1].

In male SD rats fed with HFD were investigated the effects of a high hydrostatic pressure extract of garlic (HEG) on HDL-C level and hepatic apolipoprotein A-I (apoA-I) gene expression. In animals treated with HEG, plasma TC, TG and LDL-C levels were significantly decreased, while the plasma HDL-C level and mRNA level of hepatic apoA-I were significantly increased. Furthermore, HEG upregulated the gene expression of ATP-binding cassette transporter A1 (ABCA1) and lecithin-cholesterol acyl transferase (LCAT) in obese rats [171]. LVH is a risk factor for cardiovascular morbidity and mortality [172]. The effects of three *Camellia sinensis* teas (green, red, and white) were studied on LVH and insulin resistance in LDLr$^{-/-}$ mice fed an HFD. The teas partially prevented hyperlipidemia, increased HDL-C, reduced insulin resistance and CRP levels, and completely prevented LVH in LDLr$^{-/-}$ mice fed an HFD [173]. A systematic review and meta-analysis reported that green tea extract (GTE) significantly reduced TC, LDL-C, fasting blood sugar, hemoglobin A1c (HbA1c), and DBP, while increasing HDL-C [174]. Corni Fructus extract (CFE) was administered in a rat model of diet-induced hypercholesterolemia, and the extract inhibited the elevation of both systolic and diastolic (BP), and lowered serum TC levels with a decrease in esterified cholesterol. Additionally, the protein expressions of SREBP-2 and PPARγ were elevated, indicating that CFE would activate FA oxidation [47]. *Cydonia oblonga* extract (COE) with flavonoids (>60%) from leaves and fruit was analyzed on the blood lipid and antioxidant effects using hyperlipidaemic rat models. The flavonoids from COE significantly reduced serum TC, TG, LDL-C, ALT and AST and increased HDL-C. Flavonoids improved the activity of SOD and GSH-Px in hepatic tissues and reduced malondialdehyde acid (MDA) [52]. In rats fed with HFD, *Ilex paraguariensis* (yerba mate) extract reduced serum TG and TC and decreased the atherogenic index [175]. *Ilex paraguariensis* extract from leaves was investigated on hyperlipidemia induced in hamsters by an HFD. Yerba mate extract significantly reduced body-weight gain and lowered serum lipid levels; meanwhile, Yerba mate treatment increased antioxidant enzyme activity, ameliorated LPL and hepatic lipase activities in serum and liver, upregulated mRNA expression of PPARα, and downregulated mRNA expression of SREBP-1c and ACC in the liver. Therefore, Yerba mate extract regulates the expression of genes involved in lipid oxidation and lipogenesis [176]. Moreover, Yerba mate infusions were also studied in dyslipidemic individuals over 18 years of age (men and women). Yerba mate tea showed a significant increase in ferric reducing antioxidant potential and decreased glutathione concentrations but no significant changes in lipid hydroperoxide (LOOH), protein carbonyl, and paraoxonase-1 levels; thereby, Yerba mate tea increases plasma and blood antioxidant protection in patients with dyslipidemia [177]. However, a systematic review and meta-analysis found no differences in TC, LDL-C, HDL-C, and TG levels when comparing the yerba mate and control groups. The authors concluded that because the results are based on small inconclusive studies, more research is needed to confirm these findings [178]. *Moringa oleifera* leaves are used in India as a hypocholesterolemic agent in obese patients. A study reported that administration of the crude leaf extract of *Moringa oleifera* along with HFD reduced the HFD-induced increases in serum, liver, and kidney cholesterol levels. Furthermore, the crude extract increased serum albumin [83]. *Nigella sativa* has been used for the treatment and prevention of hyperlipidemia. A study analyzed different preparations reported of *Nigella sativa* including seed powder (100 mg-20 g daily), seed oil (20–800 mg daily), thymoquinone (3.5–20 mg daily), and seed extract (methanolic extract especially), and found that these preparations of *Nigella sativa* reduce plasma concentrations of TC, LDL-C, and TG, but the effect on HDL-C was not significant. The authors concluded that lipid-modifying properties of *Nigella sativa* could be attributed to the suppression of intestinal cholesterol absorption, reduced hepatic cholesterol synthesis, and up-regulation of LDL-C receptors [85]. Cholesterol reduction is critical for the prevention of CVD. *Opuntia ficus-indica* extract (OFIE) was tested on the inhibitory activity of pancreatic lipase enzyme (in vitro) and on hypercholesterolemia induced in mice by intraperitoneal administration of Triton WR-1339 (in vivo). The extracts significantly decreased blood cholesterol levels and inhibited pancreatic lipase activity. Therefore, OFIE prevents hypercholesterolemia by pancreatic lipase inhibition, partly attributed to its polyphenolic compounds [90]. *Platycodon grandiflorus* extract (PGE) was investigated in obese mice. The extract reduced body weight gain and improved plasma lipid profiles. Furthermore, leptin was significantly reduced whereas adiponectin was elevated. PGE also downregulated lipogenic gene (LPL, ACC, and FAS) expression and increased lipolysis genes (CPT-1, HSL, and UCP2) in WAT and liver. Moreover, PGE inhibited adipogenic transcriptional factors, such as PPARγ, C/EBPα, and SREBP-1c [97]. Another study related to *Platycodon grandiflorus* root extract in HFD-induced obese mice reported that the extract exhibited antioxidant activity; meanwhile, in calf pulmonary arterial endothelial cells, both oxLDL-C-induced cell death and lactate dehydrogenase release were inhibited. In obese mice treated with *Platycodon grandiflorus* root extract, antioxidant proteins were increased, and plasma and hepatic lipid levels were reduced, thus demonstrating its beneficial effects on hyperlipidemia [98]. The representative adipokines secreted from adipose tissues with an increased plasma leptin, resistin, and TNF-α, and a reduced plasma adiponectin are related to systemic insulin resistance [1]. PGE in male ICR mice fed an HFD markedly attenuated food intake, epididymal fat weight, body weight, adipocyte size, and blood glucose levels while maintaining serum levels of adiponectin, resistin, leptin, fructosamine, and TGs. PGE also up-regulates adiponectin and down-regulates TNF-α, and leptin in fat tissue. In L6 muscle cells, the extract elevated insulin-stimulated glucose uptake [99]. Taken together, the evidence from experimental and clinical studies suggests that plant extracts have lipid-lowering effects and adipokines regulation, which may be suitable for the prevention and treatment of obesity (Table 2 and Figure 2).

Table 2. Extracts from different herbs and plants targeting dyslipidemia and adipokines in obesity.

Name of Herbs and Plants and Method of Extraction	Type of Study	Doses and Duration	Outcomes and Side Effects (Humans)
Allium sativum (garlic), high hydrostatic pressure extract. Not available with this extract method on the market.	5-week-old male Sprague Dawley rats with HFD (45% kcal from fat)	2% (*w*/*w*) of extract for 5 weeks	Decreased in plasma TG and LDL-C levels, increased in HDL-C levels, reduced hepatic TG and TC levels, upregulated hepatic apoA-I, ABCA1, and LCAT gene expression [171]. Garlic extract table may cause breath and body odor, upset stomach or heartburn.
Camellia sinensis, teas (green, red, and white). Not available on the market.	3-month-old male $LDLr^{-/-}$ mice with HFD (20% fat with 1.25% cholesterol, and 0.5% cholic acid)	25 mg/kg body weight daily for 60 days	Prevented left ventricular hypertrophy, partially prevented hyperlipidemia and insulin resistance, and reduced CRP levels [173]. Not reported side effects
Camellia sinensis, green tea extract (GTE). Extract on the market in different brands.	Systematic review and meta-analysis of randomized clinical trials	Varied dosages, some ≥1000 mg/day, others <1000 mg/day, and durations with subgroup analyses based on ≥12 weeks vs. <12 weeks	Significant reduced total cholesterol (TC) and LDL-C. Decreased fasting blood sugar, and HbA1c. Small increased HDL-C. Reduced diastolic blood pressure [174]. Green tea extracts can cause liver problems, and the symptoms can include yellowing of your skin or the whites of your eyes, stomach pain and nausea
Corni Fructus, extract produced by Tsumura Juntendo Inc. (Tokyo, Japan).	5-week-old male Wistar rats with a high cholesterol diet (1% cholesterol and 0.5% cholic acid)	50, 100, and 200 mg/kg/day for 10 days	Lowered blood pressure and serum cholesterol levels. Decreased atherogenic index, increased cholesterol and bile acid excretion. Reduced lipid peroxidation, up-regulated SREBP-2 and PPARα expression, and enhanced fatty acid oxidation [47]. No side effects have been reported
Cydonia oblonga (ethanol extract). Extract on the market in different brands.	Male Sprague Dawley rats (240 ± 20 g) induced with hyperlipidemia	Hyperlipidemia induction for 21 days and then with 40, 80, 160 mg/kg/day for 4 weeks	Reduced serum TC, TG, LDL-C, ALT, AST, increased HDL-C, reduced MDA, improved SOD and GSH-Px activity in hepatic tissues [52]. No side effects have been reported
Ilex paraguariensis (Yerba mate), hydroethanolic extract and n-butanolic fraction. Available on the market in different brands.	8-week-old male Wistar rats with HFD (60% kcal from fat) with cholesterol (2%) and cholic acid (0.2%)	Hyperlipidemia induction for 30 days and then with 200, 400, 800 mg/kg/day for 30 days	Reduced serum TG, cholesterol, and atherogenic index [175]. Yerba mate can cause insomnia, upset stomach, increased heart rate, and others.
Ilex paraguariensis (Yerba mate), aqueous extract. Available on the market in different brands.	A systematic review and meta-analysis	Various doses in included studies	No significant change in TC, LDL-C, HDL-C, and TG levels [178]. Yerba mate can cause insomnia, upset stomach, increased heart rate, and others.

Table 2. *Cont.*

Name of Herbs and Plants and Method of Extraction	Type of Study	Doses and Duration	Outcomes and Side Effects (Humans)
Ilex paraguariensis (Yerba mate), aqueous extract. Available on the market in different brands.	8-week-old male Syrian golden hamsters with HFD (15% lard and 0.2% cholesterol)	Hyperlipidemia induction for 4 weeks and then with 1%, 2%, and 4% *w/v* for 4 weeks	Decreased body weight gain, lowered serum lipid levels, increased antioxidant enzyme activity, improved lipoprotein lipase (LPL) and hepatic lipase (HL) activities, and upregulated PPARα and LDL-C receptor mRNA expression. Reduced SREBP-1c and acetyl CoA carboxylase mRNA expression [176]. Yerba mate can cause insomnia, upset stomach, increased heart rate, and others.
Ilex paraguariensis (Yerba mate), aqueous extract. Available on the market in different brands.	Randomized clinical trial with dyslipidemic individuals	1 L/day (20 mg/mL) for 90 days	Increased serum antioxidant capacity and GSH, and decreased LDL-C [177]. Mate tea did not show adverse effects in the patients.
Moringa oleifera (aqueous extract).	Male Wistar rats with HFD (3% fat)	1 mg/g for 30 days	Decreased cholesterol levels in serum, liver, And kidney. Increased serum albumin [83]. *Moringa oleifera* is likely safe when the leaves, fruit, and seeds are eaten as food.
Nigella sativa, seed powder, seed oil, and seed (methanolic extract). Available on the market in different brands.	Systematic review of experimental and clinical studies	Variable treatment time of seed powder (100 mg–20 g daily), seed oil (20–800 mg daily), and seed extract (6, 9, 14, and 21 g/kg)	Reduced TC, LDL-C, and TG. No significant effect on HDL-C [85]. *Nigella sativa* seed can cause allergic rashes, stomach upset, vomiting, or constipation.
Opuntia ficus-indica (aqueous extract). Available on the mar-ket.	Triton-induced hypercholesterolemia in male Balb-c mice	500 mg/kg in a single administration for 16 h plus fasting for 8 h	Significantly decreased cholesterol levels. Inhibited pancreatic lipase with IC50 = 588.5 µg/mL [90]. *Opuntia ficus-indica* can cause nausea, bloating, mild diarrhea, increased quantity and frequency of stools, and headache.
Platycodon grandiflorus (water extract). Extract on the market in different brands.	9-week-old male C57BL/6J mice with HFD	1 g/kg/day for 8 weeks	Reduced body weight gain by 7.5%, improved plasma lipid profiles, decreased leptin, increased adiponectin, downregulated lipogenic gene expression, increased lipolysis gene expression, and inhibited adipogenic transcription factors [97]. Side effects not reported.
Platycodon grandiflorus (70% ethanol extract). Extract on the market in different brands.	5-week-old male C57BL/6J mice with HFD (40% of fat)	Dyslipidemia induction for 5 weeks and then with 25 and 75 mg/kg/day for 4 weeks	Reduced plasma and hepatic lipid levels, upregulated antioxidant proteins, inhibited oxLDL-C-induced cell death and lactate dehydrogenase release, exhibited antioxidant activity in vitro and in vivo [98]. Side effects not reported.

Table 2. *Cont.*

Name of Herbs and Plants and Method of Extraction	Type of Study	Doses and Duration	Outcomes and Side Effects (Humans)
Platycodon grandiflorus, extract (water, 50% ethanol, and 80% ethanol). Extract on the market in different brands.	L6 muscle cells and 9-week-old male ICR mice with HFD (60% kcal from fat)	1% and 5% extract in diet for 6 weeks	Reduced food intake, body weight, epididymal fat weight, adipocyte size, and blood glucose levels. Maintained serum adiponectin, resistin, leptin, fructosamine, and triglycerides. Upregulated adiponectin mRNA, downregulated TNF-a and leptin mRNA in WAT. In L6, muscle cells increased insulin-stimulated glucose uptake [99]. Side effects not reported.

6. Plant and Herb Extracts against to Insulin Resistance, Hyperglycemia, and Diabetes

Several factors contribute to the growth of obesity and T2D, such as unhealthy eating habits, physical inactivity, sedentary lifestyle, increased stress, and environmental factors, which are typical of global urbanization and modern society in the world [1]. Increased BMI and excessive visceral adipose tissue are known to be associated with insulin resistance and beta cell dysfunction, which can lead to glucose intolerance and T2D. Obesity plays an important role in the elevated prevalence of T2D, which is characterized by insulin resistance in several tissues, including muscle, liver, and adipose tissue. T2D is manifested by low insulin secretions from β-cells and peripheral insulin resistance, including high levels of fatty acids, which promote systemic inflammation. Obesity can cause a chronic low-grade inflammatory state with high levels of cytokines such as TNF-α, IL-1β, monocyte chemoattractant protein-1 (MCP-1), and IL-6, which in part contributes to the pathogenesis of insulin resistance, promoting a reduction in glucose uptake in insulin-dependent tissues, which increases blood glucose levels, β-cell dysfunction in pancreas and results in endocrine dysfunction of adipose tissue. One of the signaling pathways involved in the inflammatory mechanisms is the activation of JNK1 by TNF-α, which results in serine phosphorylation of insulin receptor substrate 1 (IRS1) and impairs insulin signaling and subsequent insulin resistance [1,179].

In addition to obesity and T2D hyperglycemia is a known risk factor for the development of several health disorders such as oxidative stress and cardiovascular diseases. Antidiabetic effects of pregnane glycosides, alkaloids, and tannins/gallic tannins derived from *Caralluma fimbriata* have been reported [25]. The effects of *Caralluma fimbriata* extract (CFE) on insulin resistance and oxidative stress in HFD-fed Wistar male rats were investigated. The administration of CFE in obese animals resulted in a significant improvement in plasma glucose, insulin, leptin, and TGs. CFE also prevented high levels of lipid peroxidation and protein oxidation, low GSH levels, and low activities of enzymatic antioxidants [180]. Cinnamon extracts have been used to treat blood glucose. *Ceylon cinnamon* extract (CCE) was tested on carbohydrate digestion and post-meal blood glucose reduction in vitro (enzymatic assays) and in vivo (starch tolerance tests in rats), including 18 healthy female and male volunteers. In an in vitro study, CCE inhibited pancreatic α-amylase activity and reduced the glycemic response to starch in a dose-dependent manner in rats. In healthy volunteers, CCE lowered the area under the curve of glycemia with no changes in insulin secretion [30]. *Citrullus colocynthis* has been used against diabetes. Colocynth fruit extract was investigated on insulin action using 3T3-L1 adipocytes. Extracts of seed and pulp enhanced insulin-induced GLUT4 translocation and increased insulin-stimulated cellular glucose uptake. Moreover, extracts of pulp enhanced insulin-induced PKB phosphorylation without affecting phosphorylation of the insulin receptor [181]. With respect to this, compounds from *Citrullus colocynthis,* such as the 2-O-β-D-glucopyranosyl forms of cucurbitacins J/K, I, E, and B, and cucurbitacins I, B, and E, are speculated to be responsible for the insulin-enhancing activity [173]. However, a systematic review and meta-analysis in diabetic patients reported that *Citrullus colocynthis* does not have a significant effect on fasting blood sugar, HbA1c, LDL-C, TC, and TG indices, but increases HDL-C. These findings could be related to the relatively low quality of articles and the small number of included studies [33]. Corni Fructus extract (CFE) was analyzed on blood glucose and insulin resistance in db/db mice. CFE suppressed an increase in blood glucose levels during the oral glucose tolerance test. In addition, CFE lowered final fasting serum glucose and TG in diabetic mice. The mRNA expression of adiponectin, GLUT4, and PPARγ in adipose tissue was higher in diabetic mice treated with CFE [48]. In another study, Corni Fructus extract was evaluated on kidneys of diabetic db/db mice. The activities of XO and SOD were significantly higher in diabetic mice with CFE; meanwhile, the activities of CAT and GST were lowered in the diabetic mice with CFE. Additionally, the mRNA expression of eNOS in kidneys was reduced in the diabetic mice with the extract. Therefore, Corni Fructus extract has antioxidative actions that contribute to its renoprotective effects on diabetic nephropathy [182]. *Ginkgo biloba* extract (GBE) leaves (water and 12% ethanol extracts) from four different trees (1 and 2—males and 3 and 4—females) were analyzed on phenolic profile, antioxidant activity, and the potential in vitro inhibitory properties on α-amylase, α-glucosidase, and ACE enzymes, which are related to diabetes and hypertension. Aqueous extracts had higher phenolic contents than ethanolic extracts. ACE activity was only inhibited by ethanolic extracts. The results showed a strong correlation between total phenolics and α-glucosidase inhibitory activity, and to a lesser degree, a positive correlation between total phenolics and α-amylase inhibitory activity [57]. Egb761, a *Ginkgo biloba* extract, has antioxidant and antiplatelet aggregation effects. The effect of Egb761 and its major subcomponents (bilobalide, kaempferol, and quercetin) on preventing atherosclerosis was analyzed in vitro using a rat model of T2D. Egb761 dose-dependently reduced the intima–media ratio and proliferation of VSMCs and promoted greater apoptosis in obese rats with T2D. In an in vitro model, Egb761 also decreased the proliferation and migration of VSMCs. Glucose and circulating adiponectin levels were ameliorated, and plasma hs-CRP concentrations were reduced in obesogenic and diabetic rats. Moreover, caspase-3 activity and DNA fragmentation were increased while monocyte adhesion and ICAM-1/VCAM-1 levels were decreased with Egb761 in obese rats with T2D. The bioactive compounds of Egb761, kaempferol, and quercetin decreased VSMC migration and elevated caspase activity [58]. Green coffee extract (GCE) was evaluated for 10 weeks on glycemic indices, inflammation, and oxidative stress in individuals with T2D and overweight/obesity. GCE supplementation reduced body weight and BMI. In addition, patients with GCE had lower fasting blood glucose (FBG) concentration, but there was no effect on insulin levels and HOMA-IR. However, there were significant improvements in SBP, TG level, HDL-C, and TG-to-HDL-C ratio. GCE supplementation did not affect DBP, LDL-C, or TC, including MDA levels. GCE significantly decreased the hs-CRP levels in patients with T2D and overweight/obesity. Therefore, GCE possesses beneficial effects on lipid profile and inflammation in individuals with T2D and overweight/obesity [183]. *Hibiscus sabdariffa* polyphenolic extract (HPE) was analyzed on the T2D rat model. HPE decreased hyperglycemia and hyperinsulinemia, including serum TG, cholesterol, and the ratio of LDL-C/HDL-C. Moreover, HPE significantly reduced the plasma advanced glycation end product (AGE) formation and lipid peroxidation in T2D rats. Furthermore, HPE inhibits the expression of connective tissue growth factor (CTGF) and receptor of AGE (RAGE). HPE retrieved the weight loss found in T2D rats [184]. Extracts of two varieties (red and white) of *Hibiscus sabdariffa* (Roselle) calyces were evaluated on carbohydrate hydrolyzing enzymes (α-amylase and α-glucosidase). The extracts inhibited the α-amylase and α-glucosidase activities in vitro, but the red variety exhibited higher α-glucosidase inhibitory activity than the white variety, while the white variety showed higher α-amylase inhibitory activity than the red variety. Additionally, the red variety possesses higher antioxidant capacity, which appears to be more potent compared to the white variety [70]. *Hibiscus sabdariffa* extract (HSE) was evaluated on the mechanism of adipogenesis and complications of obesity-related insulin resistance in HFD-induced obese SD rats. HSE reduced food intake, body weight, lipid profiles, lipid peroxidation, inflammatory cytokines, serum leptin, insulin and duodenal glucose absorption, while it significantly elevated the glucose uptake of adipose tissue and muscle. Moreover, HSE prevents lipid accumulation by inhibiting the differentiation of 3T3-L1 adipocytes through the downregulation of genes involved in adipogenesis [69]. Roasted mate tea consumption (*Ilex paraguariensis*) was evaluated on the glycemic and lipid profiles of patients with T2D or pre-diabetes. Mate tea consumption reduced the levels of fasting glucose, HbA1c, and LDL-C of T2D patients. However, the consumption of mate tea did not change the intake of total energy, carbohydrate, protein, cholesterol, and fiber. In addition, mate tea consumption together with nutritional counseling reduced significantly the levels of LDL-C, HDL-C, and TG. Therefore, mate tea consumption ameliorated the glucose levels and lipid profile of T2D patients [77]. *Moringa oleifera* has beneficial properties to reduce the risk of chronic metabolic diseases such as T2D. One study investigated capsules of *Moringa oleifera* dry leaf powder in subjects with prediabetes for 12 weeks. *Moringa oleifera* improved FBG and HbA1c. There were no significant changes in microbiota, hepatic and renal function markers, or appetite-controlling hormones, such as glucagon-like peptide 1 (GLP-1), ghrelin, and peptide YY (PYY) [84]. *Opuntia ficus-indica* var. saboten (OFS) dried powder extract was investigated using in vitro and in vivo models. OSF inhibited α-glucosidase activity in vitro and intestinal glucose absorption in db/db mice. In L6 muscle cells, OFS elevated dose-dependent glucose uptake, stimulated AMPK and p38 MAPK phosphorylations, and increased GLUT4 translocation to the cell membrane. OFS treatment in db/db mice dose-dependently prevented hyperinsulinemia, hyperglycemia, and glucose tolerance, including insulin resistance and quantitative insulin sensitivity check index. OFS ameliorated pancreatic function through elevated β-cell mass in db/db mice [185]. Another study of *Opuntia ficus-indica* extract (OFIE) prepared from the cladodes and a proprietary stem/fruit skin-blend was tested on blood glucose and plasma insulin in normal rats. OFIE significantly lowered blood glucose levels and significantly elevated basal plasma insulin levels, suggesting a direct action on pancreatic β-cells [92]. The flowering part of *Punica granatum* has been recommended in Unani literature for the treatment of diabetes. *Punica granatum* flower extract (PGFE) was analyzed on hyperglycemia in vivo and in vitro. PGF extract markedly reduced plasma glucose levels (postprandial hyperglycemia) in non-fasted Zucker diabetic fatty rats (a genetic model of obesity and T2D). In vitro, PGFE had a potent inhibitory effect on α-glucosidase activity [105]. *Salvia miltiorrhiza* extract (SME) was investigated on the expression of VEGF induced by high concentration of glucose in HMEC-1 cells, in which mitochondrial uncoupling protein 2 (UCP2) was knocked down by using UCP2 siRNA. HMEC-1 cells with 30 mM glucose resulted in a significant increase in the expression of VEGF mRNA, and high levels of ROS. SME significantly decreased VEGF mRNA and ROS formation in HMEC-1 cells with 30 mM glucose. Interestingly, the knockdown of UCP-2 abolished the reduction in VEGF expression and ROS formation by SME. Therefore, SME has antioxidant effects and can be used for the treatment of diabetic chronic vascular complications [109]. The antidiabetic potential of fresh and shade-dried leaves of *Taraxacum officinale* was investigated. The extract of shade-dried *Taraxacum officinale* leaves demonstrated potent antidiabetic activity in a dose-dependent manner by targeting α-amylase and α-glucosidase, having great potential to suppress post-prandial glucose rise and for better management of diabetes [116]. The plant extracts described in this section have antidiabetic effects because they improve glycemic control and lipid profile, postprandial hyperglycemia, insulin resistance, inflammatory cytokines, and oxidative stress in diabetic models. Therefore, their consumption combined with nutritional intervention could be a good strategy to decrease plasma glucose levels and lipid parameters in individuals with pre-diabetes and diabetes, which may reduce their risk of developing metabolic disorders and coronary artery disease (Table 3 and Figure 2).

Table 3. Extracts from different herbs and plants targeting insulin resistance, hyperglycemia, and diabetes.

Name of Herbs and Plants and Method of Extraction	Type of Study	Doses and Duration	Outcomes and Side Effects (Humans)
Caralluma fimbriata (hydro-alcoholic extract). Extract on the market in different brands.	Male Wistar rats with HFD (60% of fat)	200 mg/kg/day for 90 days	Reduced hyperglycemia, hyperinsulinemia, hyperleptinemia, hypertriglyceridemia, oxidative stress, and improved insulin sensitivity [180]. *Caralluma fimbriata* can cause constipation and gas.
Ceylon cinnamon (hydro-alcoholic extract). Extract on the market in different brands.	Pancreatic alpha-amylase activity. 7-week-old male Wistar Han IGS rats. A randomized, placebo-controlled, cross-over clinical trial in healthy subjects.	In vitro: 0–100 μg/mL. In vivo: 6.25, 12.5, 25, 50, 100 mg/kg for 5 weeks. Humans: 1 g of extract (two 500 mg capsules), single dose post-meal.	In vitro: Inhibited pancreatic alpha-amylase (IC50 = 25 μg/mL). In vivo: Reduced glycemic response to starch. Human: Lowered postprandial glycemia by 14.8% (0–120 min) and 21.2% (0–60 min) without increasing insulin secretion [30]. No side effects were reported during the study.
Citrullus colocynthis (petroleum ether, water or 80% methanol, ethyl acetate, and n-butanol, crude aqueous extracts). Extract on the market in different brands.	3T3-L1 adipocytes	4, 20, or 100 μg/mL for 24, 48, and 96 h	Enhanced insulin-induced GLUT4 translocation and glucose uptake, and increased insulin-induced PKB phosphorylation [181]. Colocynth can cause severe irritation of the stomach and intestine lining, bloody diarrhea, bloody urine, kidney damage, and inability to urinate. Also, can cause convulsions, paralysis, and death.
Citrullus colocynthis (tablets, capsules, or oral drops). Not available on the market.	Randomized Controlled Clinical Trials	Different doses for 30 to 60 days	No significant effect on FBS, HbA1c, LDL-C, TC, and TG. Increased HDL-C levels [33]. No serious side effects of this plant were reported.
Corni Fructus (water extract). Not available on the market as extract.	7-week-old male C57BUKsJ-db/db mice and C57BL/6 mice	500 mg/kg/day for 8 weeks	Reduced blood glucose levels, improved insulin resistance, and increased glucose utilization [48]. No side effects have been reported.
Corni Fructus (aqueous extract). Extract on the market in different brands.	7-week-old male C57BL/KsJ-db/db mice	500 mg/kg/day for 8 weeks	Reduced oxidative stress, increased SOD activity, decreased XO, CAT, and GST activities. Lower mRNA expression of eNOS in kidneys [182]. No side effects have been reported.

Table 3. *Cont.*

Name of Herbs and Plants and Method of Extraction	Type of Study	Doses and Duration	Outcomes and Side Effects (Humans)
Ginkgo biloba (aqueous and 12% ethanol extracts). Extract on the market in different brands.	α-amylase and α-glucosidase activities	10, 25 and 50 mg/mL of Ginkgo leaf extract	Aqueous extracts had higher total phenolic content but only ethanolic extracts inhibited ACE, a strong correlation between total phenolics and α-glucosidase inhibitory activity, and to a lesser degree positive correlation between total phenolics and α-amylase inhibitory activity [57]. *Ginkgo biloba* can cause stomach upset, headache, dizziness, and allergic skin reactions. *Ginkgo* leaf extract might increase the risk of bruising and bleeding or cause arrhythmia.
Ginkgo biloba (Egb761). Available on the market.	RAoSMCs and HUVECs. Five-week-old male Otsuka Long-Evans Tokushima Fatty rats and five-week-old male $ApoE^{-/-}$ mice	Obesity and insulin resistance induction for 24 weeks (rats). Two months in all mice with HFD (42% fat, 1.25% cholesterol). All animals with 100 mg/kg and 200 mg/kg for 6 weeks (rats), and 2 months (mice).	Reduced intima–media ratio. Induced greater apoptosis in rats, improved glucose homeostasis and increased circulating adiponectin levels, decreased plasma hs-CRP concentrations. In vitro: Decreased VSMC proliferation and migration, Increased caspase-3 activity and DNA fragmentation, decreased monocyte adhesion and ICAM-1/VCAM-1 levels. Kaempferol and quercetin: Reduced VSMC migration and increased caspase activity and protect against atherosclerosis [58]. Ginkgo biloba can cause stomach upset, headache, dizziness, and allergic skin reactions. Ginkgo leaf extract might increase the risk of bruising and bleeding or cause arrhythmia.
Green coffee (*Coffea*), aqueous extract). Extract on the market in different brands.	A randomized, double-blind, placebo-controlled trial	400 mg (capsules) twice per day for 10 weeks	Decreased SBP, TG, hs-CRP, increased HDL-C, and marginally significant reduction in FBG. No significant changes in DBP, LDL-C, TC, insulin levels, HOMA-IR, and MDA [183]. Consuming large amounts of green coffee might cause headache, anxiety, agitation, and irregular heartbeat.
Hibiscus sabdariffa, (polyphenolic extract by methanol). Extract on the market in different brands.	8-week-old male Sprague Dawley rats with HFD and STZ	Type 2 diabetes induction: HFD for 7 weeks and then HFD and STZ for 2 weeks. Doses 100 mg/kg and 200 mg/kg for 7 weeks.	Reduced hyperglycemia, hyperinsulinemia, serum TG, cholesterol, and LDL-C/HDL-C ratio. Decreased plasma AGE formation and lipid peroxidation. Inhibited CTGF and RAGE expression in aortic regions. Improved weight loss in diabetic rats [184]. *Hibiscus sabdariffa* can cause stomach upset, gas, and constipation.

Table 3. *Cont.*

Name of Herbs and Plants and Method of Extraction	Type of Study	Doses and Duration	Outcomes and Side Effects (Humans)
Hibiscus sabdariffa (aqueous extract). Extract on the market in different brands.	α-amylase and α-glucosidase activities	Red and white varieties; IC50 values: 25.2 μg/mL (red) and 47.4 μg/mL (white) for α-glucosidase inhibition; 90.5 μg/mL (white) and 187.9 μg/mL (red) for α-amylase inhibition	Both varieties inhibited α-amylase and α-glucosidase activities, red variety exhibited higher α-glucosidase inhibitory activity, while the white variety showed higher α-amylase inhibitory activity, and strong antioxidant properties, particularly in the red variety [70]. *Hibiscus sabdariffa* can cause stomach upset, gas, and constipation.
Hibiscus sabdariffa (aqueous extract). Extract on the market in different brands.	3T3-L1 cells and male Sprague Dawley rats (100–120 g) with HFD	In vitro: 0.1, 0.5, 1 mg/mL. In vivo: 250 and 500 mg/kg/day for 8 weeks	Reduced body weight, food intake, lipid profiles, inflammatory cytokines, lipid peroxidation, serum leptin, insulin, and duodenal glucose absorption. Increased glucose uptake in adipose tissue and muscle, downregulated adipogenic Gene expression [69]. *Hibiscus sabdariffa* can cause stomach upset, gas, and constipation.
Ilex paraguariensis (Yerba mate), aqueous extract. Extract on the market in different brands.	T2DM and pre-diabetes subjects	330 mL of roasted mate tea 3 times a day for 60 days	T2DM: Significant decrease in fasting glucose, HbA1c, and LDL-C. Pre-diabetes: Significant decrease in LDL-C, non-HDL-C, and TG. Improved glycemic control and lipid profile, reduced risk of coronary disease [77]. Mate tea did not show adverse effects in the patients.
Moringa oleifera (dry leaf powder). Available on the market in different brands.	A double-blind, randomized, placebo-controlled, parallel-group clinical trial	2400 mg/day (6 capsules/day) for 12 weeks	Significant decrease in FBG and HbA1c. No significant changes in microbiota, hepatic and renal function markers, or appetite-controlling hormones [84]. *Moringa oleifera* has no side effects with supplementation [84].
Opuntia ficus-indica var. *saboten* (hot-water extract). Extract on the market in different brands.	α-Glucosidase activity. L6 muscle cells. 5-week-old male C57BL/6J db/db mice and their non-diabetic heterozygous littermates (db/-), and 9-week-old male ICR mice	α-Glucosidase activity (1, 5, 10 mg/mL). L6 muscle cells (1–200 μg/mL). db/db mice (1 and 2 g/kg BW) and db/- mice (1 g/kg BW) for 4 weeks.	Inhibited α-glucosidase activity and intestinal glucose absorption. In L6 muscle cells, increased glucose uptake, stimulated AMPK and p38 MAPK phosphorylation, and increased GLUT4. In db/db mice, improved hyperglycemia, hyperinsulinemia, glucose tolerance, and regenerated β-cells [185]. *Opuntia ficus-indica* var. *saboten* had no adverse side effects on normal mice [185].

Table 3. *Cont.*

Name of Herbs and Plants and Method of Extraction	Type of Study	Doses and Duration	Outcomes and Side Effects (Humans)
Opuntia ficus-indica (cladodes and stem/fruit skin-blend ratio 75/25) hot-water extract. Not available combined on the market.	Wistar rats either sex weighing 250–350 g	0.176–176 mg/kg for 180 min and glucose (i.p., 2 g/kg in 5 mL) 30 min after extracts administration	Both extracts lowered blood glucose levels (in doses as low as 6 mg/kg). The blend increased basal plasma insulin levels [92]. No side effects have been reported for *Opuntia ficus-indica* (cladodes and stem/fruit skin).
Punica granatum (methanolic extract). Extract on the market in different brands.	α-glucosidase activity assay. Zucker diabetic fatty (ZDF) rats and Zucker lean (ZL) rats (14–15 weeks old).	α-glucosidase activity (200 µL of extract for 5 min). 500 mg/kg body weight, oral in 5% acacia once daily for 2 weeks.	Lowered plasma glucose levels in non-fasted ZDF rats, inhibited postprandial hyperglycemia, potent inhibitory effect on α-glucosidase activity (IC50: 1.8 µg/mL) [105]. Some people have experienced sensitivity to pomegranate extract such as itching, swelling, runny nose, and difficulty breathing.
Salvia miltiorrhiza (water extract). Extract on the market in different brands.	HMEC-1 cells	10 µg/mL of extract in 30 mM glucose condition for 48 h	Decreased VEGF mRNA and ROS formation induced by high glucose, and UCP-2 siRNA abolished these effects [109]. *Salvia miltiorrhiza* can cause upset stomach, itching, and reduced appetite.
Salvia miltiorrhiza (different extracts). Extract on the market in different brands.	Review of preclinical and clinical studies on diabetes and complication	Not applicable	SM exhibits antidiabetic activities, including anti-inflammation, antioxidation, antifibrosis, and antiapoptosis. Key pathways involved are Wnt/β-catenin, TSP-1/TGF-β1/STAT3, JNK/PI3K/AKT, and others. The main compounds include salvianolic acids and diterpenoid tanshinones [107]. *Salvia miltiorrhiza* can cause upset stomach, itching, and reduced appetite.
Taraxacum officinale (aqueous extract). Extract on the market in different brands.	α-amylase and α-glucosidase activities	1, 10, 20, 30 mg/mL	Shade-dried leaves demonstrated potent antidiabetic activity via inhibiting α-amylase and α-glucosidase in a dose-dependent manner [116]. *Taraxacum officinale* can cause allergic reactions, stomach discomfort, diarrhea, or heartburn in some people.

7. Plant and Herb Extracts with Antihypertensive Effects

Obesity-associated hypertension is well documented in children and adults and in both sexes. Excess weight gain (especially increased visceral adiposity) is a major cause of hypertension and accounts for 65% to 75% of the risk for human primary hypertension and causes a cascade of associated cardiorenal and metabolic disorders. The mechanisms involved in obesity-associated hypertension are complex and include [1] physical compression of the kidneys from excess fat in and around the kidneys, [2] sympathetic nervous system (SNS) overactivation, [3] activation of the renin–angiotensin–aldosterone system (RAAS), [4] dysregulation in adipose tissue-secreted cytokines, such as leptin, insulin, resistance, TNF-α, and IL-6, [5] systemic insulin resistance, [6] endothelial dysfunction, and [7] structural and functional renal changes. In addition, SNS overactivation promotes elevations in heart rate, cardiac output, and renal tubular sodium reabsorption, which occur due to α-adrenergic and β-adrenergic receptor stimulation and indirectly through activation of other systems (e.g., RAAS) [186,187]. Weight loss is the main goal of reducing obesity-related hypertension, and current therapeutic approaches address the metabolic consequences of obesity, including dyslipidemia, inflammation, and diabetes.

The consumption of aged black garlic (ABG) is associated with improvements in several CVD risk factors. ABG extract along with dietary recommendations was analyzed on CVD risk factors in subjects with moderate hypercholesterolemia. The use of ABG extract for 6 weeks reduced DBP, particularly in men with a DBP > 75 mm Hg [188]. *Andrographis paniculata* extract (APE) was investigated using chronic intraperitoneal infusions by osmotic pumps in spontaneously hypertensive rats (SHRs) and Wistar–Kyoto (WKY) rats. APE significantly reduced the SBP of both SHRs and WKY rats. Plasma ACE activity and thiobarbituric acid (TBA) were significantly reduced in SHRs treated with APE [189]. In a meta-analysis of controlled clinical trials, berry extract from *Aronia melanocarpa* (chokeberry) was tested for an average of 6–8 weeks on TC and BP. Daily supplementation with berry extract significantly reduced SBP and TC, mainly in adults over the age of 50 years [190]. According to epidemiological studies, green tea (*Camellia sinensis*) consumption has protective effects against CVD. Green tea extract (GTE) with Ang II (induces endothelial dysfunction) were investigated for 13 days on arterial hypertension with high oxidative stress in male SD rats. GTE blunted the increased BP, LV mass index, media-to-lumen ratio, and hydroperoxide radicals, including HO-1, p22phox, and SOD-1 mRNA in the aorta caused by Ang II [191]. In a systematic review and meta-analysis of randomized clinical trials, GTE was analyzed in 20 human randomized clinical trials comprising 1536 participants. GTE significantly reduced SBP, TC, and LDL-C. Adverse events reported were elevated BP, rash, and abdominal discomfort [192]. In a crossover randomized clinical trial, green tea was analyzed on BP, endothelial function, inflammatory activity, and metabolic profile in obese prehypertensive women. Participants received three capsules daily containing 500 mg of green tea extract (GTE) for 4 weeks, with a washout period of 2 weeks between treatments. Each GTE capsule had 260 mg of polyphenols. After 4 weeks of GTE supplementation, there was a significant reduction in SBP at 24 h, daytime, and nighttime [193]. The intake of cocoa extract, which consisted of 1.4 g (415 mg flavanols) before and after 4 weeks of daily intake, was evaluated on postprandial cardiometabolic effects. The consumption of cocoa extract within an energy-restricted diet for 4 weeks showed a greater reduction in postprandial AUC of SBP compared to the control group and independently of body weight loss [41]. Leaf extract of *Ginkgo biloba* (Egb761) was investigated on hypertension with hypercholesterolemia-induced renal injury in rats. Hypertension was caused by L-N(G)-nitroarginine methyl ester (L-NAME), and hypercholesterolemia was induced by a diet with 1% cholesterol. Egb761 exhibited a progressive reduction in the SBP, and mean arterial BP. Moreover, Egb761 decreased the excess of MDA and nitrite levels and recovered the low levels of intracellular reduced glutathione (GSH) caused by hypertension with hypercholesterolemia in the renal tissue. Furthermore, hypertension with hypercholesterolemia increased the expression of TNF-α, IL-6, and IL-1β levels in renal tissues and was inhibited by treatment with Egb761. Chronic hypertension with hypercholesterolemia induced the inhibition of endothelial nitric oxide synthase (eNOS) and activation of inducible NO synthase (iNOS), but Egb761 activated eNOS and inhibited iNOS in the kidney tissues. Therefore, these findings suggest that Egb761 protects against hypertension with hypercholesterolemia-induced renal injury [59]. A new component group of *Ginkgo biloba* leaves (GBLCG), mainly composed of quercetin, kaempferol, and isorhamnetin, was investigated on reducing BP and ameliorating myocardial hypertrophy in SHRs. Total terpenoid lactones of GBLCG might be a novel cocrystal composed of Ginkgolide (A, B, C, J) and bilobalide. GBLCG had hypotensive activity and improved myocardial hypertrophy. These effects could be due to the promoting of NO synthesis and release in endothelial cells, reducing oxidative stress, and inhibiting platelet aggregation [194]. Green coffee bean extract (GCE) has protective effects against hypertension in both SHRs and humans. A study investigated the dose–response relationship of GCE in 117 male subjects with mild hypertension. After 28 days of using GCE, the decrease in SBP and DBP was statistically significant compared with the placebo group. Therefore, GCE has antihypertensive effects in patients with mild hypertension [64]. It has been reported that *Hibiscus sabdariffa* can reduce BP in human and animal studies. The extract of the dried calyx of *Hibiscus sabdariffa* (HS) and Hibiscus anthocyanins (Has) were investigated on left-ventricular myocardial capillary length and surface area in SHRs. HS consumption significantly decreased SBP, DBP, and LV mass in a dose-dependent fashion, but it did not affect the heart rate. HS also significantly increased the surface area and length density of myocardial capillaries and length density. Myocyte nuclear volume was reduced in rats with HS. There was an insignificant decrease in SBP and DBP with HA ingestion. This study showed that HS ingestion improves myocardial capillarization in SHRs through structural alterations linked to a reduction of myocardial mass and the promotion of new vessel formation [195]. *Hibiscus sabdariffa* extract (HSE) was investigated on RAAS in mild to moderate essential hypertensive Nigerian subjects. After 4 weeks of treatment with HSE (150 mg/kg/day), the extract significantly ($p < 0.001$) reduced plasma aldosterone; meanwhile, serum ACE and plasma renin activity did not change significantly. The effects observed could be related to the presence of anthocyanins in the extract [196]. *Hibiscus sabdariffa* calyces (HSC) extract was analyzed on BP, vascular function, and other cardiometabolic risk factors in men with 1% to 10% CVD risk. The consumption of aqueous extract of HSC significantly increased in % flow-mediated dilatation of the branchial artery, and there was no significant decrease in SBP and DBP, a non-significant increase in urinary and plasma nitric oxide (Nox) and reduced levels of plasma insulin and serum glucose, including TG and CRP. There was a significant improvement in the area under the systemic antioxidant response curve, and consumption of the HSC extract showed no significant changes in arterial stiffness [197]. HS extract was studied on isolated mesenteric arteries from normotensive (Wistar and WKY) and SHRs. HS extract caused a concentration-dependent relaxant effect on mesenteric artery rings of SHRs (EC50 = 0.83 $\pm$ 0.08 mg/mL), WKY (EC50 = 0.46 $\pm$ 0.04 mg/mL) and Wistar rats (EC50 = 0.44 $\pm$ 0.08 mg/mL) pre-contracted with phenylephrine (10 μM). HS extract of 2 mg/mL significantly reduced the peak of the L-type calcium current seen in cardiac myocytes by 24%. HS extract did not promote a membrane hyperpolarization of smooth muscle cells, which could suggest an absence of a direct effect on background potassium current. The authors concluded that HS extract probably implicates a vasorelaxant effect on small resistance arteries, which does not depend on the endothelium, and the reduction in L-type calcium current is part of this effect [71]. *Nigella sativa* seed extract (100 and 200 mg twice a day) supplement was evaluated in patients with mild hypertension. After 8 weeks, SBP and DBP values were statistically significantly reduced in a dose-dependent manner. The extract also caused a significant decline in the level of TC and LDL-C [87]. *Platycodon grandiflorus* (PG) is used to reduce inflammation and lower BP in the Chinese population. *Platycodon grandiflorus* root was tested for inhibiting Ang II-induced IGF-IIR activation and apoptosis pathway in H9c2 cells and SHRs. The crude extract of PG significantly inhibited the Ang II-induced IGFIIR signaling to avoid H9c2 cells apoptosis. PG extract suppressed Ang

II-dependent JNK activation and SIRT1 degradation to decrease IGF-IIR activity. Additionally, PG maintained SIRT1 stability to improve HSF1-mediated IGF-IIR suppression, which prevents H9c2 cells apoptosis. In SHRs, PG markedly decreased this apoptotic pathway in the heart tissues; thus, PG could be considered for the treatment of heart diseases in hypertensive patients [100]. According to the antioxidant properties of pomegranate, its peel extract was analyzed for damage related to hypertension and aging in a SHR model. Pomegranate peel extract showed a significant reduction in SBP and coronary ACE activity. The extract also reduced superoxide anion levels and vascular wall areas in the coronary SHRs treated with peel extract. Therefore, this study suggests that pomegranate peel extract may have beneficial effects on coronary heart disease [106]. Antioxidant properties related to leaf and root extracts of *Taraxacum officinale* were investigated in vitro and in vivo. For the in vivo model, experiments were performed on organ homogenate samples from L-NAME-induced Wistar rats. The leaf extract of *Taraxacum officinale* possessed significantly higher polyphenol and flavonoid, including free radical scavenging activity (EC50 0.37 compared to 1.34 mg/mL) and total antioxidant capacities (82.56% compared to 61.54% 3-ethylbenzothiazoline-6-sulfonic acid: ABTS, and 156 $\pm$ 5.28 compared to 40 $\pm$ 0.31 ferric reducing antioxidant power: FRAP). Both extracts significantly increased total antioxidant capacities (kidney and brain tissues) and reduced MDA levels (heart tissue) [115]. Taken together, there are several plants and herbs whose extracts have blood pressure-lowering properties in patients and animal models with hypertension. Therefore, these extracts could be used as a therapeutic strategy to prevent and treat hypertension-associated obesity (Table 4 and Figure 2).

Table 4. Extracts from different herbs and plants with antihypertensive effects.

Name of Herbs and Plants and Method of Extraction	Type of Study	Doses and Duration	Outcomes and Side Effects (Humans)
Allium sativum (aged black garlic extract). Available on the market in different brands	Randomized, crossover, double-blind, sustained, and controlled study; individuals with moderate hypercholesterolemia	250 mg (1.25 mg SAC)/tablet/day ABG for 6 weeks, with 3 weeks of washout	Significantly decreased DBP, particularly in men with a baseline DBP higher than 75 mm Hg and improved cardiovascular risk factors [188]. Garlic extract table may cause breath and body odor, upset stomach or heartburn.
Andrographis paniculata (aqueous extract). Extract on the market in different brands	Male SHR and WKY rats, aged 14–15 weeks	2.8, 1.4, 0.7 g/kg for 13 days	Lowered SBP in SHR and WKY rats, reduced plasma ACE activity and kidney TBA level in SHR. No significant effect on lung ACE activity [189]. *Andrographis* can cause side effects diarrhea, vomiting, rash, headache, runny nose, and fatigue
Aronia melanocarpa (chokeberry), berry extracts. Available on the market in different brands	Meta-analysis of controlled clinical trials, including randomized, placebo-controlled trials	Daily supplementation for an average of 6–8 weeks	Significantly reduces systolic blood pressure and TC, with stronger effects in adults over the age of 50 years [190]. Adverse effects were not found. Taking chokeberry together with drugs that slow blood clotting might increase the risk of bruising and bleeding
Camellia sinensis (Green tea), green tea extract (GTE). Extract on the market in different brands	Crossover, randomized, double-blind, placebo-controlled clinical trial	Three capsules daily, each containing 500 mg of GTE (260 mg polyphenols per capsule), for 4 weeks with a 2-week washout period between treatments	Significant decrease in SBP at 24 h, daytime, and nighttime in obese prehypertensive women. No significant changes in DBP or other metabolic parameters [193]. Green tea extracts can cause liver problems, and the symptoms can include yellowing of the skin or the whites of the eyes, stomach pain and nausea
Camellia sinensis (Green Tea), green tea extract (GTE). Extract on the market in different brands	13-week-old male Sprague Dawley rats	High dose (700 g/kg/day) or low dose (350 g/kg/day) Ang II dose for 13 days, 6 mg/mL GTE in drinking water	GTE prevented hypertension, left-ventricular hypertrophy, vascular remodeling, and endothelial dysfunction induced by high Ang II dose. It blunted increases in oxidative stress markers [191]. Green tea extracts can cause liver problems, and the symptoms can include yellowing of the skin or the whites of the eyes, stomach pain and nausea

Table 4. *Cont.*

Name of Herbs and Plants and Method of Extraction	Type of Study	Doses and Duration	Outcomes and Side Effects (Humans)
Camellia sinensis (Green tea), green tea extract (GTE). Extract on the market in different brands	A systematic review and meta-analysis of randomized clinical trials	Various doses and durations across multiple studies	Green tea epigallocatechins have ACE inhibitor properties. Green tea lowers blood pressure by suppressing NADPH oxidase activity and reducing reactive oxygen species. Some meta-analyses reported beneficial effects on blood vessel dilation and lipid profile [192]. Green tea extracts can cause constipation, abdominal discomfort, hypoglycemia, elevated BP, dyspepsia, and mild skin rash
Cocoa (flavanols-rich cocoa extract). Supplied by Nutrafur S.A. (Murcia, Spain)	Clinical trial, crossover, randomized, double-blind	1.4 g of cocoa extract (415 mg flavanols) daily for 4 weeks	Reduced postprandial SBP after daily cocoa extract intake within an energy-restricted diet [41]. Cocoa can cause allergic skin reactions, migraine headaches, nausea, stomach discomfort, constipation, and gas. Eating large amounts can cause caffeine-related side effects such as nervousness, increased urination, sleeplessness, and a fast heartbeat
Ginkgo biloba (Standardized leaf extract, Egb761). Available on the mar-ket	Male adult Wistar rats (120–160 g), hypertension induced by L-NAME and hypercholesterolemia induced by 1% cholesterol diet	100 mg/kg/day orally for 12 weeks	Reduced systolic, diastolic, and mean arterial BP. Improved serum lipid profile, protected against renal injury, reduced renal oxidative stress, nitrosative stress, and inflammation. Decreased renal TNF-α, IL-6, IL-1β, and iNOS protein expressions, and increased eNOS protein expression [59]. *Ginkgo biloba* can cause stomach upset, headache, dizziness, and allergic skin reactions. *Ginkgo* leaf extract might increase the risk of bruising and bleeding or cause arrhythmia
Ginkgo biloba (new component group of *Ginkgo biloba* leaves, GBLCG), 50% ethanol extract. Available as leaves extract in the market	Male Wistar rats and spontaneously hypertensive rats (SHRs), 200 ± 20 g	4.4, 2.2, and 1.1 mg/kg for 120 days	Reduced blood pressure and improved myocardial hypertrophy by promoting NO synthesis and release in endothelial cells, reducing oxidative stress, inhibiting platelet aggregation, and promoting lesion circulation. The hypotensive activity of GBLCG (4.4 mg/kg) was better than *Ginkgo biloba* extract [194]. *Ginkgo biloba* can cause stomach upset, headache, dizziness, and allergic skin reactions. *Ginkgo* leaf extract might increase the risk of bruising and bleeding or cause arrhythmia

Table 4. *Cont.*

Name of Herbs and Plants and Method of Extraction	Type of Study	Doses and Duration	Outcomes and Side Effects (Humans)
Coffea (green coffee bean extract, GCE) hot-water extract. Extract on the market in different brands	Healthy male volunteers (aged 30 to 50 years), with mild hypertension	46 mg, 93 mg, or 185 mg of GCE daily for 28 days	Dose-dependent reduction in SBP. Reduction in DBP was also observed [64]. Consuming large amounts of green coffee might cause headache, anxiety, agitation, and irregular heartbeat
Hibiscus sabdariffa (dried calyx and hibiscus anthocyanins), water extract. Available as dried calyces in the market	12-week-old male SHR	10%, 15%, and 20% *Hibiscus sabdariffa* for 10 weeks. 50, 100, and 200 mg/kg red anthocyanin by oral gavage for 5 days	*Hibiscus sabdariffa* reduced SBP, DBP, and LV mass; increased myocardial capillary surface area and length density. Red anthocyanin did not significantly reduce the SBP and DBP [195]. *Hibiscus sabdariffa* can cause stomach upset, gas, and constipation
Hibiscus sabdariffa (aqueous extract). Extract on the market in different brands	Wistar, Wistar-Kyoto (WKY), and SHR of about 16 weeks old	SHR (EC50 = 0.83 ± 0.08 mg/mL), WKY (EC50 = 0.46 ± 0.04 mg/mL), and Wistar rats (EC50 = 0.44 ± 0.08 mg/mL)	Concentration-dependent relaxant effect on mesenteric arteries and reduced L-type calcium current [71]. *Hibiscus sabdariffa* can cause stomach upset, gas, and constipation
Hibiscus sabdariffa calyces (HSC), aqueous extract of calyces. Available as dried calyces in the market	A randomized, controlled, single-blinded, acute, cross-over trial	7.5 g HSC in 250 mL Buxton water, at time 0 min followed by a medium fat lunch at 120 min in a random order separated by a two-week washout period	Significant increase in % flow-mediated dilatation, non-significant decrease in SBP and DBP, non-significant increase in urinary and plasma NOx, the reduced response of serum glucose, plasma insulin, serum TAG, and CRP levels. Significant improvement in systemic antioxidant response. No significant changes in arterial stiffness [197]. *Hibiscus sabdariffa* can cause stomach upset, gas, and constipation
Hibiscus sabdariffa (aqueous extract). Extract on the market in different brands	Double-blind randomized controlled trial	150 mg/kg daily for 4 weeks	Reduced plasma aldosterone, serum ACE, and increased plasma renin activity [196]. *Hibiscus sabdariffa* can cause stomach upset, gas, and constipation
Nigella sativa (seed), boiled water extract. Available on the market	A randomized, double-blind, placebo-controlled trial. Healthy male volunteers with mild hypertension	100 mg and 200 mg twice a day for 8 weeks	Significant reduction in SBP and DBP in a dose-dependent manner. Reduced TC and LDL-C levels [87]. *Nigella sativa* seed can cause allergic rashes, stomach upset, vomiting, or constipation

Table 4. *Cont.*

Name of Herbs and Plants and Method of Extraction	Type of Study	Doses and Duration	Outcomes and Side Effects (Humans)
Platycodon grandiflorus (roots) (aqueous extract). Available on the market	H9c2 myoblasts. SHRs and WKYs rats (about 300 g)	1.25, 2.5, 5 µg/µL for in vitro. 100 and 200 mg/kg/day for 50 days for in vivo	Suppressed Ang II-induced IGF-IIR signaling, reduced cardiomyocyte apoptosis, decreased SBP and DBP in SHRs [100]. Side effects not reported
Punica granatum (pomegranate peel), ethanol (95° GL) Extract. Available in the market as pomegranate peel powder	Female SHRs (4 and 28 weeks old)	25 mg/100 g rat for 30 days	Reduced SBP, coronary ACE activity, oxidative stress, and vascular remodeling in hypertensive female rats [106]. Some people have experienced sensitivity to pomegranate extract such as itching, swelling, runny nose, and difficulty breathing
Taraxacum officinale (leaves and roots), 70% ethanol extract. Available on the market	ABTS and FRAP. L-NAME-induced hypertensive Wistar rats (150 g to 200 g), both sexes	500 mg/kg/day for 21 days	Leaves possessed higher polyphenol and flavonoid, free radical scavenging activity, and total antioxidant capacities. Leaves and roots extract significantly increased total antioxidant capacities (kidney and brain tissues) and reduced MDA levels (heart tissue) [115]. *Taraxacum officinale* can cause allergic reactions, stomach discomfort, diarrhea, or heartburn in some people

8. Conclusions and Perspectives

Obesity and associated cardiovascular diseases have been recognized as a public health concern, mainly in countries where its prevalence is alarmingly high. According to the World Obesity Atlas 2023 estimation, 38% of the global population is currently overweight or obese. In Mexico, the projected trends in obesity prevalence (BMI ≥ 30 kg/m^2) will be very high by 2035, 47% in adults (https://www.worldobesity.org/resources/resource-library/world-obesity-atlas-2023, accessed on 28 June 2024). Currently, various agents are used to prevent or treat obesity and associated metabolic disorders, for instance, lowering lipids (e.g., statins, inhibitors of enzyme HMG-CoA reductase) and body weight (e.g., orlistat, an inhibitor of pancreatic lipase), and common treatment strategies employed for CVDs include a combination of anticoagulant and antithrombotic therapy such as aspirin, clopidogrel (tienopyrin), apixaban, dabigatran, rivaroxban and warfarin. Unfortunately, the use of these medications causes potentially serious side effects, including nausea, vomiting, flatulence, diarrhea, insomnia, headache, hemorrhagic, and ischemic complications. For this reason, the World Health Organization (Committee, 1980) recommended the use of herbal and plant-based medicines. Compared with pharmaceutical agents, herbs and plants extract offer similar benefits against cardiometabolic risk factors associated with obesity without the side effects. Herb and plant extracts are rich sources of various nutrients and medicinal phytochemicals, including vitamins, minerals, carotenoids, fatty acids and esters, oils, polysaccharides, proteins, polyphenols, fibers, catechins, flavonoids, terpenes, and other compounds. These bioactive phytochemicals show various beneficial properties against various human diseases. For example, polyphenols have antioxidant, anti-inflammatory, antihypertensive, and atherogenic effects, and they can inhibit platelet aggregation and activation [198], thus having a potential protective role in several diseases such as obesity, T2D, and cardiovascular disease. Although most herb and plant extracts analyzed in this review were investigated in vitro and in animal models, further future research studies in clinical trials are required to confirm the beneficial properties of these herbs and plants against cardiometabolic risk factors associated with obesity. It is well known that obesity is associated with processed foods and high-calorie diets, including a sedentary lifestyle. Therefore, healthcare systems and governments in countries with a current high prevalence of obesity must encourage people to consume healthy nutrition (vegetables and fruits), physical activity, and maintain a healthy weight to avoid obesity and CVDs, which are the main cause of mortality globally. In 2021, CVDs accounted for 20.5 million deaths, of which around 80% occurred in low- and middle-income countries [199]. Therefore, overall, the consumption of herbs and plant teas should be recommended as a possible approach to reduce cardiovascular diseases associated with obesity.

Author Contributions: J.G.-C. and J.A.-B. conceived, designed, and revised the review. J.G.-C., D.L.-C., A.S.-R. and J.G.-B. wrote the draft, reviewed it, and edited it. All authors have read and agreed to the published version of the manuscript.

Funding: This work was supported by Consejo Nacional de Humanidades, Ciencias y Tecnologías (CONAHCYT), Mexico, under grant CF-2023-I-473 to J.G.-C.

Institutional Review Board Statement: Not applicable.

Informed Consent Statement: Not applicable.

Data Availability Statement: Data sharing is not applicable.

Conflicts of Interest: The authors declare no conflicts of interest.

References

1. Gutiérrez-Cuevas, J.; Santos, A.; Armendariz-Borunda, J. Pathophysiological Molecular Mechanisms of Obesity: A Link between MAFLD and NASH with Cardiovascular Diseases. *Int. J. Mol. Sci.* **2021**, *22*, 11629. [CrossRef] [PubMed]
2. Karri, S.; Sharma, S.; Hatware, K.; Patil, K. Natural Anti-Obesity Agents and Their Therapeutic Role in Management of Obesity: A Future Trend Perspective. *Biomed. Pharmacother.* **2019**, *110*, 224–238. [CrossRef] [PubMed]

3. Gutiérrez-Cuevas, J.; Sandoval-Rodriguez, A.; Meza-Rios, A.; Monroy-Ramírez, H.C.; Galicia-Moreno, M.; García-Bañuelos, J.; Santos, A.; Armendariz-Borunda, J. Molecular Mechanisms of Obesity-linked Cardiac Dysfunction: An Up-date on Current Knowledge. *Cells* **2021**, *10*, 629. [CrossRef] [PubMed]
4. Schuster, D. Obesity and the Development of Type 2 Diabetes: The effects of Fatty Tissue Inflammation. *Diabetes Metab. Syndr. Obes. Targets Ther.* **2010**, *3*, 253–262. [CrossRef]
5. McLaughlin, T.; Lamendola, C.; Liu, A.; Abbasi, F. Preferential Fat Deposition in Subcutaneous Versus Visceral Depots Is Associated with Insulin Sensitivity. *J. Clin. Endocrinol. Metab.* **2011**, *96*, E1756–E1760. [CrossRef]
6. Konige, M.; Wang, H.; Sztalryd, C. Role of Adipose Specific Lipid Droplet Proteins in Maintaining Whole Body Energy Homeostasis. *Biochim. Biophys. Acta (BBA) Mol. Basis Dis.* **2014**, *1842*, 393–401. [CrossRef] [PubMed]
7. Garin-Shkolnik, T.; Rudich, A.; Hotamisligil, G.S.; Rubinstein, M. FABP4 Attenuates PPARγ and Adipogenesis and Is Inversely Correlated with PPARγ in Adipose Tissues. *Diabetes* **2014**, *63*, 900–911. [CrossRef] [PubMed]
8. Vincent, H.K.; Taylor, A.G. Biomarkers and Potential Mechanisms of Obesity-Induced Oxidant Stress in Humans. *Int. J. Obes.* **2006**, *30*, 400–418. [CrossRef] [PubMed]
9. Csige, I.; Ujvárosy, D.; Szabó, Z.; Lorincz, I.; Paragh, G.; Harangi, M.; Somodi, S.; Santulli, G. The Impact of Obesity on the Cardiovascular System. *J Diabetes Res* **2018**, *2018*, 3407306. [CrossRef]
10. Pi-Sunyer, X. The Medical Risks of Obesity. *Postgrad. Med.* **2009**, *121*, 21–33. [CrossRef]
11. Hossain, P.; Kawar, B.; El Nahas, M. Obesity and Diabetes in the Developing World—A Growing Challenge. *New Engl. J. Med.* **2007**, *356*, 213–215. [CrossRef]
12. Abdi Beshir, S.; Ahmed Elnour, A.; Soorya, A.; Parveen Mohamed, A.; Sir Loon Goh, S.; Hussain, N.; Al Haddad, A.H.I.; Hussain, F.; Yousif Khidir, I.; Abdelnassir, Z. A Narrative Review of Approved and Emerging Anti-Obesity Medications. *Saudi Pharm. J.* **2023**, *31*, 101757. [CrossRef] [PubMed]
13. Kang, J.G.; Park, C.-Y. Anti-Obesity Drugs: A Review about Their Effects and Safety. *Diabetes Metab. J.* **2012**, *36*, 13–25. [CrossRef] [PubMed]
14. Ahmad, M.S.; Ahmed, N. Antiglycation Properties of Aged garlic Extract: Possible Role in Prevention of Diabetic Complications. *J. Nutr.* **2006**, *136*, 796S–799S. [CrossRef] [PubMed]
15. Imaizumi, V.M.; Laurindo, L.F.; Manzan, B.; Guiguer, E.L.; Oshiiwa, M.; Otoboni, A.M.M.B.; Araujo, A.C.; Tofano, R.J.; Barbalho, S.M. Garlic: A Systematic Review of the Effects On Cardiovascular Diseases. *Crit. Rev. Food Sci. Nutr.* **2023**, *63*, 6797–6819. [CrossRef]
16. Xiong, X.J.; Wang, P.Q.; Li, S.J.; Li, X.K.; Zhang, Y.Q.; Wang, J. Garlic for hypertension: A Systematic Review and Meta-Analysis of Randomized Controlled Trials. *Phytomedicine* **2015**, *22*, 352–361. [CrossRef]
17. Nakagawa, S.; Masamoto, K.; Sumiyoshi, H.; Harada, H. Acute Toxicity Test of Garlic Extract. *J. Toxicol. Sci.* **1984**, *9*, 57–60. [CrossRef] [PubMed]
18. Fardiyah, Q.; Ersam, T.; Suyanta; Slamet, A.; Suprapto; Kurniawan, F. New Potential and Characterization of *Andrographis paniculata* L. Ness Plant Extracts as Photoprotective Agent. *Arab. J. Chem.* **2020**, *13*, 8888–8897. [CrossRef]
19. Wong, S.K.; Chin, K.-Y.; Ima-Nirwana, S. A Review on the Molecular Basis Underlying the Protective Effects of *Andrographis paniculata* and Andrographolide against Myocardial Injury. *Drug Des. Devel. Ther.* **2021**, *15*, 4615–4632. [CrossRef]
20. Kulling, S.E.; Rawel, H.M. Chokeberry (*Aronia melanocarpa*)—A Review on the Characteristic Components and Potential Health Effects. *Planta Medica* **2008**, *74*, 1625–1634. [CrossRef]
21. Banjari, I.; Misir, A.; Šavikin, K.; Jokić, S.; Molnar, M.; De Zoysa, H.K.S.; Waisundara, V.Y. Antidiabetic Effects of *Aronia melanocarpa* and Its Other Therapeutic Properties. *Front. Nutr.* **2017**, *4*, 53. [CrossRef]
22. Jurikova, T.; Mlcek, J.; Skrovankova, S.; Sumczynski, D.; Sochor, J.; Hlavacova, I.; Snopek, L.; Orsavová, J. Fruits of Black Chokeberry *Aronia melanocarpa* in the Prevention of Chronic Diseases. *Molecules* **2017**, *22*, 944. [CrossRef] [PubMed]
23. Brimson, J.M.; Prasanth, M.I.; Kumaree, K.K.; Thitilertdecha, P.; Malar, D.S.; Tencomnao, T.; Prasansuklab, A. Tea Plant (*Camellia sinensis*): A Current Update on Use in Diabetes, Obesity, and Cardiovascular Disease. *Nutrients* **2023**, *15*, 37. [CrossRef]
24. Dinh, T.C.; Phuong, T.N.T.; Minh, L.B.; Thuc, V.T.M.; Bac, N.D.; Van Tien, N.; Pham, V.H.; Show, P.L.; Tao, Y.; Ngoc, V.T.N.; et al. The Effects of Green Tea on Lipid Metabolism and Its Potential Applications for Obesity and Related Metabolic Disorders—An Existing Update. *Diabetes Metab. Syndr. Clin. Res. Rev.* **2019**, *13*, 1667–1673. [CrossRef]
25. Anwar, R.; Rabail, R.; Rakha, A.; Bryla, M.; Roszko, M.; Aadil, R.M.; Kieliszek, M. Delving the Role of *Caralluma fimbriata*: An Edible Wild Plant to Mitigate the Biomarkers of Metabolic Syndrome. *Oxidative Med. Cell. Longev.* **2022**, *2022*, 5720372. [CrossRef] [PubMed]
26. Rao, A.; Briskey, D.; dos Reis, C.; Mallard, A.R. The Effect of an Orally-Dosed *Caralluma fimbriata* Extract on Appetite Control and Body Composition in Overweight Adults. *Sci. Rep.* **2021**, *11*, 6791. [CrossRef] [PubMed]
27. Gujjala, S.; Putakala, M.; Bongu, S.B.R.; Ramaswamy, R.; Desireddy, S. Preventive Effect of *Caralluma fimbriata* against High-Fat diet Induced Injury to Heart by Modulation of Tissue Lipids, Oxidative Stress and Histological Changes in Wistar Rats. *Arch. Physiol. Biochem.* **2022**, *128*, 474–482. [CrossRef]
28. Rao, P.V.; Gan, S.H. Cinnamon: A Multifaceted Medicinal Plant. *Evid. Based Complement. Altern. Med.* **2014**, *2014*, 642942. [CrossRef]
29. Roussel, A.-M.; Hininger, I.; Benaraba, R.; Ziegenfuss, T.N.; Anderson, R.A. Antioxidant Effects of a Cinnamon Extract in People with Impaired Fasting Glucose that Are Overweight or Obese. *J. Am. Coll. Nutr.* **2009**, *28*, 16–21. [CrossRef]

30. Beejmohun, V.; Peytavy-Izard, M.; Mignon, C.; Muscente-Paque, D.; Deplanque, X.; Ripoll, C.; Chapal, N. Acute Effect of Ceylon Cinnamon Extract on Postprandial Glycemia: Alpha-Amylase Inhibition, Starch Tolerance Test in Rats, and Randomized Crossover Clinical Trial in Healthy Volunteers. *BMC Complement. Altern. Med.* **2014**, *14*, 351. [CrossRef]
31. Cheng, X.; Qin, M.; Chen, R.; Jia, Y.; Zhu, Q.; Chen, G.; Wang, A.; Ling, B.; Rong, W. *Citrullus colocynthis* (L.) Schrad.: A Promising Pharmaceutical Resource for Multiple Diseases. *Molecules* **2023**, *28*, 6221. [CrossRef] [PubMed]
32. Iftikhar, N.; Hussain, A.I.; Fatima, T.; Alsuwayt, B.; Althaiban, A.K. Bioactivity-Guided Isolation and Antihypertensive Activity of *Citrullus colocynthis* Polyphenols in Rats with Genetic Model of Hypertension. *Medicina* **2023**, *59*, 1880. [CrossRef] [PubMed]
33. Jafarizadeh, A.; Raeisi, S.A.; Ghassab-Abdollahi, N.; Yarani, R.; Araj-Khodaei, M.; Mirghafourvand, M. Effect of *Citrullus colocynthis* on Glycemic Factors and Lipid Profile in Type II Diabetic Patients: A Systematic Review and Meta-Analysis. *J. Diabetes Metab. Disord.* **2022**, *21*, 1785–1795. [CrossRef]
34. Alhawiti, N.M. Antiplatelets and Profibrinolytic Activity of *Citrullus colocynthis* in Control and High-Fat Diet-Induced Obese Rats: Mechanisms of Action. *Arch. Physiol. Biochem.* **2018**, *124*, 156–166. [CrossRef]
35. Ahmed, M.; Sajid, A.R.; Javeed, A.; Aslam, M.; Ahsan, T.; Hussain, D.; Mateen, A.; Li, X.; Qin, P.; Ji, M. Antioxidant, Antifungal, and Aphicidal Activity of the Triterpenoids Spinasterol and 22,23-Dihydrospinasterol from Leaves of *Citrullus colocynthis* L. *Sci. Rep.* **2022**, *12*, 4910. [CrossRef]
36. Marzouk, B.; Marzouk, Z.; Haloui, E.; Fenina, N.; Bouraoui, A.; Aouni, M. Screening of Analgesic and Anti-Inflammatory Activities of *Citrullus colocynthis* from Southern Tunisia. *J. Ethnopharmacol.* **2010**, *128*, 15–19. [CrossRef]
37. Alzarah, M.I.; Alaqil, A.A.; Abbas, A.O.; Nassar, F.S.; Mehaisen, G.M.K.; Gouda, G.F.; El-Atty, H.K.A.; Moustafa, E.S. Inclusion of *Citrullus colocynthis* Seed Extract into Diets Induced a Hypolipidemic Effect and Improved Layer Performance. *Agriculture* **2021**, *11*, 808. [CrossRef]
38. Rahimi, R.; Amin, G.; Ardekani, M.R.S. A Review on *Citrullus colocynthis* Schrad.: From Traditional Iranian Medicine to Modern Phytotherapy. *J. Altern. Complement. Med.* **2012**, *18*, 551–554. [CrossRef]
39. Davinelli, S.; Corbi, G.; Righetti, S.; Sears, B.; Olarte, H.H.; Grassi, D.; Scapagnini, G. Cardioprotection by Cocoa Polyphenols and ω-3 Fatty Acids: A Disease-Prevention Perspective on Aging-Associated Cardiovascular Risk. *J. Med. Food* **2018**, *21*, 1060–1069. [CrossRef]
40. Katz, D.L.; Doughty, K.; Ali, A. Cocoa and Chocolate in Human Health and Disease. *Antioxid. Redox Signal.* **2011**, *15*, 2779–2811. [CrossRef] [PubMed]
41. Ibero-Baraibar, I.; Suarez, M.; Arola-Arnal, A.; Zulet, M.A.; Martinez, J.A. Cocoa Extract Intake for 4 weeks Reduces Postprandial Systolic Blood Pressure Response of Obese Subjects, even after Following an Energy-Restricted Diet. *Food Nutr. Res.* **2016**, *60*, 30449. [CrossRef]
42. Hidalgo, I.; Ortiz, A.; Sanchez-Pardo, M.; Garduño-Siciliano, L.; Hernández-Ortega, M.; Villarreal, F.; Meaney, E.; Najera, N.; Ceballos, G.M. Obesity and Cardiovascular Risk Improvement Using Cacao By-Products in a Diet-Induced Obesity Murine Model. *J. Med. Food* **2019**, *22*, 567–577. [CrossRef]
43. Kobayashi-Hattori, K.; Mogi, A.; Matsumoto, Y.; Takita, T. Effect of Caffeine on the Body Fat and Lipid Metabolism of Rats Fed on a High-Fat Diet. *Biosci. Biotechnol. Biochem.* **2005**, *69*, 2219–2223. [CrossRef] [PubMed]
44. Olas, B. New Light on Changes in the Number and Function of Blood Platelets Stimulated by Cocoa and Its Products. *Front. Pharmacol.* **2024**, *15*, 1366076. [CrossRef]
45. Dong, Y.; Feng, Z.-L.; Chen, H.-B.; Wang, F.-S.; Lu, J.-H. *Corni fructus*: A Review of Chemical Constituents and Pharmacological Activities. *Chin. Med.* **2018**, *13*, 34. [CrossRef]
46. Gao, X.; Liu, Y.; An, Z.; Ni, J. Active Components and Pharmacological Effects of *Cornus officinalis*: Literature Review. *Front. Pharmacol.* **2021**, *12*, 633447. [CrossRef]
47. Park, C.H.; Cho, E.J.; Yokozawa, T. Protection Against Hypercholesterolemia by *Corni fructus* Extract and Its Related Protective Mechanism. *J. Med. Food* **2009**, *12*, 973–981. [CrossRef]
48. Kim, H.-J.; Kim, K.-S.; Lee, T.-J.; Kim, Y.-C. Antidiabetic Effects of *Corni fructus* Extract on Blood Glucose and Insulin Resistance in db/db Mice. *Toxicol. Res.* **2009**, *25*, 93–99. [CrossRef]
49. Amerizadeh, A.; Vaseghi, G.; Esmaeilian, N.; Asgary, S. Cardiovascular Effects of *Cydonia oblonga* Miller (Quince). *Evid. Based Complement. Altern. Med.* **2022**, *2022*, 3185442. [CrossRef]
50. Wojdyło, A.; Oszmiański, J.; Bielicki, P. Polyphenolic Composition, Antioxidant Activity, and Polyphenol Oxidase (PPO) Activity of Quince (*Cydonia oblonga* Miller) Varieties. *J. Agric. Food Chem.* **2013**, *61*, 2762–2772. [CrossRef]
51. Lee, H.S.; Jung, J.I.; Hwang, J.S.; Hwang, M.O.; Kim, E.J. *Cydonia oblonga* Miller Fruit Extract Exerts an Anti-Obesity Effect in 3T3-L1 Adipocytes by Activating the AMPK Signaling Pathway. *Nutr. Res. Pract.* **2023**, *17*, 1043–1055. [CrossRef] [PubMed]
52. Umar, A.; Iskandar, G.; Aikemu, A.; Yiming, W.; Zhou, W.; Berké, B.; Begaud, B.; Moore, N. Effects of *Cydonia oblonga* Miller Leaf and Fruit Flavonoids on Blood Lipids and Anti-Oxydant Potential in Hyperlipidemia Rats. *J. Ethnopharmacol.* **2015**, *169*, 239–243. [CrossRef] [PubMed]
53. Zhou, W.; Abdurahman, A.; Umar, A.; Iskander, G.; Abdusalam, E.; Berké, B.; Bégaud, B.; Moore, N. Effects of *Cydonia oblonga* Miller Extracts on Blood Hemostasis, Coagulation and Fibrinolysis in Mice, and Experimental Thrombosis in Rats. *J. Ethnopharmacol.* **2014**, *154*, 163–169. [CrossRef]
54. Silva, H.; Martins, F.G. Cardiovascular Activity of *Ginkgo biloba*—An Insight from Healthy Subjects. *Biology* **2023**, *12*, 15. [CrossRef]

55. Mohanta, T.K.; Tamboli, Y.; Zubaidha, P. Phytochemical and Medicinal Importance of *Ginkgo biloba* L. *Nat. Prod. Res.* **2014**, *28*, 746–752. [CrossRef] [PubMed]
56. Tao, Y.; Zhu, F.; Pan, M.; Liu, Q.; Wang, P. Pharmacokinetic, Metabolism, and Metabolomic Strategies Provide Deep Insight Into the Underlying Mechanism of *Ginkgo biloba* Flavonoids in the Treatment of Cardiovascular Disease. *Front. Nutr.* **2022**, *9*, 857370. [CrossRef] [PubMed]
57. Pinto, M.D.S.; Kwon, Y.-I.; Apostolidis, E.; Lajolo, F.M.; Genovese, M.I.; Shetty, K. Potential of *Ginkgo biloba* L. Leaves in the Management of Hyperglycemia and Hypertension Using in Vitro Models. *Bioresour. Technol.* **2009**, *100*, 6599–6609. [CrossRef] [PubMed]
58. Lim, S.; Yoon, J.W.; Kang, S.M.; Choi, S.H.; Cho, B.J.; Kim, M.; Park, H.S.; Cho, H.J.; Shin, H.; Kim, Y.-B.; et al. EGb761, a *Ginkgo biloba* Extract, Is Effective against Atherosclerosis in Vitro, and in a Rat Model of Type 2 Diabetes. *PLoS ONE* **2011**, *6*, e20301. [CrossRef] [PubMed]
59. Abdel-Zaher, A.O.; Farghaly, H.S.; El-Refaiy, A.E.; Abd-Eldayem, A.M. Protective Effect of the Standardized Extract of *Ginkgo biloba* (EGb761) against Hypertension with Hypercholesterolemia-Induced Renal Injury in Rats: Insights in the Underlying Mechanisms. *Biomed. Pharmacother.* **2017**, *95*, 944–955. [CrossRef]
60. Manach, C.; Scalbert, A.; Morand, C.; Rémésy, C.; Jiménez, L. Polyphenols: Food Sources and Bioavailability. *Am. J. Clin. Nutr.* **2004**, *79*, 727–747. [CrossRef]
61. Nunes, F.M.; Coimbra, M.A. Chemical Characterization of Galactomannans and Arabinogalactans from Two Arabica Coffee Infusions as Affected by the Degree of Roast. *J. Agric. Food Chem.* **2002**, *50*, 1429–1434. [CrossRef] [PubMed]
62. Blum, J.; Lemaire, B.; Lafay, S. Effect of a Green Decaffeinated Coffee Extract on Glycaemia. *Nutrafoods* **2007**, *6*, 13–17.
63. Asbaghi, O.; Kashkooli, S.; Mardani, M.; Rezaei Kelishadi, M.; Fry, H.; Kazemi, M.; Kaviani, M. Effect of Green Coffee Bean Extract Supplementation on Liver Function and Inflammatory Biomarkers: A Meta-Analysis of Randomized Clinical Trials. *Complement. Ther. Clin. Pract.* **2021**, *43*, 101349. [CrossRef]
64. Kozuma, K.; Tsuchiya, S.; Kohori, J.; Hase, T.; Tokimitsu, I. Antihypertensive Effect of Green Coffee Bean Extract on Mildly Hypertensive Subjects. *Hypertens. Res.* **2005**, *28*, 711–718. [CrossRef]
65. Asbaghi, O.; Sadeghian, M.; Nasiri, M.; Khodadost, M.; Shokri, A.; Panahande, B.; Pirouzi, A.; Sadeghi, O. The Effects of Green Coffee Extract Supplementation on Glycemic Indices and Lipid Profile in Adults: A Systematic Review and Dose-Response Meta-Analysis of Clinical Trials. *Nutr. J.* **2020**, *19*, 71. [CrossRef]
66. Sapian, S.; Ibrahim Mze, A.A.; Jubaidi, F.F.; Mohd Nor, N.A.; Taib, I.S.; Abd Hamid, Z.; Zainalabidin, S.; Mohamad Anuar, N.N.; Katas, H.; Latip, J.; et al. Therapeutic Potential of *Hibiscus sabdariffa* Linn. in Attenuating Cardiovascular Risk Factors. *Pharmaceuticals* **2023**, *16*, 807. [CrossRef] [PubMed]
67. Da-Costa-Rocha, I.; Bonnlaender, B.; Sievers, H.; Pischel, I.; Heinrich, M. *Hibiscus sabdariffa* L.—A Phytochemical and Pharmacological Review. *Food Chem.* **2014**, *165*, 424–443. [CrossRef]
68. Gurrola-Díaz, C.; García-López, P.; Sánchez-Enríquez, S.; Troyo-Sanromán, R.; Andrade-González, I.; Gómez-Leyva, J. Effects of *Hibiscus sabdariffa* extract powder and preventive treatment (diet) on the lipid profiles of patients with metabolic syndrome (MeSy). *Phytomedicine* **2010**, *17*, 500–505. [CrossRef] [PubMed]
69. Janson, B.; Prasomthong, J.; Malakul, W.; Boonsong, T.; Tunsophon, S. *Hibiscus sabdariffa* L. Calyx Extract Prevents the Adipogenesis of 3T3-L1 Adipocytes, and Obesity-Related Insulin Resistance in High-Fat Diet-Induced Obese Rats. *Biomed. Pharmacother.* **2021**, *138*, 111438. [CrossRef] [PubMed]
70. Ademiluyi, A.O.; Oboh, G. Aqueous Extracts of Roselle (*Hibiscus sabdariffa* Linn.) Varieties Inhibit α-Amylase and α-Glucosidase Activities in Vitro. *J. Med. Food* **2013**, *16*, 88–93. [CrossRef] [PubMed]
71. Alsayed, A.M.; Zhang, B.L.; Bredeloux, P.; Boudesocque-Delaye, L.; Yu, A.; Peineau, N.; Enguehard-Gueiffier, C.; Ahmed, E.M.; Pasqualin, C.; Maupoil, V. Aqueous Fraction from *Hibiscus sabdariffa* Relaxes Mesenteric Arteries of Normotensive and Hypertensive Rats through Calcium Current Reduction and Possibly Potassium Channels Modulation. *Nutrients* **2020**, *12*, 1782. [CrossRef]
72. de Vasconcellos, A.C.; Frazzon, J.; Noreña, C.P.Z. Phenolic Compounds Present in *Yerba mate* Potentially Increase Human Health: A Critical Review. *Plant Foods Hum. Nutr.* **2022**, *77*, 495–503. [CrossRef]
73. Paluch, E.; Okińczyc, P.; Zwyrzykowska-Wodzińska, A.; Szperlik, J.; Żarowska, B.; Duda-Madej, A.; Bąbelewski, P.; Włodarczyk, M.; Wojtasik, W.; Kupczyński, R.; et al. Composition and Antimicrobial Activity of *Ilex* Leaves Water Extracts. *Molecules* **2021**, *26*, 7442. [CrossRef] [PubMed]
74. dos Santos, T.W.; Miranda, J.; Teixeira, L.; Aiastui, A.; Matheu, A.; Gambero, A.; Portillo, M.P.; Ribeiro, M.L. *Yerba mate* Stimulates Mitochondrial Biogenesis and Thermogenesis in High-Fat-Diet-Induced Obese Mice. *Mol. Nutr. Food Res.* **2018**, *62*, e1800142. [CrossRef]
75. Arçari, D.P.; Bartchewsky, W.; Dos Santos, T.W.; Oliveira, K.A.; Funck, A.; Pedrazzoli, J.; De Souza, M.F.; Saad, M.J.; Bastos, D.H.; Gambero, A.; et al. Antiobesity Effects of *Yerba maté* Extract (*Ilex paraguariensis*) in High-Fat Diet-Induced Obese Mice. *Obesity* **2009**, *17*, 2127–2133. [CrossRef] [PubMed]
76. Kang, Y.-R.; Lee, H.-Y.; Kim, J.-H.; Moon, D.-I.; Seo, M.-Y.; Park, S.-H.; Choi, K.-H.; Kim, C.-R.; Kim, S.-H.; Oh, J.-H.; et al. Anti-Obesity and Anti-Diabetic Effects of *Yerba mate* (*Ilex paraguariensis*) in C57BL/6J Mice Fed a High-Fat Diet. *Lab. Anim. Res.* **2012**, *28*, 23–29. [CrossRef] [PubMed]

77. A Klein, G.; Stefanuto, A.; Boaventura, B.C.; De Morais, E.C.; Cavalcante, L.d.S.; De Andrade, F.; Wazlawik, E.; Di Pietro, P.F.; Maraschin, M.; da Silva, E.L. Mate Tea (*Ilex paraguariensis*) Improves Glycemic and Lipid Profiles of Type 2 Diabetes and Pre-Diabetes Individuals: A Pilot Study. *J. Am. Coll. Nutr.* **2011**, *30*, 320–332. [CrossRef]
78. Arbeláez, L.F.G.; Fantinelli, J.C.; Pardo, A.C.; Caldiz, C.I.; Ríos, J.L.; Schinella, G.R.; Mosca, S.M. Effect of an *Ilex paraguariensis* (*Yerba mate*) Extract on Infarct Size in Isolated Rat Hearts: The Mechanisms Involved. *Food Funct.* **2016**, *7*, 816–824. [CrossRef]
79. Azlan, U.K.; Mediani, A.; Rohani, E.R.; Tong, X.; Han, R.; Misnan, N.M.; Jam, F.A.; Bunawan, H.; Sarian, M.N.; Hamezah, H.S. A Comprehensive Review with Updated Future Perspectives on the Ethnomedicinal and Pharmacological Aspects of *Moringa oleifera*. *Molecules* **2022**, *27*, 5765. [CrossRef]
80. Mbikay, M. Therapeutic Potential of *Moringa oleifera* Leaves in Chronic Hyperglycemia and Dyslipidemia: A Review. *Front. Pharmacol.* **2012**, *3*, 24. [CrossRef]
81. Ezzat, S.M.; El Bishbishy, M.H.; Aborehab, N.M.; Salama, M.M.; Hasheesh, A.; Motaal, A.A.; Rashad, H.; Metwally, F.M. Upregulation of MC4R and PPAR-α Expression Mediates the Anti-Obesity Activity of *Moringa oleifera* Lam. in high-Fat Diet-Induced Obesity in Rats. *J. Ethnopharmacol.* **2020**, *251*, 112541. [CrossRef] [PubMed]
82. Xie, J.; Wang, Y.; Jiang, W.-W.; Luo, X.-F.; Dai, T.-Y.; Peng, L.; Song, S.; Li, L.-F.; Tao, L.; Shi, C.-Y.; et al. *Moringa oleifera* Leaf Petroleum Ether Extract Inhibits Lipogenesis by Activating the AMPK Signaling Pathway. *Front. Pharmacol.* **2018**, *9*, 1447. [CrossRef] [PubMed]
83. Ghasi, S.; Nwobodo, E.; Ofili, J. Hypocholesterolemic Effects of Crude Extract of Leaf of *Moringa oleifera* Lam in High-Fat Diet Fed Wistar Rats. *J. Ethnopharmacol.* **1999**, *69*, 21–25. [CrossRef] [PubMed]
84. Gómez-Martínez, S.; Díaz-Prieto, L.E.; Castro, I.V.; Jurado, C.; Iturmendi, N.; Martín-Ridaura, M.C.; Calle, N.; Dueñas, M.; Picón, M.J.; Marcos, A.; et al. *Moringa oleifera* Leaf Supplementation as a Glycemic Control Strategy in Subjects with Prediabetes. *Nutrients* **2022**, *14*, 57. [CrossRef] [PubMed]
85. Asgary, S.; Sahebkar, A.; Goli-Malekabadi, N. Ameliorative Effects of *Nigella sativa* on Dyslipidemia. *J. Endocrinol. Investig.* **2015**, *38*, 1039–1046. [CrossRef] [PubMed]
86. Derosa, G.; D'angelo, A.; Maffioli, P.; Cucinella, L.; Nappi, R.E. The Use of *Nigella sativa* in Cardiometabolic Diseases. *Biomedicines* **2024**, *12*, 405. [CrossRef] [PubMed]
87. Dehkordi, F.R.; Kamkhah, A.F. Antihypertensive Effect of *Nigella sativa* Seed Extract in Patients with Mild Hypertension. *Fundam. Clin. Pharmacol.* **2008**, *22*, 447–452. [CrossRef] [PubMed]
88. Madrigal-Santillán, E.; Portillo-Reyes, J.; Madrigal-Bujaidar, E.; Sánchez-Gutiérrez, M.; Izquierdo-Vega, J.A.; Iz-quierdo-Vega, J.; Delgado-Olivares, L.; Vargas-Mendoza, N.; Álvarez-González, I.; Morales-González, Á.; et al. *Opuntia* spp. in Human Health: A Comprehensive Summary on Its Pharmacological, Therapeutic and Preven-tive Properties. Part 2. *Plants* **2022**, *11*, 2333. [CrossRef]
89. Abbas, E.Y.; Ezzat, M.I.; El Hefnawy, H.M.; Abdel-Sattar, E. An Overview and Update on the Chemical Composi-tion and Potential Health Benefits of *Opuntia ficus-indica* (L.) Miller. *J. Food Biochem.* **2022**, *46*, e14310. [CrossRef]
90. Padilla-Camberos, E.; Flores-Fernandez, J.M.; Fernandez-Flores, O.; Gutierrez-Mercado, Y.; la Luz, J.C.-D.; Sandoval-Salas, F.; Mendez-Carreto, C.; Allen, K. Hypocholesterolemic Effect and In Vitro Pancreatic Lipase Inhibitory Activity of an *Opuntia ficus-indica* Extract. *BioMed. Res. Int.* **2015**, *2015*, 837452. [CrossRef]
91. López-Romero, P.; Pichardo-Ontiveros, E.; Avila-Nava, A.; Vázquez-Manjarrez, N.; Tovar, A.R.; Pedraza-Chaverri, J.; Torres, N. The Effect of Nopal (*Opuntia ficus indica*) on Postprandial Blood Glucose, Incretins, and Antioxidant Activity in Mexican Patients with Type 2 Diabetes after Consumption of Two Different Composition Breakfasts. *J. Acad. Nutr. Diet.* **2014**, *114*, 1811–1818. [CrossRef] [PubMed]
92. Butterweck, V.; Semlin, L.; Feistel, B.; Pischel, I.; Bauer, K.; Verspohl, E.J. Comparative Evaluation of Two Different *Opuntia ficus-indica* Extracts for Blood Sugar Lowering Effects in Rats. *Phytotherapy Res.* **2011**, *25*, 370–375. [CrossRef] [PubMed]
93. Zhang, L.; Wang, Y.; Yang, D.; Zhang, C.; Zhang, N.; Li, M.; Liu, Y. Platycodon Grandiflorus—An Ethnopharma-cological, Phytochemical and Pharmacological Review. *J. Ethnopharmacol.* **2015**, *164*, 147–161. [CrossRef] [PubMed]
94. Ji, M.-Y.; Bo, A.; Yang, M.; Xu, J.-F.; Jiang, L.-L.; Zhou, B.-C.; Li, M.-H. The Pharmacological Effects and Health Benefits of *Platycodon grandiflorus*—A Medicine Food Homology Species. *Foods* **2020**, *9*, 142. [CrossRef] [PubMed]
95. Lee, H.; Kang, R.; Kim, Y.S.; Chung, S.; Yoon, Y. Platycodin D Inhibits Adipogenesis of 3T3-L1 Cells by Modulating Kruppel-Like Factor 2 and Peroxisome Proliferator-Activated Receptor γ. *Phytotherapy Res.* **2010**, *24*, S161–S167. [CrossRef] [PubMed]
96. Kim, H.-L.; Park, J.; Jung, Y.; Ahn, K.S.; Um, J.-Y. Platycodin D, a Novel Activator of AMP-Activated Protein Kinase, Attenuates Obesity in db/db Mice via Regulation of Adipogenesis and Thermogenesis. *Phytomedicine* **2019**, *52*, 254–263. [CrossRef] [PubMed]
97. Hwang, K.-A.; Hwang, Y.-J.; Im, P.R.; Hwang, H.-J.; Song, J.; Kim, Y.-J. *Platycodon grandiflorum* Extract Reduces High-Fat Diet-Induced Obesity through Regulation of Adipogenesis and Lipogenesis Pathways in Mice. *J. Med. Food* **2019**, *22*, 993–999. [CrossRef] [PubMed]
98. Chung, M.J.; Kim, S.-H.; Park, J.-W.; Lee, Y.J.; Ham, S.-S. *Platycodon grandiflorum* Root Attenuates Vascular Endothelial Cell Injury by Oxidized Low-Density Lipoprotein and Prevents High-Fat Diet–Induced Dyslipidemia in Mice by Up-Regulating Antioxidant Proteins. *Nutr. Res.* **2012**, *32*, 365–373. [CrossRef] [PubMed]
99. Ahn, Y.-M.; Kim, S.K.; Kang, J.-S.; Lee, B.-C. *Platycodon grandiflorum* Modifies Adipokines and the Glucose Uptake in High-Fat Diet in Mice and L6 Muscle Cells. *J. Pharm. Pharmacol.* **2012**, *64*, 697–704. [CrossRef]

100. Lin, Y.-C.; Lin, C.-H.; Yao, H.-T.; Kuo, W.-W.; Shen, C.-Y.; Yeh, Y.-L.; Ho, T.-J.; Padma, V.V.; Lin, Y.-C.; Huang, C.-Y. *Platycodon grandiflorum* (PG) Reverses Angiotensin II-Induced Apoptosis by Repressing IGF-IIR Expression. *J. Ethnopharmacol.* **2017**, *205*, 41–50. [CrossRef]
101. Hou, C.; Zhang, W.; Li, J.; Du, L.; Lv, O.; Zhao, S.; Li, J. Beneficial Effects of Pomegranate on Lipid Metabolism in Metabolic Disorders. *Mol. Nutr. Food Res.* **2019**, *63*, 1800773. [CrossRef] [PubMed]
102. Maphetu, N.; Unuofin, J.O.; Masuku, N.P.; Olisah, C.; Lebelo, S.L. Medicinal Uses, Pharmacological Activities, Phytochemistry, and the Molecular Mechanisms of *Punica granatum* L. (Pomegranate) Plant Extracts: A Review. *Biomed. Pharmacother.* **2022**, *153*, 113256. [CrossRef] [PubMed]
103. Mokgalaboni, K.; Dlamini, S.; Phoswa, W.N.; Modjadji, P.; Lebelo, S.L. The Impact of *Punica granatum* Linn and Its Derivatives on Oxidative Stress, Inflammation, and Endothelial Function in Diabetes Mellitus: Evidence from Preclinical and Clinical Studies. *Antioxidants* **2023**, *12*, 1566. [CrossRef] [PubMed]
104. Reguero, M.; Gómez de Cedrón, M.; Sierra-Ramírez, A.; Fernández-Marcos, P.J.; Reglero, G.; Quintela, J.C.; Ramírez de Molina, A. Pomegranate Extract Augments Energy Expenditure Counteracting the Metabolic Stress Associated with High-Fat-Diet-Induced Obesity. *Int. J. Mol. Sci.* **2022**, *23*, 10460. [CrossRef]
105. Li, Y.; Wen, S.; Kota, B.P.; Peng, G.; Li, G.Q.; Yamahara, J.; Roufogalis, B.D. *Punica granatum* Flower Extract, a Potent α-Glucosidase Inhibitor, Improves Postprandial Hyperglycemia in Zucker Diabetic Fatty Rats. *J. Ethnopharmacol.* **2005**, *99*, 239–244. [CrossRef] [PubMed]
106. dos Santos, R.L.; Dellacqua, L.O.; Delgado, N.T.B.; Rouver, W.N.; Podratz, P.L.; Lima, L.C.F.; Piccin, M.P.C.; Meyrelles, S.S.; Mauad, H.; Graceli, J.B.; et al. Pomegranate Peel Extract Attenuates Oxidative Stress by Decreasing Coronary Angiotensin-Converting Enzyme (ACE) Activity in Hypertensive Female Rats. *J. Toxicol. Environ. Health Part A* **2016**, *79*, 998–1007. [CrossRef] [PubMed]
107. Jia, Q.; Zhu, R.; Tian, Y.; Chen, B.; Li, R.; Li, L.; Wang, L.; Che, Y.; Zhao, D.; Mo, F.; et al. *Salvia miltiorrhiza* in Diabetes: A Review of Its Pharmacology, Phytochemistry, and Safety. *Phytomedicine* **2019**, *58*, 152871. [CrossRef] [PubMed]
108. Ren, J.; Fu, L.; Nile, S.H.; Zhang, J.; Kai, G. *Salvia miltiorrhiza* in Treating Cardiovascular Diseases: A Review on Its Pharmacological and Clinical Applications. *Front. Pharmacol.* **2019**, *10*, 753. [CrossRef] [PubMed]
109. Qian, S.; Huo, D.; Wang, S.; Qian, Q. Inhibition of Glucose-Induced Vascular Endothelial Growth Factor Expression by *Salvia miltiorrhiza* Hydrophilic Extract in Human Microvascular Endothelial Cells: Evidence for Mitochondrial Oxidative Stress. *J. Ethnopharmacol.* **2011**, *137*, 985–991. [CrossRef]
110. Ai, Z.-L.; Zhang, X.; Ge, W.; Zhong, Y.-B.; Wang, H.-Y.; Zuo, Z.-Y.; Liu, D.-Y. *Salvia miltiorrhiza* Extract May Exert an Anti-Obesity Effect in Rats with High-Fat Diet-Induced Obesity by Modulating Gut Microbiome and Lipid Metabolism. *World J. Gastroenterol.* **2022**, *28*, 6131–6156. [CrossRef]
111. Kania-Dobrowolska, M.; Baraniak, J. Dandelion (*Taraxacum officinale* L.) as a Source of Biologically Active Compounds Supporting the Therapy of Co-Existing Diseases in Metabolic Syndrome. *Foods* **2022**, *11*, 2858. [CrossRef] [PubMed]
112. Olas, B. New Perspectives on the Effect of Dandelion, Its Food Products and Other Preparations on the Cardio-Vascular System and Its Diseases. *Nutrients* **2022**, *14*, 1350. [CrossRef]
113. Zhang, J.; Kang, M.-J.; Kim, M.-J.; Kim, M.-E.; Song, J.-H.; Lee, Y.-M.; Kim, J.-I. Pancreatic Lipase Inhibitory Activity of *Taraxacum officinale* in Vitro and in Vivo. *Nutr. Res. Pract.* **2008**, *2*, 200–203. [CrossRef]
114. González-Castejón, M.; García-Carrasco, B.; Fernández-Dacosta, R.; Dávalos, A.; Rodriguez-Casado, A. Reduction of Adipogenesis and Lipid Accumulation by *Taraxacum officinale* (Dandelion) Extracts in 3T3L1 Adipocytes: An in Vitro Study. *Phytotherapy Res.* **2014**, *28*, 745–752. [CrossRef] [PubMed]
115. Aremu, O.O.; Oyedeji, A.O.; Oyedeji, O.O.; Nkeh-Chungag, B.N.; Rusike, C.R.S. In Vitro and In Vivo Antioxidant Properties of *Taraxacum officinale* in Nω-Nitro-l-Arginine Methyl Ester (L-NAME)-Induced Hypertensive Rats. *Antioxidants* **2019**, *8*, 309. [CrossRef]
116. Murtaza, I.; Laila, O.; Drabu, I.; Ahmad, A.; Charifi, W.; Popescu, S.M.; Mansoor, S. Nutritional Profiling, Phytochemical Composition and Antidiabetic Potential of *Taraxacum officinale*, an Underutilized Herb. *Molecules* **2022**, *27*, 5380. [CrossRef]
117. Jo, J.; Gavrilova, O.; Pack, S.; Jou, W.; Mullen, S.; Sumner, A.E.; Cushman, S.W.; Periwal, V. Hypertrophy and/or Hyperplasia: Dynamics of Adipose Tissue Growth. *PLOS Comput. Biol.* **2009**, *5*, e1000324. [CrossRef] [PubMed]
118. Stich, V.; Berlan, M. Physiological Regulation of NEFA Availability: Lipolysis Pathway. *Proc. Nutr. Soc.* **2004**, *63*, 369–374. [CrossRef] [PubMed]
119. Frühbeck, G.; Méndez-Giménez, L.; Fernández-Formoso, J.-A.; Fernández, S.; Rodríguez, A. Regulation of Adipocyte Lipolysis. *Nutr. Res. Rev.* **2014**, *27*, 63–93. [CrossRef] [PubMed]
120. Lafontan, M.; Langin, D. Lipolysis and Lipid Mobilization in Human Adipose Tissue. *Prog. Lipid Res.* **2009**, *48*, 275–297. [CrossRef]
121. Gutiérrez-Cuevas, J.; Galicia-Moreno, M.; Monroy-Ramírez, H.C.; Sandoval-Rodriguez, A.; García-Bañuelos, J.; Santos, A.; Armendariz-Borunda, J. The Role of NRF2 in Obesity-Associated Cardiovascular Risk Factors. *Antioxidants* **2022**, *11*, 235. [CrossRef] [PubMed]
122. Xia, Y.; Zhai, X.; Qiu, Y.; Lu, X.; Jiao, Y. The Nrf2 in Obesity: A Friend or Foe? *Antioxidants* **2022**, *11*, 2067. [CrossRef] [PubMed]
123. Manna, P.; Jain, S.K. Obesity, Oxidative Stress, Adipose Tissue Dysfunction, and the Associated Health Risks: Causes and Therapeutic Strategies. *Metab. Syndr. Relat. Disord.* **2015**, *13*, 423–444. [CrossRef] [PubMed]
124. Ahima, R.S.; Flier, J.S. Adipose Tissue as an Endocrine Organ. *Trends Endocrinol. Metab.* **2000**, *11*, 327–332. [CrossRef] [PubMed]

125. Macdougall, C.E.; Wood, E.G.; Loschko, J.; Scagliotti, V.; Cassidy, F.C.; Robinson, M.E.; Feldhahn, N.; Castellano, L.; Voisin, M.-B.; Marelli-Berg, F.; et al. Visceral Adipose Tissue Immune Homeostasis Is Regulated by the Crosstalk between Adipocytes and Dendritic Cell Subsets. *Cell Metab.* **2018**, *27*, 588–601.e4. [CrossRef] [PubMed]
126. Gotoh, K.; Inoue, M.; Masaki, T.; Chiba, S.; Shimasaki, T.; Ando, H.; Fujiwara, K.; Katsuragi, I.; Kakuma, T.; Seike, M.; et al. A Novel Anti-inflammatory Role for Spleen-Derived Interleukin-10 in Obesity-Induced Inflammation in White Adipose Tissue and Liver. *Diabetes* **2012**, *61*, 1994–2003. [CrossRef] [PubMed]
127. Zhang, X.; Zhang, G.; Zhang, H.; Karin, M.; Bai, H.; Cai, D. Hypothalamic IKKβ/NF-κB and ER Stress Link Overnutrition to Energy Imbalance and Obesity. *Cell* **2008**, *135*, 61–73. [CrossRef]
128. Milanski, M.; Degasperi, G.; Coope, A.; Morari, J.; Denis, R.; Cintra, D.E.; Tsukumo, D.M.L.; Anhe, G.; Amaral, M.E.; Takahashi, H.K.; et al. Saturated Fatty Acids Produce an Inflammatory Response Predominantly through the Activation of TLR4 Signaling in Hypothalamus: Implications for the Pathogenesis of Obesity. *J. Neurosci.* **2009**, *29*, 359–370. [CrossRef] [PubMed]
129. Barale, C.; Russo, I. Influence of Cardiometabolic Risk Factors on Platelet Function. *Int. J. Mol. Sci.* **2020**, *21*, 623. [CrossRef]
130. Sivamaruthi, B.S.; Kesika, P.; Suganthy, N.; Chaiyasut, C. A Review on Role of Microbiome in Obesity and Anti-Obesity Properties of Probiotic Supplements. *Biomed. Res. Int.* **2019**, *2019*, 3291367. [CrossRef]
131. Chakraborti, C.K. New-Found Link between Microbiota and Obesity. *World J. Gastrointest. Pathophysiol.* **2015**, *6*, 110–119. [CrossRef] [PubMed]
132. Crespy, V.; Williamson, G. A Review of the Health Effects of Green Tea Catechins in In Vivo Animal Models. *J. Nutr.* **2004**, *134*, 3431S–3440S. [CrossRef] [PubMed]
133. Lin, J.; Lin-Shiau, S. Mechanisms of Hypolipidemic and Anti-Obesity Effects of Tea and Tea Polyphenols. *Mol. Nutr. Food Res.* **2006**, *50*, 211–217. [CrossRef] [PubMed]
134. Bajerska, J.; Wozniewicz, M.; Jeszka, J.; Drzymala-Czyz, S.; Walkowiak, J. Green Tea Aqueous Extract Reduces Visceral Fat and Decreases Protein Availability in Rats Fed with a High-Fat Diet. *Nutr. Res.* **2011**, *31*, 157–164. [CrossRef] [PubMed]
135. Basu, A.; Sanchez, K.; Leyva, M.J.; Wu, M.; Betts, N.M.; E Aston, C.; Lyons, T.J. Green Tea Supplementation Affects Body Weight, Lipids, and Lipid Peroxidation in Obese Subjects with Metabolic Syndrome. *J. Am. Coll. Nutr.* **2010**, *29*, 31–40. [CrossRef]
136. Kamalakkannan, S.; Rajendran, R.; Venkatesh, R.V.; Clayton, P.; Akbarsha, M.A. Antiobesogenic and Antiatherosclerotic Properties of *Caralluma fimbriata* Extract. *J. Nutr. Metab.* **2010**, *2010*, 285301. [CrossRef] [PubMed]
137. Banin, R.; Hirata, B.; Andrade, I.; Zemdegs, J.; Clemente, A.; Dornellas, A.; Boldarine, V.; Estadella, D.; Albuquerque, K.; Oyama, L.; et al. Beneficial effects of *Ginkgo biloba* Extract on Insulin Signaling Cascade, Dyslipidemia, and Body Adiposity of Diet-Induced Obese Rats. *Braz. J. Med. Biol. Res.* **2014**, *47*, 780–788. [CrossRef] [PubMed]
138. Hirata, B.K.S.; Banin, R.M.; Dornellas, A.P.S.; De Andrade, I.S.; Zemdegs, J.C.S.; Caperuto, L.C.; Oyama, L.M.; Ribeiro, E.B.; Telles, M.M. *Ginkgo biloba* Extract Improves Insulin Signaling and Attenuates Inflammation in Retroperitoneal Adipose Tissue Depot of Obese Rats. *Mediat. Inflamm.* **2015**, *2015*, 419106. [CrossRef]
139. Banin, R.M.; De Andrade, I.S.; Cerutti, S.M.; Oyama, L.M.; Telles, M.M.; Ribeiro, E.B. *Ginkgo biloba* Extract (GbE) Stimulates the Hypothalamic Serotonergic System and Attenuates Obesity in Ovariectomized Rats. *Front. Pharmacol.* **2017**, *8*, 605. [CrossRef]
140. Hirata, B.K.S.; Cruz, M.M.; De Sá, R.D.C.C.; Farias, T.S.M.; Machado, M.M.F.; Bueno, A.A.; Alonso-Vale, M.I.C.; Telles, M.M. Potential Anti-obesogenic Effects of *Ginkgo biloba* Observed in Epididymal White Adipose Tissue of Obese Rats. *Front. Endocrinol.* **2019**, *10*, 284. [CrossRef]
141. Choi, B.-K.; Park, S.-B.; Lee, D.-R.; Lee, H.J.; Jin, Y.-Y.; Yang, S.H.; Suh, J.-W. Green Coffee Bean Extract Improves Obesity by Decreasing Body Fat in High-Fat Diet-Induced Obese Mice. *Asian Pac. J. Trop. Med.* **2016**, *9*, 635–643. [CrossRef] [PubMed]
142. Seliem, E.M.; Azab, M.E.; Ismail, R.S.; Nafeaa, A.A.; Alotaibi, B.S.; Negm, W.A. Green Coffee Bean Extract Normalize Obesity-Induced Alterations of Metabolic Parameters in Rats by Upregulating Adiponectin and GLUT4 Levels and Reducing RBP-4 and HOMA-IR. *Life* **2022**, *12*, 693. [CrossRef] [PubMed]
143. Mosimann, A.L.P.; Wilhelm-Filho, D.; Da Silva, E.L. Aqueous Extract of *Ilex paraguariensis* Attenuates the Progression of Atherosclerosis in Cholesterol-Fed Rabbits. *BioFactors* **2006**, *26*, 59–70. [CrossRef] [PubMed]
144. Pang, J.; Choi, Y.; Park, T. *Ilex paraguariensis* Extract Ameliorates Obesity Induced by High-Fat Diet: Potential Role of AMPK in the Visceral Adipose Tissue. *Arch. Biochem. Biophys.* **2008**, *476*, 178–185. [CrossRef] [PubMed]
145. Lima, N.d.S.; Franco, J.G.; Peixoto-Silva, N.; Maia, L.A.; Kaezer, A.; Felzenszwalb, I.; De Oliveira, E.; De Moura, E.G.; Lisboa, P.C. *Ilex paraguariensis* (*Yerba mate*) Improves Endocrine and Metabolic Disorders in Obese Rats Primed by Early Weaning. *Eur. J. Nutr.* **2014**, *53*, 73–82. [CrossRef] [PubMed]
146. Gugliucci, A.; Bastos, D.H.M.; Schulze, J.; Souza, M.F.F. Caffeic and Chlorogenic Acids in *Ilex paraguariensis* Extracts Are the Main Inhibitors of AGE Generation by Methylglyoxal in Model Proteins. *Fitoterapia* **2009**, *80*, 339–344. [CrossRef] [PubMed]
147. Kim, S.-Y.; Oh, M.-R.; Kim, M.-G.; Chae, H.-J.; Chae, S.-W. Anti-Obesity Effects of *Yerba mate* (*Ilex Paraguariensis*): A Randomized, Double-Blind, Placebo-Controlled Clinical Trial. *BMC Complement. Altern. Med.* **2015**, *15*, 338. [CrossRef] [PubMed]
148. Kim, Y.J.; Kwon, E.-Y.; Kim, J.-W.; Lee, Y.; Ryu, R.; Yun, J.; Kim, M.; Choi, M.-S. Intervention Study on the Efficacy and Safety of *Platycodon grandiflorus* Ethanol Extract in Overweight or Moderately Obese Adults: A Single-Center, Randomized, Double-Blind, Placebo-Controlled Trial. *Nutrients* **2019**, *11*, 2445. [CrossRef]
149. Reguero, M.; De Cedrón, M.G.; Reglero, G.; Quintela, J.C.; De Molina, A.R. Natural Extracts to Augment Energy Expenditure as a Complementary Approach to Tackle Obesity and Associated Metabolic Alterations. *Biomolecules* **2021**, *11*, 412. [CrossRef]

150. Mabrouki, L.; Rjeibi, I.; Taleb, J.; Zourgui, L. Cardiac Ameliorative Effect of *Moringa oleifera* Leaf Extract in High-Fat Diet-Induced Obesity in Rat Model. *Biomed. Res. Int.* **2020**, *2020*, 6583603. [CrossRef]
151. Pimentel, G.D.; Lira, F.S.; Rosa, J.C.; Caris, A.V.; Pinheiro, F.; Ribeiro, E.B.; Nascimento, C.M.O.D.; Oyama, L.M. *Yerba mate* extract (*Ilex paraguariensis*) Attenuates Both Central and Peripheral Inflammatory Effects of Diet-Induced Obesity in Rats. *J. Nutr. Biochem.* **2013**, *24*, 809–818. [CrossRef] [PubMed]
152. Hsieh, Y.-L.; Shibu, M.A.; Lii, C.-K.; Viswanadha, V.P.; Lin, Y.-L.; Lai, C.-H.; Chen, Y.-F.; Lin, K.-H.; Kuo, W.-W.; Huang, C.-Y. *Andrographis paniculata* Extract Attenuates Pathological Cardiac Hypertrophy and Apoptosis in High-Fat Diet Fed Mice. *J. Ethnopharmacol.* **2016**, *192*, 170–177. [CrossRef] [PubMed]
153. Sikora, J.; Markowicz-Piasecka, M.; Broncel, M.; Mikiciuk-Olasik, E. Extract of *Aronia melanocarpa*-Modified Hemostasis: In Vitro Studies. *Eur. J. Nutr.* **2014**, *53*, 1493–1502. [CrossRef]
154. Sikora, J.; Broncel, M.; Markowicz, M.; Chałubiński, M.; Wojdan, K.; Mikiciuk-Olasik, E. Short-Term Supplementation with *Aronia melanocarpa* Extract Improves Platelet Aggregation, Clotting, and Fibrinolysis in Patients with Metabolic Syndrome. *Eur. J. Nutr.* **2012**, *51*, 549–556. [CrossRef] [PubMed]
155. Allison, G.L.; Lowe, G.M.; Rahman, K. Aged Garlic Extract Inhibits Platelet Activation by Increasing Intracellular cAMP and Reducing the Interaction of GPIIb/IIIa Receptor with Fibrinogen. *Life Sci.* **2012**, *91*, 1275–1280. [CrossRef]
156. Li, W.; Luo, Z.; Liu, X.; Fu, L.; Xu, Y.; Wu, L.; Shen, X. Effect of *Ginkgo biloba* Extract on Experimental Cardiac Remodeling. *BMC Complement. Altern. Med.* **2015**, *15*, 277. [CrossRef]
157. Caro-Gómez, E.; Sierra, J.A.; Escobar, J.S.; Álvarez-Quintero, R.; Naranjo, M.; Medina, S.; Velásquez-Mejía, E.P.; Tabares-Guevara, J.H.; Jaramillo, J.C.; León-Varela, Y.M.; et al. Green Coffee Extract Improves Cardiometabolic Parameters and Modulates Gut Microbiota in High-Fat-Diet-Fed ApoE$^{-/-}$ Mice. *Nutrients* **2019**, *11*, 497. [CrossRef] [PubMed]
158. Diez-Echave, P.; Vezza, T.; Rodríguez-Nogales, A.; Ruiz-Malagón, A.J.; Hidalgo-García, L.; Garrido-Mesa, J.; Molina-Tijeras, J.A.; Romero, M.; Robles-Vera, I.; Pimentel-Moral, S.; et al. The Prebiotic Properties of *Hibiscus sabdariffa* Extract Contribute to the Beneficial Effects in Diet-Induced Obesity in Mice. *Food Res. Int.* **2020**, *127*, 108722. [CrossRef] [PubMed]
159. Evseeva, M.N.; Balashova, M.S.; Kulebyakin, K.Y.; Rubtsov, Y.P. Adipocyte Biology from the Perspective of In Vivo Research: Review of Key Transcription Factors. *Int. J. Mol. Sci.* **2022**, *23*, 322. [CrossRef]
160. Sun, C.; Mao, S.; Chen, S.; Zhang, W.; Liu, C. Ppars-Orchestrated Metabolic Homeostasis in the Adipose Tissue. *Int. J. Mol. Sci.* **2021**, *22*, 8974. [CrossRef] [PubMed]
161. Savova, M.S.; Mihaylova, L.V.; Tews, D.; Wabitsch, M.; Georgiev, M.I. Targeting PI3K/AKT Signaling Pathway in Obesity. *Biomed. Pharmacother.* **2023**, *159*, 114244. [CrossRef] [PubMed]
162. Ahmad, B.; Serpell, C.J.; Fong, I.L.; Wong, E.H. Molecular Mechanisms of Adipogenesis: The Anti-Adipogenic Role of AMP-Activated Protein Kinase. *Front. Mol. Biosci.* **2020**, *7*, 76. [CrossRef] [PubMed]
163. Kim, N.-H.; Jegal, J.; Na Kim, Y.; Heo, J.-D.; Rho, J.-R.; Yang, M.H.; Jeong, E.J. Chokeberry Extract and Its Active Polyphenols Suppress Adipogenesis in 3T3-L1 Adipocytes and Modulates Fat Accumulation and Insulin Resistance in Diet-Induced Obese Mice. *Nutrients* **2018**, *10*, 1734. [CrossRef] [PubMed]
164. Oh, J.; Ahn, S.; Zhou, X.; Lim, Y.J.; Hong, S.; Kim, H.-S. Effects of Cinnamon (*Cinnamomum zeylanicum*) Extract on Adipocyte Differentiation in 3T3-L1 Cells and Lipid Accumulation in Mice Fed a High-Fat Diet. *Nutrients* **2023**, *15*, 5110. [CrossRef] [PubMed]
165. Kim, H.-L.; Jeon, Y.-D.; Park, J.; Rim, H.-K.; Jeong, M.-Y.; Lim, H.; Ko, S.-G.; Jang, H.-J.; Lee, B.-C.; Lee, K.-T.; et al. *Corni fructus* Containing Formulation Attenuates Weight Gain in Mice with Diet-Induced Obesity and Regulates Adipogenesis through AMPK. *Evid. Based Complement. Altern. Med.* **2013**, *2013*, 423741. [CrossRef] [PubMed]
166. Kim, J.-K.; So, H.; Youn, M.-J.; Kim, H.-J.; Kim, Y.; Park, C.; Kim, S.-J.; Ha, Y.-A.; Chai, K.-Y.; Kim, S.-M.; et al. *Hibiscus sabdariffa* L. Water Extract Inhibits the Adipocyte Differentiation through the PI3-K and MAPK Pathway. *J. Ethnopharmacol.* **2007**, *114*, 260–267. [CrossRef] [PubMed]
167. Kudo, M.; Gao, M.; Hayashi, M.; Kobayashi, Y.; Yang, J.; Liu, T. *Ilex paraguariensis* A.St.-Hil. Improves Lipid Metabolism in High-Fat Diet-Fed Obese Rats and Suppresses Intracellular Lipid Accumulation in 3T3-L1 Adipocytes via the AMPK-Dependent and Insulin Signaling Pathways. *Food Nutr. Res.* **2024**, *68*, 10307. [CrossRef] [PubMed]
168. Héliès-Toussaint, C.; Fouché, E.; Naud, N.; Blas-Y-Estrada, F.; del Socorro Santos-Diaz, M.; Nègre-Salvayre, A.; Barba de la Rosa, A.P.; Guéraud, F. *Opuntia* Cladode Powders Inhibit Adipogenesis in 3 T3-F442A Adipocytes and a High-Fat-Diet Rat Model by Modifying Metabolic Parameters and Favouring Faecal Fat Excretion. *BMC Complement. Med. Ther.* **2020**, *20*, 33. [CrossRef]
169. Park, Y.S. *Platycodon grandiflorum* Extract Represses Up-regulated Adipocyte Fatty Acid Binding Protein Triggered by a High Fat Feeding in Obese Rats. *World J. Gastroenterol.* **2007**, *13*, 3493–3499. [CrossRef]
170. Ezenwaka, C.E.; Okoye, O.; Esonwune, C.; Onuoha, P.; Dioka, C.; Osuji, C.; Oguejiofor, C.; Meludu, S. High Prevalence of Abdominal Obesity Increases the Risk of the Metabolic Syndrome in Nigerian Type 2 Diabetes Patients: Using the International Diabetes Federation Worldwide Definition. *Metab. Syndr. Relat. Disord.* **2014**, *12*, 277–282. [CrossRef]
171. Lee, S.; Joo, H.; Kim, C.-T.; Kim, I.-H.; Kim, Y. High Hydrostatic Pressure Extract of Garlic Increases the HDL Cholesterol Level via Up-regulation of Apolipoprotein A-I Gene Expression in Rats Fed a High-Fat Diet. *Lipids Health Dis.* **2012**, *11*, 77. [CrossRef]
172. Kannel, W.B. Prevalence and Natural History of Electrocardiographic Left Ventricular Hypertrophy. *Am. J. Med.* **1983**, *75*, 4–11. [CrossRef] [PubMed]

173. Ferreira, M.C.L.; Lima, L.N.; Cota, L.H.T.; Costa, M.B.; Orsi, P.M.E.; Espíndola, R.P.; Albanez, A.V.; Rosa, B.B.; Carvalho, M.G.S.; Garcia, J.A.D. Effect of *Camellia sinensis* Teas on Left Ventricular Hypertrophy and Insulin Resistance in Dyslipidemic Mice. *Braz. J. Med. Biol. Res.* **2020**, *53*, e9303. [CrossRef] [PubMed]
174. Zamani, M.; Kelishadi, M.R.; Ashtary-Larky, D.; Amirani, N.; Goudarzi, K.; Torki, I.A.; Bagheri, R.; Ghanavati, M.; Asbaghi, O. The Effects of Green Tea Supplementation on Cardiovascular Risk Factors: A Systematic Review and Meta-Analysis. *Front. Nutr.* **2023**, *9*, 1084455. [CrossRef]
175. Balzan, S.; Hernandes, A.; Reichert, C.L.; Donaduzzi, C.; Pires, V.A.; Gasparotto, A.; Cardozo, E.L. Lipid-Lowering Effects of Standardized Extracts of *Ilex paraguariensis* in High-Fat-Diet Rats. *Fitoterapia* **2013**, *86*, 115–122. [CrossRef]
176. Gao, H.; Long, Y.; Jiang, X.; Liu, Z.; Wang, D.; Zhao, Y.; Li, D.; Sun, B.-L. Beneficial Effects of *Yerba mate* Tea (*Ilex paraguariensis*) on Hyperlipidemia in High-Fat-Fed Hamsters. *Exp. Gerontol.* **2013**, *48*, 572–578. [CrossRef]
177. Boaventura, B.C.B.; Di Pietro, P.F.; Stefanuto, A.; Klein, G.A.; De Morais, E.C.; De Andrade, F.; Wazlawik, E.; da Silva, E.L. Association of Mate Tea (*Ilex paraguariensis*) Intake and Dietary Intervention and Effects on Oxidative Stress Biomarkers of Dyslipidemic Subjects. *Nutrition* **2012**, *28*, 657–664. [CrossRef] [PubMed]
178. Masson, W.; Barbagelata, L.; Lobo, M.; Nogueira, J.P.; Corral, P.; Lavalle-Cobo, A. Effect of *Yerba mate* (*Ilex paraguariensis*) on Lipid Levels: A Systematic Review and Meta-Analysis. *Plant Foods Hum. Nutr.* **2022**, *77*, 353–366. [CrossRef]
179. Chandrasekaran, P.; Weiskirchen, R. The Role of Obesity in Type 2 Diabetes Mellitus—An Overview. *Int. J. Mol. Sci.* **2024**, *25*, 1882. [CrossRef]
180. Sudhakara, G.; Mallaiah, P.; Sreenivasulu, N.; Sasi Bhusana, B.; Rajendran, R.; Saralakumari, D. Beneficial Effects of Hydro-Alcoholic Extract of *Caralluma fimbriata* against High-Fat Diet-Induced Insulin Resistance and Oxidative Stress in Wistar Male Rats. *J. Physiol. Biochem.* **2014**, *70*, 311–320. [CrossRef]
181. Drissi, F.; Lahfa, F.; Gonzalez, T.; Peiretti, F.; Tanti, J.-F.; Haddad, M.; Fabre, N.; Govers, R. A *Citrullus colocynthis* Fruit Extract Acutely Enhances Insulin-Induced GLUT4 Translocation and Glucose Uptake in Adipocytes by Increasing PKB Phosphorylation. *J. Ethnopharmacol.* **2021**, *270*, 113772. [CrossRef] [PubMed]
182. Kim, H.-J.; Kim, B.-H.; Kim, Y.-C. Antioxidative Action of *Corni fructus* Aqueous Extract on Kidneys of Diabetic Mice. *Toxicol. Res.* **2011**, *27*, 37–41. [CrossRef] [PubMed]
183. Khalili-Moghadam, S.; Hedayati, M.; Golzarand, M.; Mirmiran, P. Effects of Green Coffee Aqueous Extract Supplementation on Glycemic Indices, Lipid Profile, CRP, and Malondialdehyde in Patients with Type 2 Diabetes: A Randomized, Double-Blind, Placebo-Controlled Trial. *Front. Nutr.* **2023**, *10*, 1241844. [CrossRef] [PubMed]
184. Peng, C.-H.; Chyau, C.-C.; Chan, K.-C.; Chan, T.-H.; Wang, C.-J.; Huang, C.-N. *Hibiscus sabdariffa* Polyphenolic Extract Inhibits Hyperglycemia, Hyperlipidemia, and Glycation-Oxidative Stress while Improving Insulin Resistance. *J. Agric. Food Chem.* **2011**, *59*, 9901–9909. [CrossRef] [PubMed]
185. Leem, K.-H.; Kim, M.-G.; Hahm, Y.-T.; Kim, H.K. Hypoglycemic Effect of *Opuntia ficus-indica* var. *saboten is due to Enhanced Peripheral Glucose Uptake through Activation of AMPK/p38 MAPK Pathway. Nutrients* **2016**, *8*, 800. [CrossRef]
186. Hall, J.E.; do Carmo, J.M.; da Silva, A.A.; Wang, Z.; Hall, M.E. Obesity-Induced Hypertension: Interaction of neurohumoral and renal mechanisms. *Circ. Res.* **2015**, *116*, 991–1006. [CrossRef] [PubMed]
187. Shariq, O.A.; McKenzie, T.J. Obesity-Related Hypertension: A Review of Pathophysiology, Management, and the Role of Metabolic Surgery. *Gland. Surg.* **2020**, *9*, 80–93. [CrossRef]
188. Valls, R.M.; Companys, J.; Calderón-Pérez, L.; Salamanca, P.; Pla-Pagà, L.; Sandoval-Ramírez, B.A.; Bueno, A.; Puzo, J.; Crescenti, A.; Del Bas, J.M.; et al. Effects of an Optimized Aged Garlic Extract on Cardiovascular Disease Risk Factors in Moderate Hypercholesterolemic Subjects: A Randomized, Crossover, Double-Blind, Sustainedand Controlled Study. *Nutrients* **2022**, *14*, 405. [CrossRef] [PubMed]
189. Zhang, C.Y.; Tan, B.K. Hypotensive Activity of Aqueous Extract of *Andrographis paniculata* in Rats. *Clin. Exp. Pharmacol. Physiol.* **1996**, *23*, 675–678. [CrossRef]
190. Hawkins, J.; Hires, C.; Baker, C.; Keenan, L.; Bush, M. Daily Supplementation with *Aronia melanocarpa* (Chokeberry) Reduces Blood Pressure and Cholesterol: A Meta Analysis of Controlled Clinical Trials. *J. Diet. Suppl.* **2021**, *18*, 517–530. [CrossRef]
191. Antonello, M.; Montemurro, D.; Bolognesi, M.; Dipascoli, M.; Piva, A.; Grego, F.; Sticchi, D.; Giuliani, L.; Garbisa, S.; Rossi, G.P. Prevention of Hypertension, Cardiovascular Damage and Endothelial Dysfunction with Green Tea Extracts. *Am. J. Hypertens.* **2007**, *20*, 1321–1328. [CrossRef] [PubMed]
192. Onakpoya, I.; Spencer, E.; Heneghan, C.; Thompson, M. The Effect of Green Tea on Blood Pressure and Lipid Profile: A Systematic Review and Meta-Analysis of Randomized Clinical Trials. *Nutr. Metab. Cardiovasc. Dis.* **2014**, *24*, 823–836. [CrossRef] [PubMed]
193. Nogueira, L.d.P.; Neto, J.F.N.; Klein, M.R.S.T.; Sanjuliani, A.F. Short-Term Effects of Green Tea on Blood Pressure, Endothelial Function, and Metabolic Profile in Obese Prehypertensive Women: A Crossover Randomized Clinical Trial. *J. Am. Coll. Nutr.* **2017**, *36*, 108–115. [CrossRef] [PubMed]
194. Liang, H.; Yuan, X.; Sun, C.; Sun, Y.; Yang, M.; Feng, S.; Yao, J.; Liu, Z.; Zhang, G.; Li, F. Preparation of a New Component Group of *Ginkgo biloba* Leaves and Investigation of the Antihypertensive Effects in Spontaneously Hypertensive Rats. *Biomed. Pharmacother.* **2022**, *149*, 112805. [CrossRef] [PubMed]
195. Inuwa, I.; Ali, B.H.; Al-Lawati, I.; Beegam, S.; Ziada, A.; Blunden, G. Long-Term Ingestion of *Hibiscus sabdariffa* Calyx Extract Enhances Myocardial Capillarization in the Spontaneously Hypertensive Rat. *Exp. Biol. Med.* **2012**, *237*, 563–569. [CrossRef] [PubMed]

196. Nwachukwu, D.C.; Aneke, E.I.; Obika, L.F.; Nwachukwu, N.Z. Effects of Aqueous Extract of *Hibiscus sabdariffa* on the Renin-angiotensin-Aldosterone System of Nigerians with Mild to Moderate Essential Hypertension: A Comparative Study with Lisinopril. *Indian J. Pharmacol.* **2015**, *47*, 540–545. [CrossRef]
197. Abubakar, S.M.; Ukeyima, M.T.; Spencer, J.P.E.; Lovegrove, J.A. Acute Effects of *Hibiscus sabdariffa* Calyces on Postprandial Blood Pressure, Vascular Function, Blood Lipids, Biomarkers of Insulin Resistance and Inflammation in Humans. *Nutrients* **2019**, *11*, 341. [CrossRef] [PubMed]
198. Ignat, M.V.; Coldea, T.E.; Salanță, L.C.; Mudura, E. Plants of the Spontaneous Flora with Beneficial Action in the Management of Diabetes, Hepatic Disorders, and Cardiovascular Disease. *Plants* **2021**, *10*, 216. [CrossRef]
199. Di Cesare, M.; McGhie, D.V.; Perel, P.; Mwangi, J.; Taylor, S.; Pervan, B.; Kabudula, C.; Narula, J.; Bixby, H.; Pineiro, D.; et al. The Heart of the World. *Glob. Heart* **2024**, *19*, 11. [CrossRef]

pharmaceuticals

Review

White-to-Beige and Back: Adipocyte Conversion and Transcriptional Reprogramming

Stanislav Boychenko [1], Vera S. Egorova [2,*], Andrew Brovin [1] and Alexander D. Egorov [1,*]

[1] Gene Therapy Department, Center for Translational Medicine, Sirius University of Science and Technology, 354340 Sirius, Russia; bojchenko.ss@talantiuspeh.ru (S.B.); brovin.an@talantiuspeh.ru (A.B.)

[2] Biotechnology Department, Center for Translational Medicine, Sirius University of Science and Technology, 354340 Sirius, Russia

* Correspondence: egorova.vs@talantiuspeh.ru (V.S.E.); egorov.ad@talantiuspeh.ru (A.D.E.); Tel.: +7-985-4567-133 (A.D.E.)

Abstract: Obesity has become a pandemic, as currently more than half a billion people worldwide are obese. The etiology of obesity is multifactorial, and combines a contribution of hereditary and behavioral factors, such as nutritional inadequacy, along with the influences of environment and reduced physical activity. Two types of adipose tissue widely known are white and brown. While white adipose tissue functions predominantly as a key energy storage, brown adipose tissue has a greater mass of mitochondria and expresses the uncoupling protein 1 (*UCP1*) gene, which allows thermogenesis and rapid catabolism. Even though white and brown adipocytes are of different origin, activation of the brown adipocyte differentiation program in white adipose tissue cells forces them to transdifferentiate into "beige" adipocytes, characterized by thermogenesis and intensive lipolysis. Nowadays, researchers in the field of small molecule medicinal chemistry and gene therapy are making efforts to develop new drugs that effectively overcome insulin resistance and counteract obesity. Here, we discuss various aspects of white-to-beige conversion, adipose tissue catabolic re-activation, and non-shivering thermogenesis.

Keywords: adipose tissue; adipogenesis; anti-obesity; adipose browning; thermogenesis; transcription factors; PPAR gamma; phytochemicals; aryl hydrocarbon receptor; endocrine disruptors

1. Introduction

Obesity is excessive fat deposition, the primary cause of which is metabolic imbalance. According to the World Health Organization reports [1] and latest studies, the number of individuals with obesity has doubled during the last 30 years; therefore, obesity is becoming prevalent across continents and diverse ethnic groups [2]. Currently, one in eight people is obese. Obesity is a major risk factor for type 2 diabetes, which remains among the leading causes of death and disability [3,4]. During the COVID-19 pandemic, the problem of the "double burden of disease" has come to the fore: severe acute respiratory infection emerged as a leading cause of death among patients with obesity and type 2 diabetes [5,6].

From its establishment at the embryonic stage, adipose develops throughout the entire lifetime of an individual [7]. Abnormal expansion of adipose tissue relative mass results in pathologies such as obesity and cardiovascular diseases. The etiology of obesity is multifactorial and combines hereditary factors and the influence of social factors, such as malnutrition, along with reduced physical activity [8].

Adipose tissues represent a specific kind of connective tissue, considered to be a main depot for lipid accumulation, and also play a major role in the regulation of systemic metabolism [9]. Indeed, adipose sequesters the content of low-density lipoproteins, accumulates triglycerides in its lipid droplets, absorbs glucose from the bloodstream, and is able to transform it into lipids [10]. In addition to its primary function of major energy storage, adipose tissue serves as an endocrine organ; it secretes various molecules that affect systemic responses and metabolism [11].

Earlier, two canonical types of adipose tissue were described: white and brown adipose [12,13]. Unlike cells of white adipose tissue, brown adipocytes have a greater mass of mitochondria and express gene coding for uncoupling protein, which allows thermogenesis and rapid catabolism [14]. Even though white and brown adipocytes are of different origins, activation of the brown adipocyte differentiation program (e.g., as a consequence of constant sympathetic stimulation) in white adipose tissue leads to the appearance of clusters of "beige" adipocytes [15].

During chronic cold exposure, cells of white adipose tissue undergo "beigeing" and convert into beige adipocytes, characterized by thermogenesis and intensive lipolysis. Vice versa, during a prolonged positive energy balance, beige adipose can lose its thermogenic capability and undergo transdifferentiation into white adipose tissue [16,17].

A considerable time has elapsed since it was proposed that beige adipose tissue has therapeutic relevance [18]. Acknowledging the potential of molecular-based therapies in the treatment of obesity and associated diseases, we summarize the current knowledge about white-to-beige adipose conversion, discuss major transcription factors involved in the process, and focus on small molecules that participate in transdifferentiation, along with other possibilities to stimulate this conversion.

2. Types of Adipose

Adipose, comprising 20 to 25% of the total body weight in healthy individuals, reaches a considerable proportion of the body mass. Adipose tissue is composed of numerous cell types, including mature adipocytes, progenitor cells, stromal cells, and endothelial cells. In addition, adipose tissue contains a wide variety of immune cells that play a pivotal role in the homeostasis and normal functioning of adipose tissue [19]. Despite the multiplicity of cell types, the main cellular component of adipose is adipocytes.

In the early years of study, human adipose tissue was categorized into two functionally diverse types: white and brown adipose [20]. White adipose tissue is the most abundant type of adipose in adults, and the occurrence of obesity is associated with white adipose expansion [21]. White adipose tissue (WAT) resides in specific depots in the body, subcutaneous and visceral, classified based on their localization [22]. By contrast, brown adipose tissue (BAT) is predominantly present in infants and has a lesser amount in adults, concentrating mostly in the armpits, and the interscapular and supraclavicular regions [23]. Human brown adipose tissue ensures the survival of neonates during the first weeks after birth. In contrast to WAT, brown adipose tissue has a characteristic dark coloration due to the higher concentration of mitochondria. Mature brown adipocytes are characterized by thermogenin expression (uncoupling protein 1, UCP1). UCP1 is capable of transporting protons to the matrix without ATP synthesis, which leads to the release of energy in the form of heat. Since, together with the proton, UCP1 transfers free fatty acids used for oxidation in mitochondria, an increase in the concentration of free fatty acids leads to a higher conductance of protons [24]. Thus, BAT has an increased rate of catabolism, which results in non-shivering thermogenesis, and the body accesses the energy contained in deposited lipids.

Despite having many similarities in appearance and secretory activity, white and brown adipose tissues differ radically on the cellular level. In particular, brown adipocytes, having multiple lipid droplets (multilocular), are morphologically distinctive from unilocular mature white adipocytes [25]. Moreover, it is widely accepted that brown and white adipocytes originate from cells of different lineages [26]. While white adipocytes arise from multipotent progenitor cells expressing the surface marker platelet-derived growth factor receptor α (PDGFRα) [27], brown adipocytes originate from progenitors that characteristically express myogenic factor 5 (*Myf5*+), also specific to skeletal muscle cells [26]. However, there is evidence that PDGFRα+ cells participate in the development of both WAT and BAT [28], as well as that Myf5+ precursors can give rise to a broader group of cells than it was thought [29], yet the majority of brown and white adipocytes surely have distinct origins.

Brown adipose tissue was thought to be absent in adults [30], but with the efforts of nuclear medicine, thermogenic adipocytes have been found to be active in some adults [31–34]. According to the latest research, adult BAT is normally activated by cold, has a high prevalence without sexual dimorphism, and is negatively related to body fat percentage; however, it declines with age and BMI [35]. Returning to its protective role, adults with metabolically healthy overweight or obesity present higher BAT volumes and are more thermogenic compared with unhealthy obese individuals [36]. Therewith, brown adipose contributes to the enhanced consumption of glucose [37]. Together with epidemiological studies showing that the presence of brown adipose tissue correlates with lower levels of type 2 diabetes, dyslipidemia, coronary heart disease, and hypertension [38], these findings allow us to embrace the hope of a prospective drug being invented.

For all that, white and brown are not the only types of adipocytes. As was mentioned above, clusters of another kind of adipocyte tend to appear in white adipose tissue. Cold acclimation increases non-shivering thermogenesis in brown adipose and induces the appearance of brown-like loci in white adipose tissue [39,40]. Thermogenic cells isolated from the murine white fat depots occur as something in between, neither white nor brown, but "beige" cells, also called brite (brown-in-white) [41]. Similarly to white adipocytes, beige cells exhibit low basal expression of *UCP1*, but upon stimulation by cold or other stimuli, they respond by increasing the respiratory rate and *UCP1* expression [42]. Beige adipocytes originate predominantly from the Myf5-negative lineage, in contrast to brown adipocytes [43]. It was also revealed that some beige adipocytes have myosin heavy chain 11 (Myh11), which is a marker of smooth muscle cells [44]. The emergence of cold-induced thermogenic adipocytes is determined predominantly by white-to-beige adipocyte transdifferentiation. Thus, the origin of beige adipocytes is close to white, but their fate is pre-determined by the molecular factors that are able to induce this white-to-beige conversion.

There is a complex interplay in adipose tissue between adipocytes, their progenitors, and, last but not least, resident immune cells [45]. Adipocytes secrete multiple factors mediating interactions important for immune cells residing in adipose, stimulating their proliferation and possible interchange [46]. There is clear evidence that immune cells, such as adipose tissue macrophages and lymphoid cells, can influence metabolic homeostasis through adipose tissue. For instance, adipose tissue macrophages originate from yolk sac progenitors, self-renew, and become permanently resident for the rest of life [47]. Macrophages are pivotal in obesity-associated inflammation and metabolic diseases. Adipose tissue macrophages secrete small extracellular vesicles able to improve glucose tolerance and increase insulin sensitivity in adipocytes, myotubes, and primary mouse and human hepatocytes [48].

Moreover, it was revealed that another group of cells arising during fetal development from the yolk sac, innate lymphoid cells (ILC2s) [49], could promote the beigeing process in WAT [50]. It is likely that decreased ILC2 responses in human WAT is a conserved characteristic of obesity. Interleukin IL-33, critical for the maintenance of ILC2s in WAT, was associated with the recruitment of uncoupling protein 1 (UCP1)+ beige adipocytes in WAT. IL-33-induced beigeing was connected to the production by ILC2s of methionine-enkephalin peptides, which act directly to upregulate Ucp1 gene expression in adipocytes and promote beigeing in vivo [50].

Other circulating factors, such as myokines FGF21 [51], BMP7 [52,53], and exercise-induced irisin [54], are known to trigger the beigeing of WAT as well. The fact is that these molecules are also normally produced by adipose tissue and act in an autocrine manner [55–57]. There is also experimental proof that ILC2s residing in WAT produce BMP7 and are able to induce the white-to-beige transdifferentiation of adipose [58].

The present section highlights aspects related to the cellular mechanisms substantial for the normal functioning of adipose tissue, in this way determining molecular factors that can trigger white-to-beige transdifferentiation of adipose.

3. Transcriptional Events behind Adipogenesis

Adipocyte differentiation, also known as adipogenesis, is the process by which fibroblast-like precursor cells (preadipocytes) transform into mature differentiated adipocytes under the influence of adipogenic stimuli such as insulin and glucocorticoid agonists. This process may be significantly affected by an individual's genetic background and by specific small molecules, such as pharmaceuticals, phytochemicals, and pollutants.

Excessive fat accumulation is connected with both hypertrophy (an increase in adipocyte size) and hyperplasia (an increase in adipocyte numbers) and develops as a result of positive energy balance and the rate of adipocyte differentiation. The state of equilibrium between differentiated adipocytes and stromal precursor cells in adipose tissue is regulated by the zinc finger cell fate regulator Zfp521 [59]. Zinc finger protein Zfp423 influences both the early determination of preadipocytes and the terminal differentiation of adipocytes [60–62]. During differentiation of preadipocytes, Zfp423 controls the expression of key adipogenic regulators peroxisome proliferator-activated receptor γ (PPARγ) and CCAAT-enhancer-binding protein α (C/EBPα) [62,63]. However, in mature white adipocytes, Zfp423 maintains an energy-storing phenotype by suppressing the thermogenic gene program [64].

In response to adipogenic stimuli, transcription factors that regulate the expression of numerous genes involved in adipocyte differentiation are activated. The transcriptional cascade that controls differentiation has been studied extensively [12,65]. Transcription factors determine cell fate by regulating the expression of multiple genes, including genes coding for other transcription factors that determine subsequent specialization.

It was shown that the process of adipogenesis is tightly regulated by the coordinated actions of transcription factors and epigenetic regulators that determine cell fate. The peroxisome proliferator-activated receptor γ and CCAAT-enhancer-binding protein α are the main adipogenic transcription factors [66].

In recent years, numerous transcriptional and epigenetic regulators of adipogenesis have been identified in multiple studies [67]. Based on the composition of transcription complexes involved in the process and the genes they control, the adipogenic cascade is divided into two main sequential "waves" that drive the adipogenic program [68]. The "first wave" is triggered by adipogenic stimuli and includes factors such as C/EBPβ and C/EBPδ, Krüppel-like factors (KLFs), and CREB (cAMP-responsive element-binding protein). The transcription factors of the "first wave" induce the expression of the "second wave" factors, *C/EBPα* and *PPARγ*, which in turn cooperatively bind the regulatory sequences and control the expression of adipocyte-specific genes [69].

CCAAT/enhancer-binding protein β (C/EBPβ) plays an important role in the initiation and regulation of adipogenesis, acting as an early transcription factor that triggers the cascade of gene expression that is necessary for adipocyte differentiation. C/EBPβ activation is regulated by several signaling pathways, including the mitogen-activated protein kinase (MAPK) and the glycogen synthase kinase 3β (GSK3β) pathways [70]. Glucocorticoids are another important regulator of C/EBPβ. They enhance the acetylation of C/EBPβ, which increases its transcriptional activity. This effect is mediated through the interaction of C/EBPβ with acetyltransferases like p300/CBP-associated factor (PCAF) [71]. Upon activation, C/EBPβ upregulates the expression of genes of the "second wave" like a peroxisome proliferator-activated receptor gamma (PPARγ), C/EBPα, and others [72].

Another member of the C/EBP family of transcription factors, C/EBPδ, plays a significant role in adipocyte differentiation. Together with *C/EBPβ*, induction of *C/EBPδ* expression occurs at the early stages of adipocyte differentiation. Moreover, C/EBPβ and C/EBPδ have a synergistic role in adipocyte differentiation both in vitro and in vivo. Primary embryonic fibroblasts from both C/EBPβ (−/−) and C/EBPδ (−/−) mice were not able to differentiate into mature adipocytes and lacked the capacity to express *PPARγ* and *C/EBPα* [73].

Our previous study revealed another transcription factor that negatively controls the adipogenic differentiation. The knockdown of Prep1 gene expression was shown to affect the conversion of murine preadipocytes from the 3T3-L1 cell line into adipocytes [74]. Decreased expression of Prep1 resulted in enhanced adipogenic differentiation and a significant increase in the insulin-sensitive glucose carrier Glut4 gene expression [75]. Prep1 downregulation resulted in a significant improvement in the ex vivo adipogenic differentiation of both adipose-derived mesenchymal stromal cells (MSCs) [76] and bone marrow-derived MSCs [77]. Presumably, the absence of Prep1 increased the binding of C/EBPβ to chromatin, as it did not affect the C/EBPβ level nor phosphorylation in 3T3-L1 cells [77]. Single cell transcriptomics revealed the increase in cells with the Brown Fat Cell Differentiation pattern of gene expression in hypomorphic $Prep1^{i/i}$ mice suggesting that a lower dosage of Prep1 results in adipose "browning" in vivo [78].

The "first wave" of the adipogenic cascade also includes Krüppel-like factors that are involved not only in adipogenesis but also in the processes of cellular growth and apoptosis. KLFs are characterized by their ability to bind to CACCC-box and GC-rich regions of DNA, through which they regulate the transcription of target genes. Several KLFs are known for their ability to promote adipogenesis. For example, KLF4 is induced by cAMP and promotes adipogenesis by controlling *C/EBPβ* expression [79]. KLF5 facilitates adipogenesis through the activation of main adipogenic transcription factors such as PPARγ and C/EBPα [80]. KLF6 promotes preadipocyte differentiation (Figure 1) by repressing a gene coding for preadipocyte factor named Delta-like 1 (Dlk1, or Pref1), which is a well-known autocrine suppressor of adipogenesis [81]. On the other hand, several KLF factors suppress adipogenesis: KLF2 inhibits the *Pparg* gene expression [82], KLF3 represses the transcription of *C/EBPα* by recruiting C-terminal binding protein (CtBP) corepressors [83], and KLF7 inhibits adipogenesis by decreasing the expression of both *PPARγ* and *C/EBPα* [84]. Importantly, there is a member of the KLF family, KLF11, that acts specifically to promote white-to-beige transdifferentiation by altering the "superenhancers" bound by PPARγ towards the set selective for beige adipocytes [85].

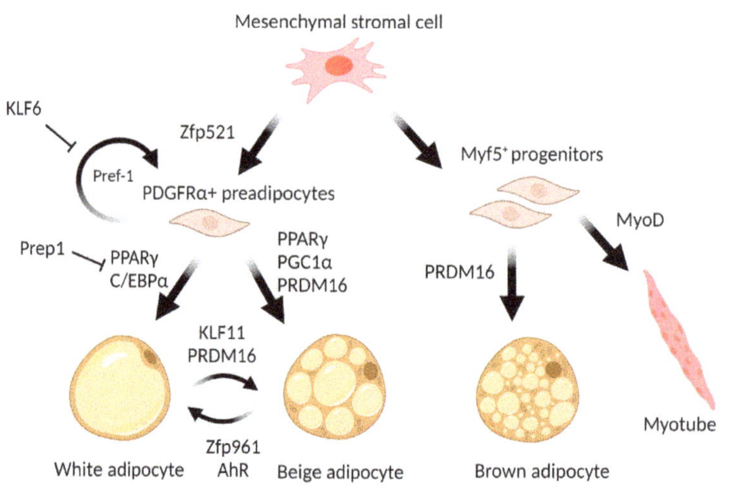

Figure 1. The scheme of adipocyte differentiation.

There were ~12,000 transcription factor hotspots identified in the early phase of adipogenesis, characterized by simultaneous and sequential binding of transcription factors [86]. These hotspots are highly enriched in superenhancer regions (expanding to several kilobases) that drive the adipogenic reprogramming of gene expression. Specifically, it was revealed that the binding of transcription factors to these superenhancers defines the process of white-to-beige transdifferentiation [85]. Apparently, the role of superenhancers in adipose beigeing highlights the importance of the mediator complex. Superenhancers are characterized by the immense binding of Mediator subunit 1 (MED1). Although MED1 is not required for the survival of embryos or for the proliferation of embryonic stem cells, it fulfills essential roles during the terminal differentiation of adipocytes. Ablation of MED1 leads to defects in the development of both brown and white adipocytes and lipodystrophy [87].

Cyclin C (CCNC) is one of the subunits of the Mediator complex, which has demonstrated its importance for adipogenic regulation. CCNC deficiency impaired the proliferation of brown fat progenitors during embryogenesis. But its ablation did not affect either brown adipogenesis or cell death. Moreover, the deficiency of CCNC was shown to reduce the accumulation of lipids in differentiated brown adipocytes age-dependently. CCNC in adipocytes is required for lipogenic gene expression through the activation of the C/EBPα/GLUT4/ChREBP axis [88].

CREB-TF (CREB, cAMP response element-binding protein) is a transcription factor that binds to cAMP response elements, specific DNA sequences found upstream of genes induced after cAMP elevation. Activation of CREB is predominantly mediated by the cAMP signaling pathway. Once activated, CREB promotes adipogenesis by enhancing the transcription of *C/EBPβ* by binding to its promoter [89]. Moreover, CREB activation is both necessary and sufficient to initiate adipogenesis in the 3T3-L1 model cell line of preadipocytes. *CREB* expression is stimulated by several adipogenesis-inducing agents, such as insulin, dexamethasone, and dibutyryl cAMP. In addition to C/EBPβ, CREB directly binds to the promoters of adipocyte-specific genes such as peroxisome proliferator-activated receptor gamma 2 (*PPARγ2*, the shorter isoform of *PPARγ*) and fatty acid-binding protein 4 (*FABP4*) [90]. Depletion of CREB and its closely related ATF-1 (Activating Transcription Factor 1, cyclic AMP-dependent transcription factor) expression in 3T3-L1 preadipocytes leads to their inability to differentiate into mature adipocytes [91].

The "second wave" of differentiation includes major factors such as PPARγ and C/EBPα. It is widely accepted that the main role in the execution of an adipogenic program belongs to the nuclear receptor PPARγ. Its expression is a necessary and sufficient requirement for differentiation towards the mature adipocyte state [92]. Ectopic expression of *PPARγ* is sufficient to induce adipocyte differentiation in fibroblasts, and so far, no transcription factor has been identified that is able to promote adipogenesis in the absence of PPARγ [93,94]. Furthermore, PPARγ not only triggers adipocyte differentiation but also modulates the metabolic functions of mature adipocytes. It plays a crucial role in lipid uptake and storage, and its activity is modulated by various post-translational modifications, which affect its stability and interaction with coactivators and corepressors. Upon activation, PPARγ forms heterodimers with the retinoid X receptor (RXR) and binds to specific DNA sequences known as peroxisome proliferator response elements (PPREs) within the regulatory regions of target genes. It upregulates the expression of key transcription factors such as *C/EBPα* (CCAAT/enhancer-binding protein alpha) and *C/EBPβ*, which initiate the differentiation cascade. In addition, PPARγ directly stimulates the expression of adipocyte-specific genes, including those of adiponectin, leptin, and fatty acid-binding protein 4 (*FABP4*) [95]. These genes are essential for lipid transport and accumulation, regulation of homeostasis, systemic insulin sensitivity, and adipocyte function. More than 60% of the genes upregulated during the process of adipogenesis have binding sites for both *PPARγ* and *C/EBPα* within 50 kb of the transcription start site [96]. It was defined that the total number of PPARγ-binding sites exceeds 52,000, of which 4439 were attributed either to white or beige adipocytes (2228 white-selective and 2211 beige-selective) [85].

Although PPARγ has an effect on the expression of a large number of genes, much attention has been paid to the study of the interaction between PPARγ and the transcriptional regulator PR domain-containing protein 16 (PRDM16). PPARγ directly recruits PRDM16 to form a transcriptionally active complex that triggers a browning program in WAT. PPARγ also recruits other factors such as Histone-lysine N-methyltransferase (EHMT1) and Early B-cell factor (EBF2) that can be present in the PPARγ/PRDM16 complex and enhance its function [97]. Transcriptional complexes formed by PPARγ with PRDM16, EBF2, and EHMT1 determine the beigeing of white adipose tissue, and maintain the unique functions of adaptive thermogenesis and energy homeostasis controlled by the PPARγ/PRDM16/PGC1α complexes in the brown/beige cells.

PRDM16 plays a pivotal role in the determination and differentiation of brown and beige adipocytes. During transdifferentiation of myoblasts into brown adipocytes, PRDM16 serves as a molecular switch, and its PR domain determines alterations in CpG methylation of myogenic factors [98]. PRDM16 enhances transdifferentiation into BAT by interacting with PPARγ and activating its transcriptional function. Loss of *PRDM16* expression in BAT precursors promotes muscle differentiation [26]. *PRDM16* expression in subcutaneous white adipocytes is a determinant of a brown fat-like gene program and thermogenesis in these tissues [99]. The *Prdm16* gene is required in young mice to suppress the expression of white adipocyte-selective genes in BAT through recruitment of the histone methyltransferase Ehmt1 (G9a-like protein), the enzyme that provides repressive modifications of chromatin [100]. Loss of *EHMT* leads to a brown fat deficiency and induces muscle differentiation in vivo through demethylation of histone 3 lysine 9 of the muscle-selective gene promoters [97]. In order to ensure the induction of browning, PRDM16 should form a transcriptional complex with C/EBPβ. This complex enhances the function of C/EBPβ as a transcriptional activator, inducing the expression of other transcription factors and coactivators, such as *PPARγ* and *PGC1α* [101]. As well, PRDM16 physically binds to MED1 (Mediator Complex Subunit 1) and recruits it to PPARγ superenhancers at beige-selective genes [102]. Other proteins can regulate PRDM16 stability. For example, in [103], it was demonstrated that the CUL2–APPBP2 ubiquitin E3 ligase complex catalyzes the polyubiquitination and degradation of PRDM16 protein. Inhibition of this complex extends the PRDM16 protein half-life and stimulates adipocyte browning. On the other hand, CBX4 (Chromobox 4), a polycomb group protein, is a SUMO E3 ligase for Prdm16 [104]. An increased expression level of CBX4 in adipose tissue during cold exposure leads to sumoylation of Prdm16 at the lysine 917 residue and thus blocks its ubiquitination-mediated degradation. Regulating the interaction between PRDM16 and PPARγ is one of the ways for cells to enhance or suppress a WAT browning. Qi-Xiang Ma and colleagues showed [105] that knockout of *Bcat2* (Branched Chain Aminotransferase 2) leads to an increase in inguinal WAT browning and thermogenesis through the suppression of acetylation of PRDM16 at K915. This modification disrupts the interaction between PRDM16 and PPARγ. PexRAP is a peroxisomal lipid synthetic enzyme interacting both with PPARγ and PRDM16 that can disrupt the PRDM16-PPARγ complex [106]. Transcription factor Hlx (H2.0-Like Homeobox) through Prdm16-mediated co-activation drives WAT browning [107]. It was described that Prdm16 interacts with the transcription factor Hlx, which increases the expression of genes specific to thermogenic adipocytes by stabilizing Prdm16 in response to β3-adrenergic signaling. Hlx is involved in the regulation of white adipose tissue beigeing, and may be seen as a possible molecular target.

Peroxisome proliferator-activated receptor gamma coactivator 1-alpha (PGC-1α) is a key regulator of energy metabolism in a cell. PGC-1α is activated by the action of the cAMP signaling pathway (PKA-p38/MAPK) and physically interacts with PPARγ, PPARα, and other nuclear factors. PGC-1α influences genes related to energy metabolism, including mitochondrial biogenesis, oxidative phosphorylation, and gluconeogenesis, and it is expressed mostly in tissues that require an elevated amount of energy. Adipose-specific overexpression of PGC-1α promotes the browning of white adipose tissue and enhances mitochondrial biogenesis and respiration [108].

EBF2 is a member of the early B-cell factor family of transcription factors and is known to play critical roles in B-cell development, neuronal development, and immune cell function. Several studies have highlighted the importance of EBF2 in adipocyte differentiation [109,110]. *EBF2* is highly expressed in brown adipose. It has been demonstrated that EBF2 promotes the expression of genes associated with mitochondrial biogenesis and thermogenesis (*UCP1*). Suzanne Shapira and her colleagues demonstrated that EBF2 functions as a transcriptional activator of the histone acetylation and methylation reader DPF3 (double PHD fingers 3), which recruits the BAF chromatin remodeling complex to brown adipocyte-specific gene promoters [111]. This mechanism leads to the induction of brown adipocyte genes' expression and the acquisition of a brown-like phenotype in white adipocytes. Additionally, EBF2 binds to PPARγ target genes, reprogramming cells to brown adipocytes when expressed in myoblasts [110]. Both EBF1 and EBF2 cooperate with estrogen-related receptor α and PGC-1 α to promote Ucp1 transcription [112].

It is known that members of the forkhead box factors (Fox) family are largely involved in adipose tissue functioning. In particular, the main intracellular target of insulin signaling, FoxO1, inhibits the expression of *UCP1* [113]. In a quite recent study, it was demonstrated that hepatic FoxO1 suppresses systemic Fgf21 secretion, promotes the whitening of brown/beige adipose tissue, and impairs glucose metabolism [114]. Most recently, an in vivo study utilizing post-developmental adipose-specific conditional deletion of FoxO1 in mice showed an increase in lineage plasticity and adipose browning [115]. Another member of the forkhead box family, FoxP1, inhibits brown/beige adipocyte differentiation and thermogenesis by repressing the transcription of the β3-adrenergic receptor (β3-AR) [116].

Conversely, FoxA3 contributes positively to adipocyte differentiation, modulating *PPARγ* expression both in vitro and in vivo [117]. Lately, it has been shown that FoxP4 is expressed in adipose tissue and directly regulates the *UCP1* expression level via binding to the response element upstream of the *UCP1* transcription start site [118]. The binding sites of *FoxP4* were also identified upstream of the promoter region of the *Ppargc1a* gene, which codes for PGC1α [119]. Importantly, the FoxP4 level correlates with the expression level of such BAT marker genes as PRDM16, PGC1α, and Elovl3 [119].

Cell death-inducing DNA fragmentation factor-like effector A (CIDEA) is a member of the CIDE family of proteins, which are characterized by the presence of a conserved CIDE-N domain. In adipocytes, CIDEA is a protein associated with lipid droplets that promotes lipid droplet fusion in brown adipocytes [120]. In beige adipocytes, CIDEA transcriptionally regulates UCP1 by inhibiting LXRα repression of UCP1 enhancer activity and increasing PPARγ binding to the UCP1 enhancer [121].

Understanding the role of miRNAs in transcriptional regulation of adipocyte browning could offer new opportunities for drug development.

Some miRNAs serve as positive regulators of browning. miR-455 promotes brown adipocyte differentiation and thermogenesis by activating AMPKα1 and targeting adipogenic suppressors Necdin and Runx1t1 [122]. Runx1t1 is also the target for another miRNA—miR-193b [123]. Overexpression of miR-30b/c stimulates UCP1 expression through the suppression of transcriptional corepressor receptor-interacting protein 140 (Rip140) [124] and mediating PPARγ activity [125]. Transducer of ErbB-2.1 (Tob1) repression by miR-32 results in increased serum Fibroblast Growth Factor 21 (FGF21) levels that stimulate browning of scWAT in the response to prolonged cold exposure [126]. Inhibition of miR-182 or miR-203 results in a reduction in brown adipocyte marker mRNAs, such as Ucp1, Pgc1a, Cidea, and Ppara [127]. The expression of miR-129 results in an increase in UCP1 expression through the targeting of its inhibitors—Igf2 (insulin-like growth factor 2) and Egr1 (Early growth factor response 1) [128]. MiR-669a-5p mimic significantly enhances the expression of Pgc-1α and Ucp1 in 3T3-L1 cells and promotes adipogenic differentiation of C3H10T1/2 cells [129].

Other miRNAs act as negative regulators of browning. Overexpression of miR-27 in brown preadipocytes suppresses the expression of *Prdm16, Ucp1, Creb, and Pparα* by targeting the 3′ UTR of *Prdm16* and *Pparα* [130]. miR-34a attenuates FGF21 signaling through the downregulation of FGFR1 and SIRT1 that increases PGC-1α acetylation, which results in the suppression of PGC-1α activity [131]. miR-155 suppresses the development of adipogenic and thermogenic programs by targeting Cebpβ [132]. miR-133 downregulates *PRDM16* expression, thereby suppressing the brown fat differentiation and browning [133].

Inhibition of miR-143-3p protected against the development of insulin resistance by targeting insulin-like growth factor 2 receptor (IGF2R) [134]. MiR-93 serves as a negative regulator of adipogenesis by targeting transcription factor T-box 3 (Tbx3) and Sirtuin-7 (Sirt7) [135]. MiR-378 has a dual role as an inhibitor of browning and as positive regulator of BAT [136].

Summarizing the description of transcription factors involved in adipogenesis and WAT browning, it can be concluded that increased activation and expression of genes involved in thermogenesis, the specific transcriptional pattern of brown and beige adipocytes, is an important feature of browning in WAT. This pattern includes PPARα and PPARγ, as well as their coactivators PRDM16 and PGC1-α, CIDEA, and major functional proteins such as type II iodothyronine deiodinase (DIO2) and uncoupling protein 1 (UCP1). Most of the chemicals that affect the process of transdifferentiation act upon the transcription factors involved in the white-to-beige adipose conversion.

4. Small Molecule Compounds and Dietary Molecules

Reprogramming of adipose cells using small molecules that act upon (activate or inhibit) molecular targets involved in BAT biogenesis is a simple, noninvasive intervention technique that is currently being actively studied [137]. This approach enables an opportunity to counteract obesity and related diseases such as type 2 diabetes mellitus, hyperlipidemia, dyslipidemia, cardiovascular disease, etc. With the use of small molecules, not only adipocytes but also fibroblasts [138], endothelial cells [139], and myoblasts [140] can be transformed into beige adipocytes.

Here, we provide a brief retrospective of the small molecules that induce adipose tissue browning via their effect on the respective transcription factors.

4.1. PPARs

PPARγ is able to bind numerous compounds, including its natural ligand (15-deoxy-Δ12,14 prostaglandin J2) and synthetic anti-diabetic thiazolidinediones; this binding promotes heterodimerization of PPARγ with RXR and activation of PPAR-dependent genes. Full agonism of PPARγ ligands has been shown to activate the brown adipose transcriptional program in subcutaneous white adipose tissue [141]. However, due to the specific structure of the ligand-binding site, PPARγ is able to interact both with synthetic ligands, such as rosiglitazone and pioglitazone, and many natural compounds (with lower affinity), including the flavonoids quercetin [142], kaempferol [143], and carotenoid lycopene [144,145]. The effects of the above substances include activation and upregulation of PPAR-dependent genes in various cell types: macrophages, salivary gland cells, prostate tumor cells, and adipose tissue.

Synthetic PPARγ activators, in particular rosiglitazone (Figure 2), increase the expression levels of brown adipocyte-specific genes (*UCP1*, *CIDEA*, *ELOVL3*, and *DIO2*) in white adipocytes via SIRT1-, PRDM16-, C/EBPα-, and PGC1α-mediated mechanisms [85]. In [85], using human white adipocytes (human multipotent adipose-derived stem (hMADS) cells) in vitro, it was demonstrated that once induced, the expression of brown adipocyte marker genes is maintained for a period up to one week independently of continued rosiglitazone administration; hence, the compound administration switches on a stable beige adipocyte gene program. However, browning induced by thiazolidinedione treatment in vivo was not associated with increased energy expenditure or weight loss [146].

Recently, dual PPARα/γ activation was described, which also promotes browning of adipose tissue in vivo and is superior to selective PPARγ activation due to a concomitant PPARα-mediated upregulation of fibroblast growth factor 21 (FGF21), which also plays an important role in adipogenesis. The most active substance of dual PPARα/γ activators, tesaglitazar, increased the *UCP1* expression level in mouse preadipocytes (up to 1700-fold) and adipocytes (up to 80-fold). Two-week long in vivo experiments proved that tesaglitazar treatment resulted in an increase in Ucp1, Pgc1a, and Cidea mRNA levels in WAT and, most importantly, in increased energy expenditure in contrast to rosiglitazone treatment.

Additional benefits of tesaglitazar treatment were increased insulin sensitivity, improved dyslipidemia (2-fold reduction in both plasma triglycerides and total cholesterol levels), and improved hepatic steatosis (liver triglyceride content reduced by more than 80% in the high-dose tesaglitazar group compared to controls) [147].

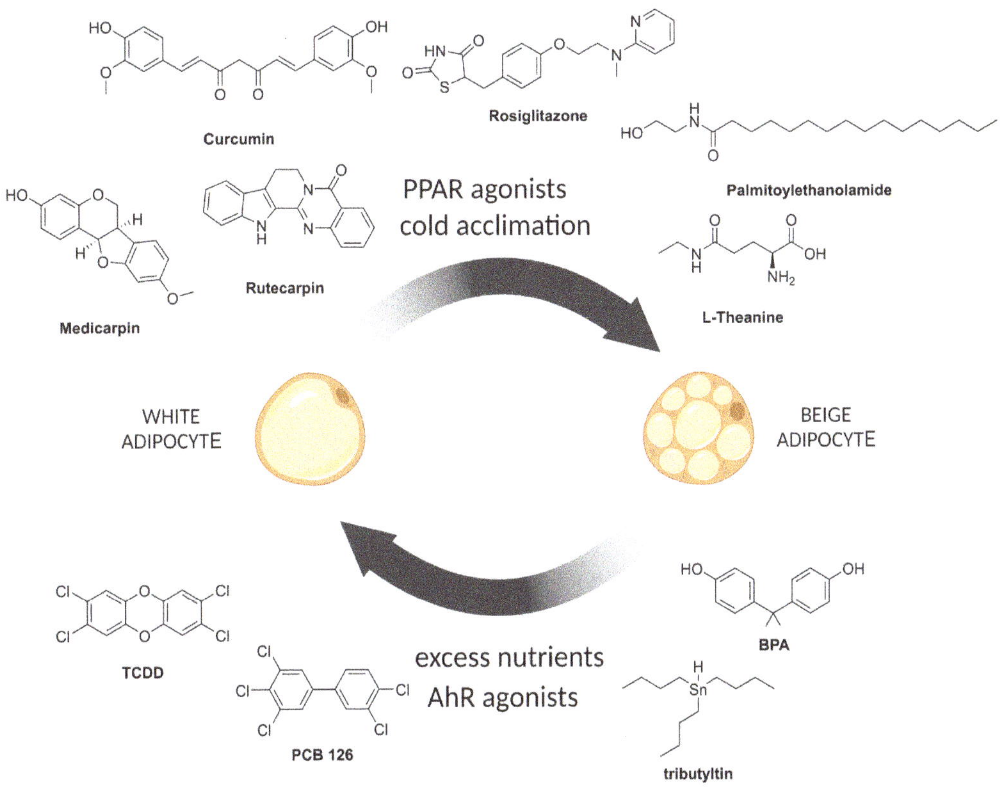

Figure 2. Chemical substances that affect white-to-beige adipocyte conversion.

It is worth noting that PRDM16 knockout significantly inhibited rosiglitazone-induced browning and completely abolished rosiglitazone-induced increases in uncoupled respiration in adipocytes. Rosiglitazone significantly increased PRDM16 protein levels in vivo both in BAT and inguinal WAT from wild type mice, and from PRDM16 transgenic mice in contrast to a non-significant or no effect on PRDM16 mRNA levels. Therefore, rosiglitazone revealed itself to be a potent stabilizer of the PRDM16 protein [141].

Sesaminol, a lignan extracted from the seeds of sesame (*Sesamum indicum*), increased expression levels of *Ucp1*, *Fabp4*, and *Pparγ*, and mitochondrial-specific genes such as Cidea, Pgc1α, Pparα, Cox8b, and Dio2 in mouse primary white adipocytes in vitro. In vivo intraperitoneal administration of sesaminol promoted the formation of multilocular lipid droplets, reduced the size of lipid droplets, and reduced the lipid content by ~43% in the adipose tissue of mice. Sesaminol also increased the expression levels of BAT-specific genes *Cidea* (~4-fold), *Elovl3* (~7-fold), and *Ucp1* (~6.5-fold). The BAT tissue of sesaminol-treated mice demonstrated ~1.5× higher rates of basal respiration compared to the untreated control animals. In high-fat diet (HFD)-fed mice, sesaminol treatment decreased weight gain by ~6% as compared to HFD control mice and enhanced glucose clearance and insulin sensitivity [148].

4.2. PRDM16

L-Theanine is a nonproteinogenic amino acid, a component of green tea (*Camelia sinensis*) extract, able to promote the browning of WAT by enhancing adaptive thermogenesis and increasing the expression of thermogenic genes such as *Prdm16* and *Ucp1*. Treatment of the C3H10T1/2 cell line with L-theanine in vitro induced upregulation of *Prdm16*, *PGC1a*, and *Ucp1* in a dose-dependent manner. This process is mediated through the AMPK/α-Ketoglutarate/PRDM16 axis.

In vivo, L-theanine increased the oxygen consumption rate and, consequently, enhanced mitochondrial function in WAT compared to mice in the control group. L-theanine induced the expression of the brown fat-specific genes in inguinal WAT (iWAT), epidydimal WAT (eWAT), and BAT and increased the protein levels of Prdm16, Ucp1, and PGC1α, according to immunoblotting results. In HFD-fed obese mice, L-theanine induced about a two-fold reduction in iWAT and eWAT tissue weight and, consequently, reduced body weight gain. L-theanine-treated mice also exhibited improved glucose tolerance and insulin sensitivity [149]. It is worth noting that PRDM16 knockout abolished L-theanine-induced BAT-specific gene overexpression in vitro and resulted in impaired cold tolerance both in L-theanine-treated and control mice in vivo [149]. Administration of L-theanine also increases energy expenditure, improves glucose tolerance, and enhances insulin sensitivity in mice [149].

Bexarotene (Bex) is a specific agonist of retinoid X receptors (RXR), which act downstream of PPARγ in adipogenesis. In vitro, Bex induced expression of brown adipocyte-specific genes, including *Pparg*, *Prdm16*, *Ppargc1a*, and *Ucp1*, and promoted brown adipogenic differentiation in C2C12 cells. At the same time, HX531 (an antagonist of RXR) inhibited both basal and Bex-induced brown adipogenic differentiation in C2C12 cells. In vivo, Bex at 50 mg/kg/day was orally administered to mice for 4 weeks along with a high-fat diet. Bex upregulated *Ucp1*, *Ppargc1a*, *Prdm16*, *Ppara*, *Pparg*, and *Ppard* in the adipose tissue of mice. Bex treatment reduced body weight gain in comparison with HFD-fed control mice despite similar food consumption, suggesting that Bex likely increases energy expenditure; moreover, Bex increased heat production and improved glucose sensitivity and insulin resistance, and enhanced cold tolerance [140].

Dietary long-chain omega-3 polyunsaturated fatty acids (PUFAs), in particular eicosapentaenoic acid (EPA), which is the main compound of fish oil, have an anti-inflammatory bioactive effect and potentially induce browning of adipose tissue [150]. It was shown that EPA upregulates browning markers such as *PGC1α* and *PRDM16* in a UCP1-independent manner [151–153]. Administration of EPA to WT and UCP-1 knockout mice resulted in improvements in insulin resistance and inflammation; however, EPA did not affect body weight or adiposity [151].

4.3. SIRT1/AMPK/PGC1α Axis

Curcumin is a natural curcuminoid of turmeric (*Curcuma longa*), which is safe and tolerable even at high doses (12 g/day) in humans [154]. Curcumin displays beneficial health effects, prevents weight gain, and is related to obesity and inflammation in animal models [155]. In vitro, curcumin significantly increased the expression of brown fat markers (PGC-1α, PPARγ, and UCP1) in 3T3-L1 cells and primary white adipocytes in a dose-dependent manner. Curcumin treatment enhanced mitochondrial biogenesis: the density of mitochondria and, moreover, mRNA and protein levels of PGC-1α, a key player in mitochondrial biogenesis, were markedly elevated. Curcumin treatment increased both total AMPK and phosphorylated AMPK levels; therefore, the authors hypothesized that curcumin induces browning via the AMPK-mediated pathway. This hypothesis was proved in an experiment with the treatment of adipocytes with AICAR (an activator of AMPK) and dorsomorphin (an inhibitor of AMPK). Dorsomorphin treatment abolished overexpression of *UCP1*, *PRDM16*, and *PGC-1α*, while the activator AICAR treatment resulted in elevated expression of these brown marker proteins [156]. In vivo, curcumin induced the expression of a number of brown fat-specific genes in iWAT, including *Ucp1*, *Ppargc1a*, *Prdm16*, *Dio2*,

Ppara, and *Cidea*, and increased mitochondrial biogenesis as determined by mtDNA copy number. Curcumin reduced weight gain in C57BL/6 mice but did not affect food intake, i.e., increased energy expenditure. Curcumin-treated mice exhibited increased cold tolerance compared with control mice [154,157].

Medicarpin is a natural pterocarpan found in *Swartzia madagascariensis* and *Medicago truncatula* [158], which demonstrates different biological effects, including stimulation of bone regeneration, inhibition of osteoclastogenesis, and induction of apoptosis [159]. In vitro medicarpin treatment increased brown- and beige-fat marker expression in C3H10T1/2 cells, including *Ucp1* (2.6-fold), *Ppargc1a* (4.5-fold), *Prdm16* (2-fold), *Ppara* (2.3-fold), *Cidea* (1.9-fold), and *Elovl3* (4.8-fold). Medicarpin significantly increased the expression of certain mitochondrial genes (*Cox7a*, *Cox8b*, *Tfam*, and key mitochondrial biogenesis marker *Sirt1* (four-fold)) and increased mitochondrial mass compared to rosiglitazone. Medicarpin treatment induced AMPKα activation in a dose-dependent manner. To confirm the mechanism of medicarpin action via AMPK, a specific AMPK inhibitor, dorsomorphin, was used that abrogated medicarpin-mediated upregulation of *Pparc*, *Prdm16*, *Ppargc1a*, and *Ucp1* [160].

Palmitoylethanolamide (PEA) is a natural endocannabinoid-like lipid mediator, an amide of palmitic acid. PEA has been shown to promote the conversion of white adipose tissue to beige. PEA is able to restore sensitivity to leptin and tissue hormones [161]. The activity of PEA evaluated in 3T3-L1 cells showed increased expression of such genes specific for thermogenic adipocytes as *Ucp1*, *Ppargc1a*, *Prdm16*, and *Cox8b*. Leptin and adiponectin levels increased after PEA treatment, along with decreased secretion of the proinflammatory cytokines IL-6 and TNF-α [161].

Caffeine, often consumed in combination with other related compounds such as catechins, theobromine, and quercetin, promotes the browning of white adipocytes by upregulating the expression of brown adipocyte-specific genes and inducing lipolysis. Treatment of differentiated 3T3-L1 cells with caffeine and catechins results in suppression of lipid accumulation coupled by enhanced expression of genes coding for PPARγ, GLUT4, HSL, UCP1, and TMEM26 [162]. In addition, caffeine was shown to inhibit 3T3-L1 differentiation by disrupting mitotic clonal expansion in 3T3-L1 preadipocytes and inhibiting AKT/GSK3β signaling in differentiating 3T3-L1 preadipocytes [163]. Caffeine was able to promote *Ucp1* gene expression and enhance mitochondrial biogenesis in mouse mesenchymal stem cells [164]. In vivo studies demonstrate that caffeine consumption upregulates the expression of genes coding for UCP1, UCP2, and UCP3 in BAT and UCP2 and UCP3 in skeletal muscle, thereby promoting thermogenesis in obese yellow KK mice [165]. Ingestion of 4.5 mg$\cdot$kg^{-1} of caffeine raises 3 hr postexercise energy expenditure by up to 15% [166]. Theobrownin (TB) is a main active ingredient found in pu-erh tea (*Camelia sinensis*), which stimulates lipid metabolism and, as such, contributes to body weight reduction [167]. It was shown that TB regulates lipolysis in rats and prevents the increase in serum cholesterol levels in rats on a high-fat diet [168].

Theobromine, a methylxanthine derived from cocoa beans, is known for its various health-promoting properties. Theobromine suppresses adipocyte differentiation by causing the degradation of the C/EBPβ protein through the ubiquitin-proteasome pathway. This process is mediated by the interaction with adenosine receptor A1 (AR1) and increased sumoylation of C/EBPβ [169]. Moreover, theobromine inhibits lipid accumulation and the expression of *PPARγ*, *C/EBPα*, *aP2*, and *leptin* in 3T3-L1 cells. Disruption of 3T3-L1 differentiation by theobromine is carried out through the AMPK and ERK/JNK signaling pathways [170]. In vivo administration of theobromine in HFD-fed mice leads to increased expression of key browning markers such as PRDM16 and UCP1, leading to the browning of iWAT and activating BAT [171]. Theobromine upregulates the expression of UCP1 in a PPARγ ligand-dependent manner [172].

Coffee, tea, and cocoa-derived bioactive components possessing anti-obesity effects include chlorogenic acid, trigonelline, kahweol, catechins, epigallocatechin gallate, theaflavins, thearubigins, and quercetin [173].

Quercetin, a bioactive compound present in the extract of onion peel (*Allium cepa*), contributes to adipose tissue browning via the SIRT1/AMPK signaling pathway [174,175]. Treatment of 3T3-L1 cells with quercetin derivatives in concentrations up to 25 μg/mL induced cell browning [176]. Administration of onion peel extract or 0.1% (*w*/*w*) quercetin along with HFD to C57Bl/6J mice induced upregulation of brown fat markers, such as PRDM16, UCP1, Cidea, and PGC-1α in WAT. Quercetin treatment also resulted in a reduction in plasma triglyceride levels; however, it did not affect body composition or energy expenditure in mice [176,177].

Phytol, the most abundant acyclic isoprenoid, used as a precursor for synthetic vitamin E production, was able to decrease the body weight gain in mice through stimulation of inguinal WAT browning [178]. At the same time, phytol administration led to an increase in the expression of genes characteristic for brown adipocyte (*UCP1*, *PRDM16*, *PGC1α*). Thorough in vitro studies demonstrated that a 100 μM phytol solution increased mitochondria content and oxygen consumption in the differentiated 3T3-L1. It also stimulated brown adipogenic differentiation and the formation of brown-like adipocytes by promoting mRNA and/or protein expression of brown adipocyte markers (UCP1, PRDM16, PGC1α, Cidea, and Elovl3) and beige adipocyte markers (CD137 and TMEM26). Meanwhile, inhibition of AMPKα with Compound C abolished phytol-stimulated brown adipogenic differentiation and the formation of brown-like adipocytes, confirming that phytol is acting through the AMPKα signaling pathway in 3T3-L1.

Previously discovered activities of small molecules, in particular micronutrients and phytochemicals, on browning of adipose tissue confirm their contribution to the formation and functioning of beige adipose tissue in adults. It is worth noting that the molecular mechanisms described above explain many but not all observed effects.

5. Disruption of White-to-Beige Transdifferentiation

There is a group of chemical compounds that have been shown to disrupt the normal functioning of endocrine regulation. Their specific ability to distort the regulatory function is linked to their hormone-like structure [179]. Some endocrine-disrupting chemicals are known to derail adipogenesis and inhibit the browning of adipose tissue [180]. Most of the discussed compounds are environmental contaminants and industrial pollutants described as endocrine disruptors for their ability to impair processes of systemic regulation [181]. More than twenty years ago, Jerrold Heindel reasonably hypothesized the influence of endocrine-disrupting chemicals (EDCs) on obesity, as nearly every aspect of metabolism is regulated by the endocrine system [182]. Endocrine disruptors act explicitly or implicitly as obesogens by defecting adipogenesis and fostering lipid accumulation [183].

EDCs interact with nuclear hormone receptors important for the development of white adipocytes. One of the first well-studied endocrine disruptors was the drug diethylstilbestrol, a synthetic estrogen widely prescribed from the 1940s through to the 1970s. It was also the first chemical to confirm the proposed theory of obesogens in vivo, as neonatal exposure caused an increase in body fat [184]. These effects of pharmaceutical estrogens selectively binding the estrogen receptors are mediated through downstream-regulated genes and are predominantly sex-dependent [185]. Activation of ERα led to murine adipose-derived stromal cell differentiation towards the white adipocyte lineage; instead, ERα deficiency determined the cell fate towards smooth muscle or brown adipocytes [186]. The latter is possibly the mechanism underlying the sex-dependent manner of adiposity and, specifically, adipocyte proliferation differences.

Compounds widely used for plastic production, such as bisphenol A (BPA), were shown to alter the adipose tissue metabolism as well [187]. BPA is found in plastic bottles and food containers, as it is used for the production of polycarbonate plastics and epoxy resins [188]. It is one of the main obesogens, which means it can disrupt normal metabolic processes and contribute to obesity.

Studies have shown that exposure to BPA can induce preadipocyte differentiation, therefore promoting adipocyte hypertrophy and leading to increased fat accumulation [189].

Exposure to BPA disrupts normal adipocyte development by inducing differentiation through a non-classical estrogen receptor pathway rather than through glucocorticoid stimulation. This leads to an increase in adipose tissue mass in vivo and hypertrophic adipocytes in males, which results in increased body weight [190]. Moreover, BPA has been linked to the induction of proinflammatory pathways and upregulation of the expression of cytokine genes such as IL1β, IL6, and TNFα. Thus, BPA can exert effects associated with a chronic low-grade inflammatory state of adipose tissue [191].

The reported xenoestrogenic effect of BPA largely impairs development and leads to adverse effects in reproduction [192]. The mechanism of endocrine disruption exerted by BPA in most conditions results in transgenerational effects [193]. Recently, BPA was considered particularly dangerous by the Committee of the Member States of the European Chemicals Agency because of its reproductive toxicity and its endocrine-disrupting properties for human health and the environment. Since then, it has been substituted by other compounds from the bisphenol family, such as BPS, BPF, and BPAF [194].

New BPA-replacement compounds may be even more harmful than the original BPA. For example, most highly prevalent "BPA-free" plastics contain bisphenol S (BPS). It has been reported that the presence of BPAF and BPS is associated with such metabolic disorders as gestational diabetes [195]. The evidence is clear that the xenoestrogenic activity of bisphenols leads to suppression of beige adipocyte formation, which is important for thermogenesis and energy expenditure [196,197]. By inhibiting the formation of beige adipocytes (Figure 2), bisphenols disrupt the important metabolic function of beige adipose, contributing to weight gain and systemic metabolism.

Peroxisome proliferator-activated receptors are hormone receptors, described earlier as molecular targets for synthetic thiazolidinediones. Some EDCs were demonstrated to have effects on PPAR activity. Organotin compounds used in antifouling paints and as stabilizers in plastics can disrupt adipocyte differentiation and function. In particular, organic derivatives of tin (IV), tributyltin (TBT), and triphenyltin (TPT), having a completely different structure from that of 9-cis retinoic acid (9cisRA), the endogenous ligand of the Retinoid X Receptor, mimic its action and induce heterodimerization of PPARγ:RXR complexes [198,199]. Organotins have been shown to induce PPAR activity showing the absence of specific transcriptional marks characteristic for thermogenesis [200,201]—they inhibit the browning of white adipose tissue [202].

Another group of pollutants that pose a threat to adipose tissue health are phthalates. Phthalates are a group of chemicals used in plastics, personal care products, and food packaging. Bis(2-ethylhexyl)phthalate (DEHP) is the plasticizer most widely used to manufacture various soft poly(vinylchloride) plastics, especially tubes for medical equipment, while mono(2-ethylhexyl)-phthalate (MEHP) is its metabolite [203]. Both MEHP and DEHP were shown to disturb adipogenesis in cell culture models by hyper-activating PPARγ [204,205]. Phthalates can activate PPAR:RXR heterodimerization [206]. Moreover, it was demonstrated that the synergy of both MEHP and 9-*cis*-RA and a combination of suboptimal concentrations of MEHP and a natural ligand of PPAR (15d-PGJ2) resulted in activation of the PPARγ:RXR dimer towards PPRE-DNA binding greater than that of either compound alone [207]. Structural studies show that the MEHP molecule binds the activating function-2 (AF-2) sub-pocket and the hydrophobic ligand-binding pocket [208], resembling interactions between PPARγ and endogenous fatty acids binding. Thus, the contribution of phthalates to activation of the nuclear receptor PPARγ is undeniable and often leads to disruption of regulation. Apart from adipose tissue, PPARs are expressed in the central nervous system and in organs of the reproductive system, i.e., the gonads (testis and ovary), uterus, prostate, mammary gland, and pituitary gland [209]. Even so, some researchers still raise the question of whether phthalates have a beneficial or malicious effect on thermogenic adipose tissues [210]. It turns out that there is a need for careful interpretation of ambiguous moments, as it was reported that there was an increase in browning marker gene expression (*Pparg*, *Ppargc1a*, and *Ucp1*) in WAT and higher amounts of BAT [211], but at the same time, increased body weight gain in HFD-fed mice [212].

Therefore, disrupting the normal activity of PPAR phthalates can cause excess adiposity in childhood and later in life [213,214]. Developmental exposure to phthalates has been shown to decrease UCP1 protein expression and BAT activity, inducing significant hypothermia and leading to hyperphagia in male mice [215]. This observation confirms that EDCs such as phthalates inhibit the beigeing of white adipose tissue.

Compounds that counteract the beigeing process include polychlorinated biphenyls and dioxins. Polychlorinated biphenyls (PCBs) are a group of industrial chemicals that were banned in the 1970s but are still present in the environment due to their persistence. Exposure to PCB126 was shown to impair adipogenesis and alter adipocyte metabolism [216]. PCB126-induced disruption resulted in a significant reduction in fully differentiated adipocytes due to PPARγ inhibition. The reduction in PPARγ transcript levels observed was accompanied by the activation of AhR by PCB126. PCBs have a dioxin-like structure and therefore bind to and activate the aryl hydrocarbon receptor (AhR). Moreover, when the cells were exposed to PCB126 during differentiation, the browning of white adipose tissue was inhibited by disrupting mitochondrial uncoupling and energy expenditure [217]. Differentiated adipocytes exposed to PCB126 had a reduced ability for UCP1-related uncoupling.

Dioxins are far beyond other xenobiotics in their toxic effects, specifically those related to metabolic disorders like obesity, diabetes, and metabolic syndrome [218]. This is aggravated by the fact that dioxins accumulate in the adipose tissue of mammals due to their high lipophilicity. 2,3,7,8-Tetrachlorodibenzo-*p*-dioxin (TCDD) is one of the most potent compounds of the dioxin class, and the spectra of its toxicity include metabolic disorders emerging through direct action on adipocytes or the induction of local inflammation of the adipose tissue [219].

Brown adipose tissue was identified as a target tissue for TCDD almost 40 years ago, and the direct effects of dioxins were studied in rats [220]. Thereafter, the experiments with TCDD were limited due to its high toxicity, but a model was established to study the effects of dioxins' release from adipose. The epididymal fat pads of dioxin-exposed mice were collected and grafted on the back skin of untreated recipient animals [221]. Redistribution of TCDD to other tissues led to massive changes in gene expression and was found to be completely dependent on AhR activation.

AhR

The aryl hydrocarbon receptor belongs to the Per-ARNT-Sim (PAS) family of transcription factors, known as sensors of environmental signals [222]. AhR is a transcription factor that was originally identified as a sensor of dioxins [223].

AhR resides in the cytoplasm when not activated in a majority of cell types forming the complex with HSP90 (Heat Shock Protein 90), co-chaperone p23 and its partner, the aryl hydrocarbon receptor-interacting protein (AIP also known as ARA9) [224,225]. The AIP protein, structurally related to the FK506-binding protein class of immunophilins, acts as a chaperone, presumably maintaining properly folded AhR in the cytosol and improving the stability, subcellular localization, recognition of ligand and, subsequently, efficient translocation.

When AhR binds a ligand, it translocates into the nucleus, where, in the form of a heterodimer with AhR nuclear translocator (ARNT) induces the expression of genes involved in various biological responses. Specifically, the AhR:ARNT heterodimer binds enhancers known as dioxin-responsive elements (DREs or XREs) in order to induce the expression of genes encoding xenobiotic-metabolizing enzymes [226]. This pathway represents an adaptive response that allows for the detoxification of a wide variety of compounds with polycyclic aromatic structures by xenobiotic-metabolizing enzymes. Therefore, the number of AhR-induced genes includes *Cyp1a1*, *Cyp1a2*, *Cyp1b1*, and a negative regulator of AhR signaling known as the AhR repressor (AhRR), which competes with ARNT in the process of heterodimerization and represses the activation of AhR-dependent genes [227].

TCDD binds to the AhR, inducing the transcription of xenobiotic-metabolizing enzymes as well. Despite the induction of these enzymes, the TCDD and other persistent organic pollutants are metabolized insufficiently, and their elimination or degradation is slow; therefore, the accumulation in adipose is observed [228].

AhR is expressed in adipocytes [229], and specifically, in the model cell line 3T3-L1. The level of AhR was shown to decrease in 3T3-L1 cells during differentiation, as well as its binding activity towards the response elements and the response to TCDD. AhR has earned increased attention for its possible involvement in the regulation of body weight, adipose tissue expansion, and lipid homeostasis in vivo [230,231]. Although some data showed that activation of AhR led to lipogenesis suppression, mouse embryonic fibroblasts isolated from AhR-deficient mice displayed enhanced synthesis of triacylglycerols [232]. TCDD-induced activation of AhR was able to inhibit adipogenesis by suppressing PPARγ activity and impairing the adipogenesis of 3T3-L1 in vitro. The absence of such an effect in mouse embryonic fibroblasts isolated from AhR−/− mice highlighted the role of AhR in hormone-induced adipogenesis, suggesting its role as an early regulator of adipocyte differentiation.

Recent in vitro experiments demonstrated that AhR overexpression suppressed adipocyte differentiation through reduced PPARγ stability and, on the contrary, siRNA-mediated Ahr gene silencing led to adipocyte differentiation in 3T3-L1 cells [233]. Furthermore, it was found that AhR functions as the substrate receptor in CUL4B-RING E3 ubiquitin ligase targeting PPARγ ubiquitination by binding two lysine sites on residues 268 and 293.

Animal research unexpectedly revealed an increased body weight in mice with adipocyte-specific AhR deficiency compared to wild type mice. The phenotype demonstrated an increased fat mass and adipose tissue inflammation, accompanied by a decreased glucose tolerance when fed a high-fat diet [234]. Instead, the whole-body deficiency of AhR protected mice from high-fat diet-induced obesity through increased energy expenditure [230]. Moreover, AhR deficiency did not alter insulin sensitivity in adipose or muscle tissues. The expression of the major thermogenic gene, uncoupling protein 1 (*Ucp1*), in brown adipose tissue and genes responsible for mitochondrial β-oxidation in muscle were significantly higher in AhR (−/−) and AhR (+/−) mice compared with wild type mice. Another study recently revealed a sex-dependent phenotype of AhR depletion specific for mature adipose tissue (CadKO) cells [235]. CadKO females had a lean phenotype and healthy adipose–hypothalamic crosstalk. Interestingly, HFD-induced leptin rise was reduced in CadKO females, while the leptin receptor was increased in the energy regulatory regions of the hypothalamus, suggesting an increase in leptin sensitivity. The expression level of estrogen receptor α (ERα) was increased in CadKO female adipose tissue and the hypothalamus. CadKO males displayed a delayed progression of obesity and insulin resistance. In males, beneficial effects of adipose-specific AhR depletion were mediated through the maintenance of healthy crosstalk between adipocytes and immune cells: proinflammatory adipocytokines' (such as TNFα, IL1β, IL6) secretion was improved and inflammatory macrophage infiltration into adipose was reduced. Overall, adipose-specific knockout of AhR gene improved weight control and systemic glucose homeostasis in a high-fat-diet-induced condition with more pronounced effects in females.

We suppose that AhR can regulate the browning of adipose through tissue-resident immune cells. This suggestion was confirmed by experimental data showing that AhR plays an important role in regulating ILCs. *AhR* is expressed in ILC2s at the highest levels, and its pharmacological activation could suppress the function of this distinct population of lymphoid cells [236]. Remembering that ILC2s regulate adipose function and metabolic homeostasis through the induction of beigeing [50] it is highly likely that AhR depletion in these cells may prevent obesity.

Several phytochemical and dietary compounds are able to modulate physiological processes by antagonizing AhR signaling [237]. In particular, isoprenoids and phenylpropanoids [238], quercetin, kaempferol [239], curcuminoids, and coumarins [240], were demonstrated to antagonize aryl hydrocarbon receptor. A number of AhR ligands, such as curcumin [241,242], resveratrol [243–245], and quercetin [246], repeatedly demonstrated inhibition of TCDD-induced gene expression. A specific group of monoterpenoids, carvones, the constituents of essential oils of dill, caraway, and spearmint, was reported to be noncompetitive, insurmountable antagonists of AhR [247]. Binding of such natural ligands inhibits the heterodimerization of AhR with ARNT and does not lead to *Cyp1a1* gene induction [247]. In addition, synthetic small molecules were developed that act as powerful AhR antagonists: CH-223191 [248], 6,2,4-trimethoxyflavone [249], and GNF351 [250], including two molecules being tested in clinical trials BAY2416964 [251] and IK-175 [252].

This section is an example that one can be convinced that something "bad", exhibiting direct toxic activity, can be turned into "good"—a tool for studying the molecular mechanisms of the regulation of inflammation in adipose tissue. The critical role of AhR in PPARγ stability represents the potential of AhR as a therapeutic target for metabolic disease treatment. A multitude of AhR natural antagonists have been described, encouraging the development of new small molecule compounds exerting antagonism of AhR. We think that the discussed compounds and molecular mechanisms can possibly give a clearer insight into the nature of the problem.

6. Methods of White-to-Beige Conversion

White-to-beige conversion occurs naturally, but also can be induced artificially in many ways and approaches. As was already noted, the most common methods are based on the application of small molecules that initialize tissue reprogramming. Bexarotene and rosiglitazone are the most used and well-known agonists of PPARγ and its partner retinoid X receptor that regulate the transformation of C2C12 cells to beige fat tissue [140]. Discovering new agonists of this receptor can be a perspective for future research. In addition to RXR agonists, several small molecules such as rosiglitazone, BMP7, and forskolin can be used as a part of a "chemical cocktail" that allows the enforcing of the overexpression of transcriptional factors such as C/EBP-β, C-MYC [253].

In a similar way, the "gene cocktail" PRDM16, BMP7, and PGC1A can be applied for transfection with ultrasound-targeted microbubble destruction methods [254]. In this method, lipid microbubbles are filled with a plasmid mixture burst under ultrasonication of target tissue and gas carries DNA to cells. The potency effect of such gene delivery was measured with RT-PCR by the overexpression of *UCP1* gene after 24 h. The authors note that the level of UCP1 expression with three genes is higher than with PRDM16 alone, but a single gene can also be used for gene therapy applications.

Viral gene delivery is the most common type of gene therapy approach used to convert WAT into beige adipose, to achieve stable ubiquitous or tissue-specific overexpression of target genes and increase energy expenditure. Different types of noninfective recombinant viruses, including adenovirus, retrovirus, lentivirus, and adeno-associated virus (AAV) were used to direct the transgene expression in adipose tissue [255]. However, it was shown, that adenovirus, retrovirus, and lentivirus are immunogenic and do not provide the long-term transgene expression [256–259]. Moreover, gamma-retroviruses and lentiviruses are characterized by an increased risk of carcinogenicity and genomic instability due to their ability to integrate into the host genome [260,261]. In contrast, AAV vectors (Figure 3) are characterized by low immunogenicity, low toxicity, and carcinogenicity risk, are present in the nucleus in the form of episomes, and provide stable and long-term transgene expression [255,262].

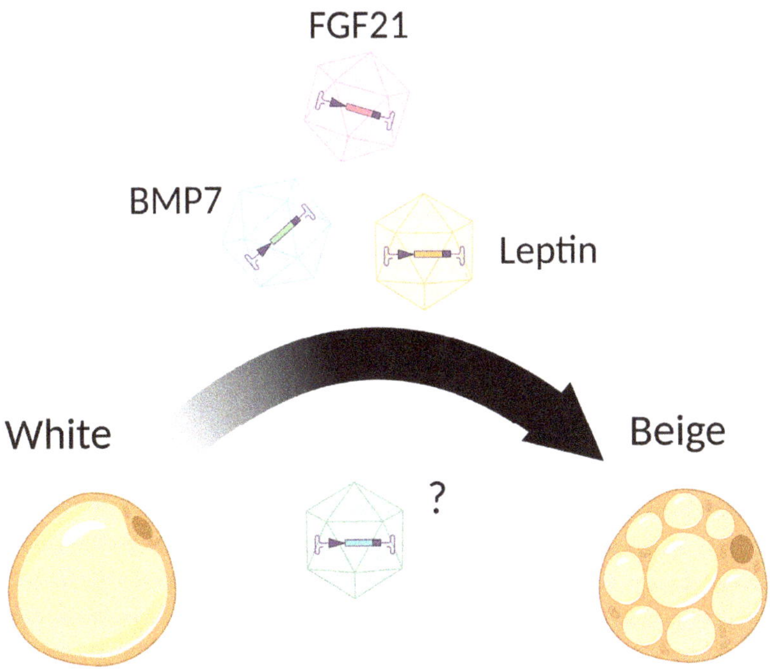

Figure 3. AAV vectors in white-to-beige conversion.

AAV vectors could be injected intravenously [263,264] or locally (for example, into WAT depot [265], intracranial [266]). Systemic delivery requires a higher dose than is used when the virus is injected locally [262,264,267]. Moreover, local injection or tissue-specific expression is associated with fewer adverse events. Targeting WAT provides an opportunity for surgical removal of this organ in case some severe adverse events happen [268]. Tissue-specific expression is achieved by using tissue-specific promoters (i.e., the adipose tissue-specific adiponectin promoter [264], the liver-specific human α1-antitrypsin (hAAT) promoter [262], the liver-specific albumin promoter [267]). However, the disadvantage of tissue-specific promoters is that they are weaker in terms of achieving high transgene expression than ubiquitous (hybrid cytomegalovirus enhancer/chicken-actin (CBA or CAG)) or cytomegalovirus promoters (CMV). Moreover, due to the limited capacity of AAV, mini-versions of the promoters are used (adipocyte protein 2 promoter (mini/aP2) for WAT and uncoupling protein 1 promoter (mini/UCP1) for BAT) [269]. Moreover, to de-target viral vector expression from the liver or heart in order to mitigate the risk of adverse events, target sequences for local miR-122a or miR-1 are introduced into the 3′-UTR of the AAV expression cassette [264,265]. One of the first attempts at adeno-associated virus application for adipose tissue transfection was performed in 2006 by Mizukami [268]. In this work, the delivery of the erythropoietin gene into adipose cells using different AAV serotypes (AAV1–5) was studied. As a result, the AAV1 serotype demonstrated the highest transduction efficiency, which was evaluated according to the erythropoietin expression level in the blood measured using qPCR. The removal of transduced adipose tissue resulted in normalization of the erythropoietin level in the blood; this result supported the efficiency and safety of the approach. A number of experiments with the new generation of recombinant serotypes (AAV5–9) showed the highest transduction efficiency of AAV8, which resulted in the highest level of GFP expression under the control of the adiponectin promoter in brown adipose that was visualized with immunoblotting and fluorescent microscopy [264]. When the most efficient AAV serotype was found, researchers made a successful attempt to deliver the leptin gene to the adipose tissue of ob/ob mice as an approach to correct congenital generalized lipodystrophy, associated with severe metabolic imbalance, the virtual lack of adipose tissue, hepatic steatosis, and related cardiovascular conditions. The AAV vector encoding leptin gene under the control of adiponectin gene promoter was constructed. Moreover, to decrease non-specific transgene expression in liver, the sequence of miR-122 was introduced to the construction. I.v. injection of 1×10^{12} vg of the obtained vector to ob/ob leptin-deficient mice resulted in a decrease in weight gain, and an improvement in hyperinsulinemia and glucose tolerance. Therefore, the authors proved the concept that adipose-specific leptin overexpression can correct gene deficiency and related disease in a mouse model [264].

In another study, intraperitoneal injection of AAV vector, encoding the gene of leptin under the control of a potent CBA promoter (dose: 4×10^{10} vg), resulted in high level of transgene expression in visceral adipose tissue. AAV also contained the second expression cassette encoding miRNA targeting the woodchuck posttranscriptional regulatory element (WPRE) sequence, which was present only in the transgene expression cassette, under the control of the liver-specific albumin promoter. This miRNA enabled the restriction of off-target leptin overexpression in the liver. The injection of AAV, encoding the leptin gene, to ob/ob mice resulted in a sharp decrease in food intake, the normalization of body weight, complete rescue of the impaired glycemic control, and an increase in oxygen consumption and locomotor activity [267].

Another attempt at a gene replacement strategy using AAV8 was utilized in a mouse model with congenital lypodistrophy caused by seipin knockout [263]. This disease is associated with mutations in the BSCL2 gene (from the alternative name of congenital lypodistrophy: Berardinelli-Seip syndrome), which is coding for the protein seipin. A single i.p. injection of 1×10^{12} vg AAV, encoding GFP under the constitutive CMV promoter, resulted in GFP expression in WAT and BAT. The treatment of seipin knockout mice with 1×10^{12} vg AAV8, encoding human BSCL2 gene (AAV8-CMV-hBSCL2), resulted in an increase in body weight gain, the recovery of hyperglycemia, hepatomegaly, and insulin resistance, and the partial restoration of adipose tissue.

Fibroblast growth factor 21 (FGF21) is a peptide hormone contributing to energy homeostasis regulation. FGF21 was shown to be a promising compound for diabetes mellitus therapy [270]. AAV vectors encoding the FGF21 gene under the control of the liver-specific hAAT promoter were constructed [271]. A total of 5×10^{10} vg of the resulting vector or non-coding AAV vector was iv injected into ob/ob and HFD-fed mice. The treatment of HFD-fed mice with 5×10^{10} vg AAV8-hAAT-FGF21 resulted in progressive weight loss (the body weight at the end of the study was similar to the baseline values measured before the initiation of HFD), and improvements in HFD-associated WAT hypertrophy and inflammation, hepatic steatosis, and fibrosis. AAV8-hAAT-FGF21 treatment induced BAT activation, which was demonstrated by a dose-dependent increase in UCP1 level. However, the authors did not observe the appearance of multilocular adipocytes (i.e., browning) in WAT. Treated with 5×10^{11} vg AAV8-hAAT-FGF21, ob/ob mice also demonstrated decreased WAT inflammation, an improvement in hepatic steatosis, and a marked reduction in the total liver triglyceride and cholesterol content.

A few successful attempts at BMP7 overexpression using viral vectors were made [259, 262,265]. Bone morphogenic protein 7 (BMP7) belongs to the superfamily of transforming growth factors β, which contribute to such vital processes as cell proliferation, differentiation, and apoptosis [272]. BMP7 was shown to promote brown adipocyte differentiation from multipotent mesenchymal stem cells [259]. The first attempts of BMP7 overexpression were made using adenovirus (Ad) vectors [259]; Ad vector transduction resulted in an increase in brown adipose tissue mass, increase in energy expenditure, and weight gain reduction. However, due to the high immunogenicity of Ad vectors, long-term transgene overexpression could not be reached.

A number of works on the overexpression of BMP7 were conducted in the scientific group of Prof. Fatima Bosch [262,265]. First, AAV8 vectors encoding BMP7 gene under the control of the ubiquitous CAG promoter and under the control of the liver-specific hAAT promoter were created [265]. To de-target transgene expression from the liver and heart, target sequences for miR-122a and miR-1 were introduced into the 3′-UTR of AAV vector expression cassettes. Injection of the obtained vectors (1×10^{12} vg) into the epidymal WAT of ob/ob mice reduced WAT inflammation, and improved hepatic steatosis and insulin resistance, but did not induce brown adipogenesis, as was shown by the unchanged level of expression of *Ucp1* and *Ppargc1a* in iBAT and iWAT.

In another work [262], an AAV8 vector encoding the BMP7 gene under the control of a synthetic hybrid liver-specific promoter composed of the hepatocyte control region enhancer from the apolipoprotein E gene (ApoE) and the hAAT promoter was constructed. Intravenous injection of 1×10^{12} vg AAV-BMP7 vector into HFD-fed obese mice resulted in the normalization of body weight and liver weight within a few weeks. Upregulation of thermogenic markers *Ucp1*, *Cidea*, and *Ppargc1a* was demonstrated in iWAT of AAV-BMP7-treated animals, which indicated the activation of non-shivering thermogenesis. Moreover, hepatic steatosis and insulin resistance were mitigated in AAV-BMP7-treated mice. The induction of non-shivering thermogenesis and improvement in insulin sensitivity were also demonstrated in ob/ob mice after treatment with AAV-BMP7.

Anderson et al. [266] performed a study on the overexpression of the hypotalamic protein TrkB.FL, related to metabolic homeostasis and autism spectrum disorder (ASD) development, in the hypothalamus of BTBRT+Itpr3tf/J mice (on a normal chow diet and HFD-fed), which serve as the model of ASD. In this study, an AAV2 vector containing CMV enhancer, chicken β-actin (CBA) promoter, and the TrkB.FL gene was injected intracranially (into the hypothalamus) at a dose of 2.5×10^9 vg/side to obtain a high level of constitutive TrkB.FL overexpression. As a result, transgenic mice both on NCD and HFD demonstrated a decreased percent body weight gain compared to normal BTBRT+Itpr3tf/J mice, despite the fact that they consumed significantly more food. AAV2-TrkB.FL-transfected NCD mice also showed improved glucose tolerance.

Despite that fact, the majority of studies were focused on the overexpression of brown adipose tissue activators, and in the last few years, a number of experiments have been performed where gene knockout resulted in an increase in energy expenditure and an improvement in metabolic outcomes. A number of reports were published demonstrating that gene knockout results in the activation of the browning program and an increase in energy expenditure. For example, knockout of NAD^+-dependent deacylase sirtuin 7 (SIRT7) resulted in the upregulation of UCP1, and an increase in body temperature and energy expenditure in mice [273]. Selective knockout of Rbm43 in mouse adipocytes increased PGC1α translation, mitochondrial biogenesis, and adipose thermogenesis [274]. Genetic or pharmacological inactivation of key upstream kinases of the Hippo signaling pathway, STK3 and STK4, increased the expression level of UCP1 in BAT and WAT, increased mitochondrial mass and conferred resistance to metabolic dysfunction induced by HFD, and increased mitochondrial content in adipose tissue and mitochondrial oxidative respiration [275]. Ablation of Sam68 (Src-associated-in-mitosis-of-68 kDa) in adult mice led to body weight reduction [276]. Adipose thermogenesis and energy expenditure were also increased after knockout of the Krüppel-associated box (KRAB) domain-containing zinc finger protein ZFP961, which serves as a potent repressor of the thermogenic program [277].

From the presented data, we anticipate the use of AAVs as one of the safest known vectors for gene therapy [278]. Most of the experimental studies show the effectiveness of AAV usage (Table 1), but regarding the limitations of the study, these findings should be viewed with caution. It is known that even adeno-associated viral vectors have unintended side effects [279]. In order to weaken these adverse events and improve the scientific significance of the experiments, we expect the utilization of different optogenetic switches developed earlier [280]. Currently, we are developing AAVs coding for transcription factors able to stimulate white-to-beige conversion both in vitro and in vivo.

Table 1. Gene therapy and genetic models (KO) targeting adipose tissue.

	Target Gene	AAV Serotype (Genetic Therapy Tool)	Expression Cassette	Dose	Administration Route	Outcome	Reference
Overexpression	Erythropoietin	AAV1–5	CMV-Epo	6×10^{11} vg	s.c.	Efficient delivery of the erythropoietin gene into adipose tissue resulted in an increase in blood Epo level.	[268]
	Leptin	AAV2/8	Adipo-Lep-miR122 (8x)	1×10^{12} vg	i.v.	Successful delivery of the leptin gene to AT of ob/ob mice, decrease in weight gain, an improvement in hyperinsulinemia, and glucose tolerance.	[264]
	Leptin	AAVRec2	Albumin promoter-Lep-miR-WPRE-CBA-leptin-WRPE	4×10^{10} vg	i.p.	Decrease in food intake, normalization of body weight, normalization of glycemic control, increase in oxygen consumption, and locomotor activity in ob/ob mice.	[267]
	BSCL2	AAV8	CMV-hBSCL2	1×10^{12} vg	i.v.	Normalization of hyperglycemia and severe insulin resistance in seipin-deficient mice.	[263]
	FGF21	AAV8	hAAT-FGF21	5×10^{10}–5×10^{11} vg	i.v.	Weight loss, improvement of WAT inflammation, hepatic steatosis, and fibrosis in HFD-fed mice; improvement of WAT inflammation, hepatic steatosis, and reduction in the total liver triglyceride and cholesterol content in ob/ob mice.	[271]
	BMP7	AAV8	CAG-BMP7; hAAT-BMP7	1×10^{12} vg	Intra eWAT injection	Efficient de-targeting of the transgene from liver and heart; improvement of hepatic steatosis and insulin sensitivity in ob/ob mice. BMP7 overexpression in WAT did not induce brown adipogenesis.	[265]
	BMP7	AAV8	Hybrid hAAT-BMP7	1×10^{12} vg	i.v.	Upregulation of brown fat markers, induction of non-shivering thermogenesis, normalization of body weight, improvement of hepatic steatosis and insulin resistance in HFD-fed and ob/ob mice.	[265]
	TrkB.FL	AAV2	CBA-TrkB.FL	2.5×10^{9} vg/ side of hypothalamus	i.c.	Decrease in percent body weight gain and improvement of glucose tolerance in BTBRT+Itpr3tf/J mice in NCD and HFD.	[266]

Table 1. *Cont.*

	Target Gene	AAV Serotype (Genetic Therapy Tool)	Expression Cassette	Dose	Administration Route	Outcome	Reference
Knockout	*SIRT7*					Upregulation of UCP1, increase in body temperature, and energy expenditure.	[273]
	STK3 and *STK4*					Increased *UCP1* expression level in BAT and WAT, increase in mitochondrial mass, and mitochondrial oxidative respiration in adipose tissue.	[275]
	Rbm43					Upregulation of PGC1α, increase in mitochondrial biogenesis and adipose thermogenesis.	[274]
	Sam68					Prevention of high-fat-diet-induced weight gain and insulin resistance.	[276]
	ZFP961					Increase in adipose thermogenesis and energy expenditure.	[277]

7. Conclusions

Obesity, one of the major problems of modern medicine, has a multifactorial pathogenesis. At the moment, a large number of small molecules have been evaluated for their ability to trigger different mechanisms of adipocyte conversion through indirect activation of signaling and transcriptional cascades, including the activation of pivotal regulators of transcription that control important metabolic pathways. In order to identify possible factors influencing white-to-beige conversion occurring in adipose tissue, we examined a variety of cellular and molecular determinants. Additionally, we described the action of phytochemical and dietary molecules affecting the transdifferentiation process in connection with molecular targets, with a specific focus on transcription factors. We spotted that the influence of pollutants and environmental disruptors on adipose tissue, which is relevant in the modern postindustrial milieu, is based on their activity towards transcription factors. Additionally, we noticed that some of the reported natural ligands antagonizing AhR were previously discussed in the "Small Molecule Compounds" section as known white-to-beige inducers. It is possible that the phenomenon of these natural phytochemicals and dietary molecules is based on their ability to suppress the transcriptional activity of AhR:ARNT and, in consequence, stabilize PPARγ. Specifically, we highlighted the possible use of AhR as a therapeutic target for metabolic disease treatment.

Existing state-of-the-art gene therapy offers several opportunities to stimulate the conversion of WAT into beige adipose tissue. As we noticed, most of the anti-obesity gene therapy approaches exploit the possibility of inducing white-to-beige adipose transition by overexpressing the genes coding for secreted factors, such as leptin, FGF21, or BMP7. However, gene therapy drugs based on the induction of single transcription factors may have fundamentally different features. Firstly, the use of AAV coding for transcription factors expands the scope of the drug effects, and since the transcription factors stimulating white-to-beige conversion are well-known, it makes it possible to exert a high-precision impact on cells. Secondly, the use of nucleic acid-based drugs changes the functioning of the cell at the level of mRNA transcripts, which are regulated by intracellular mechanisms, and has fewer off-target effects compared to the use of secreted proteins and small molecules.

Another protective mechanism that controls the process of adipogenesis at the systemic level is endocrine regulation, which is much more susceptible to influence from xenobiotic substances. In this case, adipogenesis is influenced not only by small-molecule-based drugs but also by other substances from the external environment. The influence of bisphenols, phthalates, and, widely used in modern industry and agriculture, dioxin-like compounds, poses a great threat to health. In addition to the generally recognized toxic effects known for each of these substances, we think that their intake with food, air, and water results in further problems. The accumulation of these substances in adipose, leading to prolonged adipogenesis impairment, can also affect other processes in the organism, resulting in chronic intoxication. Nevertheless, both adipocytes and adipose tissue-resident immune cells express AhR, which is responsible for dioxin sensing. Targeted ablation of this transcription factor can normalize the process of adipogenesis and suppress the proinflammatory activity of resident immune cells. Thus, gene therapy drugs that target transcription processes open up broad prospects for obesity treatment and metabolic improvement, including the reduction in the harmful effects of environmental factors.

Hereby, we summarize the current knowledge about white-to-beige adipose conversion, concluding that both small molecule medicinal chemistry and gene therapy are perspectives for the development of new strategies to overcome insulin resistance and counteract obesity.

Author Contributions: Conceptualization, S.B. and A.D.E.; scientific data search and original draft preparation, S.B., V.S.E., A.B. and A.D.E.; draft review and editing, A.D.E.; visualization, A.D.E.; supervision, A.D.E.; funding acquisition, A.D.E. All authors have read and agreed to the published version of the manuscript.

Funding: This research was funded by the Russian Science Foundation and Kuban Science Foundation (project no. 22-14-20046).

Acknowledgments: The authors gratefully acknowledge the support of Russian Science Foundation and Kuban Science Foundation, administrative support of Anna Ryzhova and Marina Predeina, and the friendly and extensive endorsement of Alexander Karabelsky, Roman Ivanov, and Andrey Kuzovlev, who performed the visualization of chemical structures.

Conflicts of Interest: The authors declare no conflicts of interest.

References

1. At Least One in Eight People Now Obese. Available online: https://news.un.org/en/story/2024/02/1147107 (accessed on 10 May 2024).
2. Phelps, N.H.; Singleton, R.K.; Zhou, B.; Heap, R.A.; Mishra, A.; Bennett, J.E.; Paciorek, C.J.; Lhoste, V.P.; Carrillo-Larco, R.M.; Stevens, G.A.; et al. Worldwide Trends in Underweight and Obesity from 1990 to 2022: A Pooled Analysis of 3663 Population-Representative Studies with 222 Million Children, Adolescents, and Adults. *Lancet* **2024**, *403*, 1027–1050. [CrossRef] [PubMed]
3. Di Angelantonio, E.; Bhupathiraju, S.N.; Wormser, D.; Gao, P.; Kaptoge, S.; de Gonzalez, A.B.; Cairns, B.J.; Huxley, R.; Jackson, C.L.; Joshy, G.; et al. Body-Mass Index and All-Cause Mortality: Individual-Participant-Data Meta-Analysis of 239 Prospective Studies in Four Continents. *Lancet* **2016**, *388*, 776–786. [CrossRef] [PubMed]
4. Ong, K.L.; Stafford, L.K.; McLaughlin, S.A.; Boyko, E.J.; Vollset, S.E.; Smith, A.E.; Dalton, B.E.; Duprey, J.; Cruz, J.A.; Hagins, H.; et al. Global, Regional, and National Burden of Diabetes from 1990 to 2021, with Projections of Prevalence to 2050: A Systematic Analysis for the Global Burden of Disease Study 2021. *Lancet* **2023**, *402*, 203–234. [CrossRef] [PubMed]
5. Sawadogo, W.; Tsegaye, M.; Gizaw, A.; Adera, T. Overweight and Obesity as Risk Factors for COVID-19-Associated Hospitalisations and Death: Systematic Review and Meta-Analysis. *BMJ Nutr. Prev. Health* **2022**, *5*, 10–18. [CrossRef] [PubMed]
6. Russo, A.; Pisaturo, M.; Zollo, V.; Martini, S.; Maggi, P.; Numis, F.G.; Gentile, I.; Sangiovanni, N.; Rossomando, A.M.; Bianco, V.; et al. Obesity as a Risk Factor of Severe Outcome of COVID-19: A Pair-Matched 1:2 Case–Control Study. *J. Clin. Med.* **2023**, *12*, 4055. [CrossRef]
7. Arner, P. Fat Tissue Growth and Development in Humans. In *Recent Research in Nutrition and Growth*; Colombo, J., Koletzko, B., Lampl, M., Eds.; Karger Publishers: Basel, Switzerland, 2018; pp. 37–45.
8. Hruby, A.; Hu, F.B. The Epidemiology of Obesity: A Big Picture. *Pharmacoeconomics* **2015**, *33*, 673–689. [CrossRef] [PubMed]
9. Luo, L.; Liu, M. Adipose Tissue in Control of Metabolism. *J. Endocrinol.* **2016**, *231*, R77–R99. [CrossRef]
10. Morigny, P.; Boucher, J.; Arner, P.; Langin, D. Lipid and Glucose Metabolism in White Adipocytes: Pathways, Dysfunction and Therapeutics. *Nat. Rev. Endocrinol.* **2021**, *17*, 276–295. [CrossRef] [PubMed]
11. Liu, Y.; Qian, S.-W.; Tang, Y.; Tang, Q.-Q. The Secretory Function of Adipose Tissues in Metabolic Regulation. *Life Metab.* **2024**, *3*, loae003. [CrossRef]
12. Rosen, E.D.; Spiegelman, B.M. What We Talk about When We Talk about Fat. *Cell* **2014**, *156*, 20–44.
13. Frontini, A.; Cinti, S. Distribution and Development of Brown Adipocytes in the Murine and Human Adipose Organ. *Cell Metab.* **2010**, *11*, 253–256. [CrossRef] [PubMed]
14. Ricquier, D. Uncoupling Protein 1 of Brown Adipocytes, the Only Uncoupler: A Historical Perspective. *Front. Endocrinol.* **2011**, *2*, 85. [CrossRef]
15. Cinti, S.; Frederich, R.C.; Zingaretti, M.C.; De Matteis, R.; Flier, J.S.; Lowell, B.B. Immunohistochemical Localization of Leptin and Uncoupling Protein in White and Brown Adipose Tissue. *Endocrinology* **1997**, *138*, 797–804. [CrossRef] [PubMed]
16. Rosenwald, M.; Perdikari, A.; Rülicke, T.; Wolfrum, C. Bi-Directional Interconversion of Brite and White Adipocytes. *Nat. Cell Biol.* **2013**, *15*, 659–667. [CrossRef]
17. Zhu, Y.; Liu, W.; Qi, Z.; Qi, Z.; Liu, W. Adipose Tissue Browning and Thermogenesis under Physiologically Energetic Challenges: A Remodelled Thermogenic System Corresponding Authors. *J. Physiol.* **2024**, *602*, 23–48.
18. Koksharova, E.O.; Mayorov, A.Y.; Shestakova, M.V.; Dedov, I.I. Metabolic Characteristics and Therapeutic Potential of Brown and ?Beige? Adipose Tissues. *Diabetes Mellit.* **2014**, *17*, 5–15. [CrossRef]
19. Theret, M.; Mounier, R.; Rossi, F. The Origins and Non-Canonical Functions of Macrophages in Development and Regeneration. *Development* **2019**, *146*, dev156000. [CrossRef]
20. Feyrter, F. About the Diversity of Human Adipose Tissue. *Wien. Klin. Wochenschr.* **1947**, *59*, 477–480.
21. White, U. Adipose Tissue Expansion in Obesity, Health, and Disease. *Front. Cell Dev. Biol.* **2023**, 11. [CrossRef]
22. Marcadenti, A.; de Abreu-Silva, E.O. Different Adipose Tissue Depots: Metabolic Implications and Effects of Surgical Removal. *Endocrinol. Y Nutr. (Engl. Ed.)* **2015**, *62*, 458–464. [CrossRef]
23. Vosselman, M.J.; van Marken Lichtenbelt, W.D.; Schrauwen, P. Energy Dissipation in Brown Adipose Tissue: From Mice to Men. *Mol. Cell Endocrinol.* **2013**, *379*, 43–50. [CrossRef]
24. Fedorenko, A.; Lishko, P.V.; Kirichok, Y. Mechanism of Fatty-Acid-Dependent UCP1 Uncoupling in Brown Fat Mitochondria. *Cell* **2012**, *151*, 400–413. [PubMed]
25. Haugen, F.; Drevon, C.A. The Interplay between Nutrients and the Adipose Tissue: Plenary Lecture. *Proc. Nutr. Soc.* **2007**, *66*, 171–182. [CrossRef]

26. Seale, P.; Bjork, B.; Yang, W.; Kajimura, S.; Chin, S.; Kuang, S.; Scimè, A.; Devarakonda, S.; Conroe, H.M.; Erdjument-Bromage, H.; et al. PRDM16 Controls a Brown Fat/Skeletal Muscle Switch. *Nature* **2008**, *454*, 961–967. [CrossRef] [PubMed]
27. Berry, R.; Rodeheffer, M.S. Characterization of the Adipocyte Cellular Lineage In Vivo. *Nat. Cell Biol.* **2013**, *15*, 302–308. [CrossRef]
28. Lee, Y.-H.; Granneman, J.G. Seeking the Source of Adipocytes in Adult White Adipose Tissues. *Adipocyte* **2012**, *1*, 230–236. [CrossRef]
29. Sanchez-Gurmaches, J.; Hung, C.M.; Sparks, C.A.; Tang, Y.; Li, H.; Guertin, D.A. PTEN Loss in the Myf5 Lineage Redistributes Body Fat and Reveals Subsets of White Adipocytes That Arise from Myf5 Precursors. *Cell Metab.* **2012**, *16*, 348–362. [CrossRef]
30. Nedergaard, J.; Bengtsson, T.; Cannon, B. Unexpected Evidence for Active Brown Adipose Tissue in Adult Humans. *Am. J. Physiol. Endocrinol. Metab.* **2007**, *293*, 444–452.
31. van Marken Lichtenbelt, W.D.; Vanhommerig, J.W.; Smulders, N.M.; Drossaerts, J.M.A.F.L.; Kemerink, G.J.; Bouvy, N.D.; Schrauwen, P.; Teule, G.J.J. Cold-Activated Brown Adipose Tissue in Healthy Men. *N. Engl. J. Med.* **2009**, *360*, 1500–1508. [CrossRef]
32. Cypess, A.M.; Lehman, S.; Williams, G.; Tal, I.; Rodman, D.; Goldfine, A.B.; Kuo, F.C.; Palmer, E.L.; Tseng, Y.-H.; Doria, A.; et al. Identification and Importance of Brown Adipose Tissue in Adult Humans. *N. Engl. J. Med.* **2009**, *360*, 1509–1517. [CrossRef]
33. Virtanen, K.A.; Lidell, M.E.; Orava, J.; Heglind, M.; Westergren, R.; Niemi, T.; Taittonen, M.; Laine, J.; Savisto, N.-J.; Enerbäck, S.; et al. Functional Brown Adipose Tissue in Healthy Adults. *N. Engl. J. Med.* **2009**, *360*, 1518–1525. [CrossRef] [PubMed]
34. Cypess, A.M.; White, A.P.; Vernochet, C.; Schulz, T.J.; Xue, R.; Sass, C.A.; Huang, T.L.; Roberts-Toler, C.; Weiner, L.S.; Sze, C.; et al. Anatomical Localization, Gene Expression Profiling and Functional Characterization of Adult Human Neck Brown Fat. *Nat. Med.* **2013**, *19*, 635–639. [CrossRef]
35. van Marken Lichtenbelt, W.D. Human Brown Adipose Tissue—A Decade Later. *Obesity* **2021**, *29*, 1099–1101. [CrossRef]
36. Jurado-Fasoli, L.; Sanchez-Delgado, G.; Alcantara, J.M.A.; Acosta, F.M.; Sanchez-Sanchez, R.; Labayen, I.; Ortega, F.B.; Martinez-Tellez, B.; Ruiz, J.R. Adults with Metabolically Healthy Overweight or Obesity Present More Brown Adipose Tissue and Higher Thermogenesis than Their Metabolically Unhealthy Counterparts. *EBioMedicine* **2024**, *100*, 104948. [CrossRef]
37. Maliszewska, K.; Kretowski, A. Brown Adipose Tissue and Its Role in Insulin and Glucose Homeostasis. *Int. J. Mol. Sci.* **2021**, *22*, 1530. [CrossRef] [PubMed]
38. Becher, T.; Palanisamy, S.; Kramer, D.J.; Eljalby, M.; Marx, S.J.; Wibmer, A.G.; Butler, S.D.; Jiang, C.S.; Vaughan, R.; Schöder, H.; et al. Brown Adipose Tissue Is Associated with Cardiometabolic Health. *Nat. Med.* **2021**, *27*, 58–65. [CrossRef] [PubMed]
39. Young, P.; Arch, J.R.S.; Ashwell, M. Brown Adipose Tissue in the Parametrial Fat Pad of the Mouse. *FEBS Lett.* **1984**, *167*, 10–14. [CrossRef] [PubMed]
40. Hanssen, M.J.W.; van der Lans, A.A.J.J.; Brans, B.; Hoeks, J.; Jardon, K.M.C.; Schaart, G.; Mottaghy, F.M.; Schrauwen, P.; van Marken Lichtenbelt, W.D. Short-Term Cold Acclimation Recruits Brown Adipose Tissue in Obese Humans. *Diabetes* **2016**, *65*, 1179–1189. [CrossRef]
41. Barbatelli, G.; Murano, I.; Madsen, L.; Hao, Q.; Jimenez, M.; Kristiansen, K.; Giacobino, J.P.; De Matteis, R.; Cinti, S. The Emergence of Cold-Induced Brown Adipocytes in Mouse White Fat Depots Is Determined Predominantly by White to Brown Adipocyte Transdifferentiation. *Am. J. Physiol. Endocrinol. Metab.* **2010**, *298*, E1244–E1253. [CrossRef]
42. Wu, J.; Boström, P.; Sparks, L.M.; Ye, L.; Choi, J.H.; Giang, A.-H.; Khandekar, M.; Virtanen, K.A.; Nuutila, P.; Schaart, G.; et al. Beige Adipocytes Are a Distinct Type of Thermogenic Fat Cell in Mouse and Human. *Cell* **2012**, *150*, 366–376.
43. Shan, T.; Liang, X.; Bi, P.; Zhang, P.; Liu, W.; Kuang, S. Distinct Populations of Adipogenic and Myogenic Myf5-Lineage Progenitors in White Adipose Tissues. *J. Lipid Res.* **2013**, *54*, 2214–2224. [CrossRef] [PubMed]
44. Long, J.Z.; Svensson, K.J.; Tsai, L.; Zeng, X.; Roh, H.C.; Kong, X.; Rao, R.R.; Lou, J.; Lokurkar, I.; Baur, W.; et al. A Smooth Muscle-Like Origin for Beige Adipocytes. *Cell Metab.* **2014**, *19*, 810–820. [CrossRef]
45. An, S.-M.; Cho, S.-H.; Yoon, J.C. Adipose Tissue and Metabolic Health. *Diabetes Metab. J.* **2023**, *47*, 595–611. [CrossRef] [PubMed]
46. Chazenbalk, G.; Bertolotto, C.; Heneidi, S.; Jumabay, M.; Trivax, B.; Aronowitz, J.; Yoshimura, K.; Simmons, C.F.; Dumesic, D.A.; Azziz, R. Novel Pathway of Adipogenesis through Cross-Talk between Adipose Tissue Macrophages, Adipose Stem Cells and Adipocytes: Evidence of Cell Plasticity. *PLoS ONE* **2011**, *6*, e17834. [CrossRef] [PubMed]
47. Schulz, C.; Perdiguero, E.G.; Chorro, L.; Szabo-Rogers, H.; Cagnard, N.; Kierdorf, K.; Prinz, M.; Wu, B.; Jacobsen, S.E.W.; Pollard, J.W.; et al. A Lineage of Myeloid Cells Independent of Myb and Hematopoietic Stem Cells. *Science* **2012**, *336*, 86–90. [CrossRef] [PubMed]
48. Rohm, T.V.; Castellani Gomes Dos Reis, F.; Isaac, R.; Murphy, C.; Cunha e Rocha, K.; Bandyopadhyay, G.; Gao, H.; Libster, A.M.; Zapata, R.C.; Lee, Y.S.; et al. Adipose Tissue Macrophages Secrete Small Extracellular Vesicles That Mediate Rosiglitazone-Induced Insulin Sensitization. *Nat. Metab.* **2024**, *6*, 880–898. [CrossRef] [PubMed]
49. Ricardo-Gonzalez, R.R.; Molofsky, A.B.; Locksley, R.M. ILC2s—Development, Divergence, Dispersal. *Curr. Opin. Immunol.* **2022**, *75*, 102168. [CrossRef] [PubMed]
50. Brestoff, J.R.; Kim, B.S.; Saenz, S.A.; Stine, R.R.; Monticelli, L.A.; Sonnenberg, G.F.; Thome, J.J.; Farber, D.L.; Lutfy, K.; Seale, P.; et al. Group 2 Innate Lymphoid Cells Promote Beiging of White Adipose Tissue and Limit Obesity. *Nature* **2015**, *519*, 242–246. [CrossRef] [PubMed]
51. Fisher, F.M.; Kleiner, S.; Douris, N.; Fox, E.C.; Mepani, R.J.; Verdeguer, F.; Wu, J.; Kharitonenkov, A.; Flier, J.S.; Maratos-Flier, E.; et al. FGF21 Regulates PGC-1α and Browning of White Adipose Tissues in Adaptive Thermogenesis. *Genes Dev.* **2012**, *26*, 271–281. [CrossRef]

52. Schulz, T.J.; Tseng, Y.-H. Emerging Role of Bone Morphogenetic Proteins in Adipogenesis and Energy Metabolism. *Cytokine Growth Factor Rev.* **2009**, *20*, 523–531. [CrossRef]
53. Elsen, M.; Raschke, S.; Tennagels, N.; Schwahn, U.; Jelenik, T.; Roden, M.; Romacho, T.; Eckel, J. BMP4 and BMP7 Induce the White-to-Brown Transition of Primary Human Adipose Stem Cells. *Am. J. Physiol. Cell Physiol.* **2014**, *306*, C431–C440. [CrossRef] [PubMed]
54. Boström, P.; Wu, J.; Jedrychowski, M.P.; Korde, A.; Ye, L.; Lo, J.C.; Rasbach, K.A.; Boström, E.A.; Choi, J.H.; Long, J.Z.; et al. A PGC1-α-Dependent Myokine That Drives Brown-Fat-like Development of White Fat and Thermogenesis. *Nature* **2012**, *481*, 463–468. [CrossRef] [PubMed]
55. Lopez-Legarrea, P.; de la Iglesia, R.; Crujeiras, A.B.; Pardo, M.; Casanueva, F.F.; Zulet, M.A.; Martinez, J.A. Higher Baseline Irisin Concentrations Are Associated with Greater Reductions in Glycemia and Insulinemia after Weight Loss in Obese Subjects. *Nutr. Diabetes* **2014**, *4*, e110. [CrossRef] [PubMed]
56. Shaw, A.; Tóth, B.B.; Arianti, R.; Csomós, I.; Póliska, S.; Vámos, A.; Bacso, Z.; Győry, F.; Fésüs, L.; Kristóf, E. BMP7 Increases UCP1-Dependent and Independent Thermogenesis with a Unique Gene Expression Program in Human Neck Area Derived Adipocytes. *Pharmaceuticals* **2021**, *14*, 1078. [CrossRef] [PubMed]
57. Abu-Odeh, M.; Zhang, Y.; Reilly, S.M.; Ebadat, N.; Keinan, O.; Valentine, J.M.; Hafezi-Bakhtiari, M.; Ashayer, H.; Mamoun, L.; Zhou, X.; et al. FGF21 Promotes Thermogenic Gene Expression as an Autocrine Factor in Adipocytes. *Cell Rep.* **2021**, *35*, 109331. [CrossRef] [PubMed]
58. Miyajima, Y.; Ealey, K.N.; Motomura, Y.; Mochizuki, M.; Takeno, N.; Yanagita, M.; Economides, A.N.; Nakayama, M.; Koseki, H.; Moro, K. Effects of BMP7 Produced by Group 2 Innate Lymphoid Cells on Adipogenesis. *Int. Immunol.* **2020**, *32*, 407–419. [CrossRef] [PubMed]
59. Sun, C.; Berry, W.L.; Olson, L.E. PDGFRα Controls the Balance of Stromal and Adipogenic Cells during Adipose Tissue Organogenesis. *Development* **2017**, *144*, 83–94. [CrossRef] [PubMed]
60. Shao, M.; Hepler, C.; Vishvanath, L.; MacPherson, K.A.; Busbuso, N.C.; Gupta, R.K. Fetal Development of Subcutaneous White Adipose Tissue Is Dependent on Zfp423. *Mol. Metab.* **2017**, *6*, 111–124. [CrossRef]
61. Gupta, R.K.; Mepani, R.J.; Kleiner, S.; Lo, J.C.; Khandekar, M.J.; Cohen, P.; Frontini, A.; Bhowmick, D.C.; Ye, L.; Cinti, S.; et al. Zfp423 Expression Identifies Committed Preadipocytes and Localizes to Adipose Endothelial and Perivascular Cells. *Cell Metab.* **2012**, *15*, 230–239. [CrossRef]
62. Gupta, R.K.; Arany, Z.; Seale, P.; Mepani, R.J.; Ye, L.; Conroe, H.M.; Roby, Y.A.; Kulaga, H.; Reed, R.R.; Spiegelman, B.M. Transcriptional Control of Preadipocyte Determination by Zfp423. *Nature* **2010**, *464*, 619–623. [CrossRef]
63. Huang, Y.; Das, A.K.; Yang, Q.-Y.; Zhu, M.-J.; Du, M. Zfp423 Promotes Adipogenic Differentiation of Bovine Stromal Vascular Cells. *PLoS ONE* **2012**, *7*, e47496. [CrossRef] [PubMed]
64. Shao, M.; Ishibashi, J.; Kusminski, C.M.; Wang, Q.A.; Hepler, C.; Vishvanath, L.; MacPherson, K.A.; Spurgin, S.B.; Sun, K.; Holland, W.L.; et al. Zfp423 Maintains White Adipocyte Identity through Suppression of the Beige Cell Thermogenic Gene Program. *Cell Metab.* **2016**, *23*, 1167–1184. [CrossRef] [PubMed]
65. Shapira, S.N.; Seale, P. Transcriptional Control of Brown and Beige Fat Development and Function. *Obesity* **2019**, *27*, 13–21. [CrossRef] [PubMed]
66. Farmer, S.R. Transcriptional Control of Adipocyte Formation. *Cell Metab.* **2006**, *4*, 263–273. [CrossRef] [PubMed]
67. Lee, J.-E.; Schmidt, H.; Lai, B.; Ge, K. Transcriptional and Epigenomic Regulation of Adipogenesis. *Mol. Cell Biol.* **2019**, *39*, e00601-18. [CrossRef] [PubMed]
68. Siersbæk, R.; Nielsen, R.; Mandrup, S. Transcriptional Networks and Chromatin Remodeling Controlling Adipogenesis. *Trends Endocrinol. Metab.* **2012**, *23*, 56–64. [CrossRef] [PubMed]
69. Siersbæk, R.; Baek, S.; Rabiee, A.; Nielsen, R.; Traynor, S.; Clark, N.; Sandelin, A.; Jensen, O.N.; Sung, M.-H.; Hager, G.L.; et al. Molecular Architecture of Transcription Factor Hotspots in Early Adipogenesis. *Cell Rep.* **2014**, *7*, 1434–1442. [CrossRef]
70. Park, B.-H.; Qiang, L.; Farmer, S.R. Phosphorylation of C/EBPβ at a Consensus Extracellular Signal-Regulated Kinase/Glycogen Synthase Kinase 3 Site Is Required for the Induction of Adiponectin Gene Expression during the Differentiation of Mouse Fibroblasts into Adipocytes. *Mol. Cell Biol.* **2004**, *24*, 8671–8680. [CrossRef]
71. Abdou, H.S.; Atlas, E.; Haché, R.J.G. A Positive Regulatory Domain in CCAAT/Enhancer Binding Protein β (C/EBPβ) Is Required for the Glucocorticoid-Mediated Displacement of Histone Deacetylase 1 (HDAC1) from the C/Ebpα Promoter and Maximum Adipogenesis. *Endocrinology* **2013**, *154*, 1454–1464. [CrossRef]
72. Zuo, Y.; Qiang, L.; Farmer, S.R. Activation of CCAAT/Enhancer-Binding Protein (C/EBP) α Expression by C/EBPβ during Adipogenesis Requires a Peroxisome Proliferator-Activated Receptor-γ-Associated Repression of HDAC1 at the C/Ebpα Gene Promoter. *J. Biol. Chem.* **2006**, *281*, 7960–7967. [CrossRef]
73. Tanaka, T.; Yoshida, N.; Kishimoto, T.; Akira, S. Defective Adipocyte Differentiation in Mice Lacking the C/EBPβ and/or C/EBPδ Gene. *EMBO J.* **1997**, *16*, 7432–7443. [CrossRef] [PubMed]
74. Egorov, A.D.; Penkov, D.N.; Tkachuk, V.A. Molecular and Cellular Mechanisms of Adipogenesis. *Diabetes Mellit.* **2015**, *18*, 12–19. [CrossRef]
75. Penkov, D.N.; Akopyan, Z.A.; Kochegura, T.N.; Egorov, A.D. Transcriptional Control of Insulin-Sensitive Glucose Carrier Glut4 Expression in Adipose Tissue Cells. *Dokl. Biochem. Biophys.* **2016**, *467*, 145–149. [CrossRef] [PubMed]

76. Pen'kov, D.N.; Egorov, A.D.; Tkachuk, V.A. Rol' Faktora Transkriptsii PREP1 v Protsesse Differentsirovki Mezenkhimal'nykh Stromal'nykh Kletok v Adipotsity. *Genes Cells* **2017**, *12*, 192.
77. Maroni, G.; Tkachuk, V.A.; Egorov, A.; Morelli, M.J.; Luongo, R.; Levantini, E.; Blasi, F.; Magli, M.C.; Penkov, D. Prep1 Prevents Premature Adipogenesis of Mesenchymal Progenitors. *Sci. Rep.* **2017**, *7*, 15573. [CrossRef] [PubMed]
78. Maroni, G.; Panetta, D.; Luongo, R.; Krishnan, I.; La Rosa, F.; Campani, D.; Salvadori, P.; Iozzo, P.; Blasi, F.; Penkov, D.; et al. The Role of Prep1 in the Regulation of Mesenchymal Stromal Cells. *Int. J. Mol. Sci.* **2019**, *20*, 3639. [CrossRef] [PubMed]
79. Birsoy, K.; Chen, Z.; Friedman, J. Transcriptional Regulation of Adipogenesis by KLF4. *Cell Metab.* **2008**, *7*, 339–347. [CrossRef] [PubMed]
80. Oishi, Y.; Manabe, I.; Tobe, K.; Tsushima, K.; Shindo, T.; Fujiu, K.; Nishimura, G.; Maemura, K.; Yamauchi, T.; Kubota, N.; et al. Krüppel-like Transcription Factor KLF5 Is a Key Regulator of Adipocyte Differentiation. *Cell Metab.* **2005**, *1*, 27–39. [CrossRef]
81. Li, D.; Yea, S.; Li, S.; Chen, Z.; Narla, G.; Banck, M.; Laborda, J.; Tan, S.; Friedman, J.M.; Friedman, S.L.; et al. Krüppel-like Factor-6 Promotes Preadipocyte Differentiation through Histone Deacetylase 3-Dependent Repression of DLK1. *J. Biol. Chem.* **2005**, *280*, 26941–26952. [CrossRef]
82. Sen Banerjee, S.; Feinberg, M.W.; Watanabe, M.; Gray, S.; Haspel, R.L.; Denkinger, D.J.; Kawahara, R.; Hauner, H.; Jain, M.K. The Krüppel-like Factor KLF2 Inhibits Peroxisome Proliferator-Activated Receptor-γ Expression and Adipogenesis. *J. Biol. Chem.* **2003**, *278*, 2581–2584. [CrossRef]
83. Sue, N.; Jack, B.H.A.; Eaton, S.A.; Pearson, R.C.M.; Funnell, A.P.W.; Turner, J.; Czolij, R.; Denyer, G.; Bao, S.; Molero-Navajas, J.C.; et al. Targeted Disruption of the Basic Krüppel-Like Factor Gene (Klf3) Reveals a Role in Adipogenesis. *Mol. Cell Biol.* **2008**, *28*, 3967–3978. [CrossRef] [PubMed]
84. Kawamura, Y.; Tanaka, Y.; Kawamori, R.; Maeda, S. Overexpression of Kruppel-like Factor 7 Regulates Adipocytokine Gene Expressions in Human Adipocytes and Inhibits Glucose-Induced Insulin Secretion in Pancreatic β-Cell Line. *Mol. Endocrinol.* **2006**, *20*, 844–856. [CrossRef] [PubMed]
85. Loft, A.; Forss, I.; Siersbæk, M.S.; Schmidt, S.F.; Larsen, A.-S.B.; Madsen, J.G.S.; Pisani, D.F.; Nielsen, R.; Aagaard, M.M.; Mathison, A.; et al. Browning of Human Adipocytes Requires KLF11 and Reprogramming of PPARγ Superenhancers. *Genes Dev.* **2015**, *29*, 7–22. [CrossRef] [PubMed]
86. Siersbæk, R.; Rabiee, A.; Nielsen, R.; Sidoli, S.; Traynor, S.; Loft, A.; Poulsen, L.L.C.; Rogowska-Wrzesinska, A.; Jensen, O.N.; Mandrup, S. Transcription Factor Cooperativity in Early Adipogenic Hotspots and Super-Enhancers. *Cell Rep.* **2014**, *7*, 1443–1455. [CrossRef] [PubMed]
87. Ito, K.; Schneeberger, M.; Gerber, A.; Jishage, M.; Marchildon, F.; Maganti, A.V.; Cohen, P.; Friedman, J.M.; Roeder, R.G. Critical Roles of Transcriptional Coactivator MED1 in the Formation and Function of Mouse Adipose Tissues. *Genes Dev.* **2021**, *35*, 729–748. [CrossRef] [PubMed]
88. Song, Z.; Xiaoli, A.M.; Li, Y.; Siqin, G.; Wu, T.; Strich, R.; Pessin, J.E.; Yang, F. The Conserved Mediator Subunit Cyclin C (CCNC) Is Required for Brown Adipocyte Development and Lipid Accumulation. *Mol. Metab.* **2022**, *64*, 101548. [CrossRef] [PubMed]
89. Zhang, J.W.; Klemm, D.J.; Vinson, C.; Lane, M.D. Role of CREB in Transcriptional Regulation of CCAAT/Enhancer-Binding Protein β Gene during Adipogenesis. *J. Biol. Chem.* **2004**, *279*, 4471–4478. [CrossRef] [PubMed]
90. Reusch, J.E.B.; Colton, L.A.; Klemm, D.J. CREB Activation Induces Adipogenesis in 3T3-L1 Cells. *Mol. Cell. Biol.* **2000**, *20*, 1008–1020. [CrossRef]
91. Fox, K.E.; Fankell, D.M.; Erickson, P.F.; Majka, S.M.; Crossno, J.T.; Klemm, D.J. Depletion of CAMP-Response Element-Binding Protein/ATF1 Inhibits Adipogenic Conversion of 3T3-L1 Cells Ectopically Expressing CCAAT/Enhancer-Binding Protein (C/EBP) α, C/EBP β, or PPARγ2. *J. Biol. Chem.* **2006**, *281*, 40341–40353. [CrossRef]
92. Rosen, E.D.; Sarraf, P.; Troy, A.E.; Bradwin, G.; Moore, K.; Milstone, D.S.; Spiegelman, B.M.; Mortensen, R.M. Farber, DPPARγ Is Required for the Differentiation of Adipose Tissue In Vivo and In Vitro. *Mol. Cell* **1999**, *4*, 611–617. [CrossRef]
93. Tontonoz, P.; Spiegelman, B.M. Fat and beyond: The Diverse Biology of PPARγ. *Annu. Rev. Biochem.* **2008**, *77*, 289–312. [CrossRef] [PubMed]
94. Tontonoz, P.; Hu, E.; Spiegelman, B.M. Stimulation of Adipogenesis in Fibroblasts by PPARy2, a Lipid-Activated Transcription Factor. *Cell* **1994**, *79*, 1147–1156. [CrossRef] [PubMed]
95. Ma, X.; Wang, D.; Zhao, W.; Xu, L. Deciphering the Roles of PPARγ in Adipocytes via Dynamic Change of Transcription Complex. *Front. Endocrinol.* **2018**, *9*, 473. [CrossRef] [PubMed]
96. Lefterova, M.I.; Zhang, Y.; Steger, D.J.; Schupp, M.; Schug, J.; Cristancho, A.; Feng, D.; Zhuo, D.; Stoeckert, C.J.; Liu, X.S.; et al. PPARγ and C/EBP Factors Orchestrate Adipocyte Biology via Adjacent Binding on a Genome-Wide Scale. *Genes Dev.* **2008**, *22*, 2941–2952. [CrossRef] [PubMed]
97. Ohno, H.; Shinoda, K.; Ohyama, K.; Sharp, L.Z.; Kajimura, S. EHMT1 Controls Brown Adipose Cell Fate and Thermogenesis through the PRDM16 Complex. *Nature* **2013**, *504*, 163–167. [CrossRef] [PubMed]
98. Li, X.; Wang, J.; Jiang, Z.; Guo, F.; Soloway, P.D.; Zhao, R. Role of PRDM16 and Its PR Domain in the Epigenetic Regulation of Myogenic and Adipogenic Genes during Transdifferentiation of C2C12 Cells. *Gene* **2015**, *570*, 191–198. [CrossRef] [PubMed]
99. Seale, P.; Conroe, H.M.; Estall, J.; Kajimura, S.; Frontini, A.; Ishibashi, J.; Cohen, P.; Cinti, S.; Spiegelman, B.M. Prdm16 Determines the Thermogenic Program of Subcutaneous White Adipose Tissue in Mice. *J. Clin. Investig.* **2011**, *121*, 96–105. [CrossRef] [PubMed]

100. Harms, M.J.; Ishibashi, J.; Wang, W.; Lim, H.W.; Goyama, S.; Sato, T.; Kurokawa, M.; Won, K.J.; Seale, P. Prdm16 Is Required for the Maintenance of Brown Adipocyte Identity and Function in Adult Mice. *Cell Metab.* **2014**, *19*, 593–604. [CrossRef]
101. Chi, J.; Cohen, P. The Multifaceted Roles of PRDM16: Adipose Biology and Beyond. *Trends Endocrinol. Metab.* **2016**, *27*, 11–23. [CrossRef]
102. Harms, M.J.; Lim, H.W.; Ho, Y.; Shapira, S.N.; Ishibashi, J.; Rajakumari, S.; Steger, D.J.; Lazar, M.A.; Won, K.J.; Seale, P. PRDM16 Binds MED1 and Controls Chromatin Architecture to Determine a Brown Fat Transcriptional Program. *Genes Dev.* **2015**, *29*, 298–307. [CrossRef]
103. Wang, Q.; Li, H.; Tajima, K.; Verkerke, A.R.P.; Taxin, Z.H.; Hou, Z.; Cole, J.B.; Li, F.; Wong, J.; Abe, I.; et al. Post-Translational Control of Beige Fat Biogenesis by PRDM16 Stabilization. *Nature* **2022**, *609*, 151–158. [CrossRef] [PubMed]
104. Chen, Q.; Huang, L.; Pan, D.; Zhu, L.J.; Wang, Y.X. Cbx4 Sumoylates Prdm16 to Regulate Adipose Tissue Thermogenesis. *Cell Rep.* **2018**, *22*, 2860–2872. [CrossRef] [PubMed]
105. Ma, Q.X.; Zhu, W.Y.; Lu, X.C.; Jiang, D.; Xu, F.; Li, J.T.; Zhang, L.; Wu, Y.L.; Chen, Z.J.; Yin, M.; et al. BCAA–BCKA Axis Regulates WAT Browning through Acetylation of PRDM16. *Nat. Metab.* **2022**, *4*, 106–122. [CrossRef] [PubMed]
106. Lodhi, I.J.; Dean, J.M.; He, A.; Park, H.; Tan, M.; Feng, C.; Song, H.; Hsu, F.F.; Semenkovich, C.F. PexRAP Inhibits PRDM16-Mediated Thermogenic Gene Expression. *Cell Rep.* **2017**, *20*, 2766–2774. [CrossRef] [PubMed]
107. Huang, L.; Pan, D.; Chen, Q.; Zhu, L.J.; Ou, J.; Wabitsch, M.; Wang, Y.X. Transcription Factor Hlx Controls a Systematic Switch from White to Brown Fat through Prdm16-Mediated Co-Activation. *Nat. Commun.* **2017**, *8*, 68. [CrossRef] [PubMed]
108. Shen, S.H.; Singh, S.P.; Raffaele, M.; Waldman, M.; Hochhauser, E.; Ospino, J.; Arad, M.; Peterson, S.J. Adipocyte-Specific Expression of PGC1α Promotes Adipocyte Browning and Alleviates Obesity-Induced Metabolic Dysfunction in an HO-1-Dependent Fashion. *Antioxidants* **2022**, *11*, 1147. [CrossRef] [PubMed]
109. Jimenez, M.A.; Åkerblad, P.; Sigvardsson, M.; Rosen, E.D. Critical Role for Ebf1 and Ebf2 in the Adipogenic Transcriptional Cascade. *Mol. Cell Biol.* **2007**, *27*, 743–757. [CrossRef] [PubMed]
110. Rajakumari, S.; Wu, J.; Ishibashi, J.; Lim, H.W.; Giang, A.H.; Won, K.J.; Reed, R.R.; Seale, P. EBF2 Determines and Maintains Brown Adipocyte Identity. *Cell Metab.* **2013**, *17*, 562–574. [CrossRef] [PubMed]
111. Shapira, S.N.; Lim, H.W.; Rajakumari, S.; Sakers, A.P.; Ishibashi, J.; Harms, M.J.; Won, K.J.; Seale, P. EBF2 Transcriptionally Regulates Brown Adipogenesis via the Histone Reader DPF3 and the BAF Chromatin Remodeling Complex. *Genes Dev.* **2017**, *31*, 660–673. [CrossRef]
112. Angueira, A.R.; Shapira, S.N.; Ishibashi, J.; Sampat, S.; Sostre-Colón, J.; Emmett, M.J.; Titchenell, P.M.; Lazar, M.A.; Lim, H.W.; Seale, P. Early B Cell Factor Activity Controls Developmental and Adaptive Thermogenic Gene Programming in Adipocytes. *Cell Rep.* **2020**, *30*, 2869–2878.e4. [CrossRef]
113. Liu, L.; Tao, Z.; Zheng, L.D.; Brooke, J.P.; Smith, C.M.; Liu, D.; Long, Y.C.; Cheng, Z. FoxO1 Interacts with Transcription Factor EB and Differentially Regulates Mitochondrial Uncoupling Proteins via Autophagy in Adipocytes. *Cell Death Discov.* **2016**, *2*, 16066. [CrossRef] [PubMed]
114. Stöhr, O.; Tao, R.; Miao, J.; Copps, K.D.; White, M.F. FoxO1 Suppresses Fgf21 during Hepatic Insulin Resistance to Impair Peripheral Glucose Utilization and Acute Cold Tolerance. *Cell Rep.* **2021**, *34*, 108893. [CrossRef] [PubMed]
115. Shi, L.; Tao, Z.; Zheng, L.; Yang, J.; Hu, X.; Scott, K.; de Kloet, A.; Krause, E.; Collins, J.F.; Cheng, Z. FoxO1 Regulates Adipose Transdifferentiation and Iron Influx by Mediating Tgfβ1 Signaling Pathway. *Redox Biol.* **2023**, *63*, 102727. [CrossRef] [PubMed]
116. Liu, P.; Huang, S.; Ling, S.; Xu, S.; Wang, F.; Zhang, W.; Zhou, R.; He, L.; Xia, X.; Yao, Z.; et al. Foxp1 Controls Brown/Beige Adipocyte Differentiation and Thermogenesis through Regulating B3-AR Desensitization. *Nat. Commun.* **2019**, *10*, 5070. [CrossRef]
117. Xu, L.; Panel, V.; Ma, X.; Du, C.; Hugendubler, L.; Gavrilova, O.; Liu, A.; McLaughlin, T.; Kaestner, K.H.; Mueller, E. The Winged Helix Transcription Factor Foxa3 Regulates Adipocyte Differentiation and Depot-Selective Fat Tissue Expansion. *Mol. Cell Biol.* **2013**, *33*, 3392–3399. [CrossRef] [PubMed]
118. Perie, L.; Verma, N.; Mueller, E. The Forkhead Box Transcription Factor FoxP4 Regulates Thermogenic Programs in Adipocytes. *J. Lipid Res.* **2021**, *62*, 100102. [CrossRef] [PubMed]
119. Wang, F.; Xu, S.; Chen, T.; Ling, S.; Zhang, W.; Wang, S.; Zhou, R.; Xia, X.; Yao, Z.; Li, P.; et al. FOXP4 Differentially Controls Cold-Induced Beige Adipocyte Differentiation and Thermogenesis. *Development* **2022**, *149*, dev200260. [CrossRef] [PubMed]
120. Young, S.G.; Barneda, D.; Planas-Iglesias, J.; Gaspar, M.L.; Mohammadyani, D.; Prasannan, S.; Dormann, D.; Han, G.-S.; Jesch, S.A.; Carman, G.M.; et al. The Brown Adipocyte Protein CIDEA Promotes Lipid Droplet Fusion via a Phosphatidic Acid-Binding Amphipathic Helix. *Elife* **2015**, *4*, e07485. [CrossRef]
121. Jash, S.; Banerjee, S.; Lee, M.J.; Farmer, S.R.; Puri, V. CIDEA Transcriptionally Regulates UCP1 for Britening and Thermogenesis in Human Fat Cells. *iScience* **2019**, *20*, 73–89. [CrossRef]
122. Zhang, H.; Guan, M.; Townsend, K.L.; Huang, T.L.; An, D.; Yan, X.; Xue, R.; Schulz, T.J.; Winnay, J.; Mori, M.; et al. Micro RNA-455 Regulates Brown Adipogenesis via a Novel HIF 1an-AMPK-PGC 1α Signaling Network. *EMBO Rep.* **2015**, *16*, 1378–1393. [CrossRef]
123. Sun, L.; Xie, H.; Mori, M.A.; Alexander, R.; Yuan, B.; Hattangadi, S.M.; Liu, Q.; Kahn, C.R.; Lodish, H.F. Mir193b–365 Is Essential for Brown Fat Differentiation. *Nat. Cell Biol.* **2011**, *13*, 958–965. [CrossRef]
124. Hu, F.; Wang, M.; Xiao, T.; Yin, B.; He, L.; Meng, W.; Dong, M.; Liu, F. MiR-30 Promotes Thermogenesis and the Development of Beige Fat by Targeting RIP140. *Diabetes* **2015**, *64*, 2056–2068. [CrossRef] [PubMed]

125. Saha, P.K.; Hamilton, M.P.; Rajapakshe, K.; Putluri, V.; Felix, J.B.; Masschelin, P.; Cox, A.R.; Bajaj, M.; Putluri, N.; Coarfa, C.; et al. MiR-30a Targets Gene Networks That Promote Browning of Human and Mouse Adipocytes. *Am. J. Physiol. Endocrinol. Metab.* **2020**, *319*, E667–E677. [CrossRef]
126. Ng, R.; Hussain, N.A.; Zhang, Q.; Chang, C.; Li, H.; Fu, Y.; Cao, L.; Han, W.; Stunkel, W.; Xu, F. MiRNA-32 Drives Brown Fat Thermogenesis and Trans-Activates Subcutaneous White Fat Browning in Mice. *Cell Rep.* **2017**, *19*, 1229–1246. [CrossRef]
127. Kim, H.-J.; Cho, H.; Alexander, R.; Patterson, H.C.; Gu, M.; Lo, K.A.; Xu, D.; Goh, V.J.; Nguyen, L.N.; Chai, X.; et al. MicroRNAs Are Required for the Feature Maintenance and Differentiation of Brown Adipocytes. *Diabetes* **2014**, *63*, 4045–4056. [CrossRef] [PubMed]
128. Gharanei, S.; Shabir, K.; Brown, J.E.; Weickert, M.O.; Barber, T.M.; Kyrou, I.; Randeva, H.S. Regulatory MicroRNAs in Brown, Brite and White Adipose Tissue. *Cells* **2020**, *9*, 2489. [CrossRef] [PubMed]
129. Tan, X.; Zhu, T.; Zhang, L.; Fu, L.; Hu, Y.; Li, H.; Li, C.; Zhang, J.; Liang, B.; Liu, J. MiR-669a-5p Promotes Adipogenic Differentiation and Induces Browning in Preadipocytes. *Adipocyte* **2022**, *11*, 120–132. [CrossRef] [PubMed]
130. Sun, L.; Trajkovski, M. MiR-27 Orchestrates the Transcriptional Regulation of Brown Adipogenesis. *Metabolism* **2014**, *63*, 272–282. [CrossRef]
131. Fu, T.; Seok, S.; Choi, S.; Huang, Z.; Suino-Powell, K.; Xu, H.E.; Kemper, B.; Kemper, J.K. MicroRNA 34a Inhibits Beige and Brown Fat Formation in Obesity in Part by Suppressing Adipocyte Fibroblast Growth Factor 21 Signaling and SIRT1 Function. *Mol. Cell Biol.* **2014**, *34*, 4130–4142. [CrossRef]
132. Chen, Y.; Siegel, F.; Kipschull, S.; Haas, B.; Fröhlich, H.; Meister, G.; Pfeifer, A. MiR-155 Regulates Differentiation of Brown and Beige Adipocytes via a Bistable Circuit. *Nat. Commun.* **2013**, *4*, 1769. [CrossRef]
133. Trajkovski, M.; Ahmed, K.; Esau, C.C.; Stoffel, M. MyomiR-133 Regulates Brown Fat Differentiation through Prdm16. *Nat. Cell Biol.* **2012**, *14*, 1330–1335. [CrossRef] [PubMed]
134. Xihua, L.; Shengjie, T.; Weiwei, G.; Matro, E.; Tingting, T.; Lin, L.; Fang, W.; Jiaqiang, Z.; Fenping, Z.; Hong, L. Circulating MiR-143-3p Inhibition Protects against Insulin Resistance in Metabolic Syndrome via Targeting of the Insulin-like Growth Factor 2 Receptor. *Transl. Res.* **2019**, *205*, 33–43. [CrossRef] [PubMed]
135. Cioffi, M.; Vallespinos-Serrano, M.; Trabulo, S.M.; Fernandez-Marcos, P.J.; Firment, A.N.; Vazquez, B.N.; Vieira, C.R.; Mulero, F.; Camara, J.A.; Cronin, U.P.; et al. MiR-93 Controls Adiposity via Inhibition of Sirt7 and Tbx3. *Cell Rep.* **2015**, *12*, 1594–1605. [CrossRef] [PubMed]
136. Pan, D.; Mao, C.; Quattrochi, B.; Friedline, R.H.; Zhu, L.J.; Jung, D.Y.; Kim, J.K.; Lewis, B.; Wang, Y.-X. MicroRNA-378 Controls Classical Brown Fat Expansion to Counteract Obesity. *Nat. Commun.* **2014**, *5*, 4725. [CrossRef] [PubMed]
137. Armani, A.; Feraco, A.; Camajani, E.; Gorini, S.; Lombardo, M.; Caprio, M. Nutraceuticals in Brown Adipose Tissue Activation. *Cells* **2022**, *11*, 3996. [CrossRef] [PubMed]
138. Tu, W.; Fu, Y.; Xie, X. RepSox, a Small Molecule Inhibitor of the TGFβ Receptor, Induces Brown Adipogenesis and Browning of White Adipocytes. *Acta Pharmacol. Sin.* **2019**, *40*, 1523–1531. [CrossRef] [PubMed]
139. Haynes, B.A.; Huyck, R.W.; James, A.J.; Carter, M.E.; Gaafar, O.U.; Day, M.; Pinto, A.; Dobrian, A.D. Isolation, Expansion, and Adipogenic Induction of CD34+CD31+ Endothelial Cells from Human Omental and Subcutaneous Adipose Tissue. *J. Vis. Exp.* **2018**, *137*, e57804. [CrossRef] [PubMed]
140. Nie, B.; Nie, T.; Hui, X.; Gu, P.; Mao, L.; Li, K.; Yuan, R.; Zheng, J.; Wang, H.; Li, K.; et al. Brown Adipogenic Reprogramming Induced by a Small Molecule. *Cell Rep.* **2017**, *18*, 624–635. [CrossRef] [PubMed]
141. Ohno, H.; Shinoda, K.; Spiegelman, B.M.; Kajimura, S. PPARγ Agonists Induce a White-to-Brown Fat Conversion through Stabilization of PRDM16 Protein. *Cell Metab.* **2012**, *15*, 395–404. [CrossRef]
142. Lee, S.-M.; Moon, J.; Cho, Y.; Chung, J.H.; Shin, M.-J. Quercetin Up-Regulates Expressions of Peroxisome Proliferator-Activated Receptor γ, Liver X Receptor α, and ATP Binding Cassette Transporter A1 Genes and Increases Cholesterol Efflux in Human Macrophage Cell Line. *Nutr. Res.* **2013**, *33*, 136–143. [CrossRef]
143. Beekmann, K.; Rubió, L.; de Haan, L.H.J.; Actis-Goretta, L.; van der Burg, B.; van Bladeren, P.J.; Rietjens, I.M.C.M. The Effect of Quercetin and Kaempferol Aglycones and Glucuronides on Peroxisome Proliferator-Activated Receptor-Gamma (PPAR-γ). *Food Funct.* **2015**, *6*, 1098–1107. [CrossRef]
144. Selim, M.A.; Mosaad, S.M.; El-Sayed, N.M. Lycopene Protects against Bisphenol A Induced Toxicity on the Submandibular Salivary Glands via the Upregulation of PPAR-γ and Modulation of Wnt/β-Catenin Signaling. *Int. Immunopharmacol.* **2022**, *112*, 109293. [CrossRef]
145. Yang, C.-M.; Lu, I.-H.; Chen, H.-Y.; Hu, M.-L. Lycopene Inhibits the Proliferation of Androgen-Dependent Human Prostate Tumor Cells through Activation of PPARγ-LXRα-ABCA1 Pathway. *J. Nutr. Biochem.* **2012**, *23*, 8–17. [CrossRef]
146. Wang, H.; Liu, L.; Lin, J.Z.; Aprahamian, T.R.; Farmer, S.R. Browning of White Adipose Tissue with Roscovitine Induces a Distinct Population of UCP1 + Adipocytes. *Cell Metab.* **2016**, *24*, 835–847. [CrossRef]
147. Kroon, T.; Harms, M.; Maurer, S.; Bonnet, L.; Alexandersson, I.; Lindblom, A.; Ahnmark, A.; Nilsson, D.; Gennemark, P.; O'Mahony, G.; et al. PPARγ and PPARα Synergize to Induce Robust Browning of White Fat in Vivo. *Mol. Metab.* **2020**, *36*, 100964. [CrossRef] [PubMed]
148. Divakaran, S.J.; Srivastava, S.; Jahagirdar, A.; Rajendran, R.; Sukhdeo, S.V.; Rajakumari, S. Sesaminol Induces Brown and Beige Adipocyte Formation through Suppression of Myogenic Program. *FASEB J.* **2020**, *34*, 6854–6870. [CrossRef]

149. Peng, W.-Q.; Xiao, G.; Li, B.-Y.; Guo, Y.-Y.; Guo, L.; Tang, Q.-Q. L-Theanine Activates the Browning of White Adipose Tissue Through the AMPK/α-Ketoglutarate/Prdm16 Axis and Ameliorates Diet-Induced Obesity in Mice. *Diabetes* **2021**, *70*, 1458–1472. [CrossRef] [PubMed]
150. Kalupahana, N.S.; Claycombe, K.; Newman, S.J.; Stewart, T.; Siriwardhana, N.; Matthan, N.; Lichtenstein, A.H.; Moustaid-Moussa, N. Eicosapentaenoic Acid Prevents and Reverses Insulin Resistance in High-Fat Diet-Induced Obese Mice via Modulation of Adipose Tissue Inflammation1–3. *J. Nutr.* **2010**, *140*, 1915–1922. [CrossRef] [PubMed]
151. Zu, Y.; Pahlavani, M.; Ramalingam, L.; Jayarathne, S.; Andrade, J.; Scoggin, S.; Festuccia, W.T.; Kalupahana, N.S.; Moustaid-Moussa, N. Temperature-Dependent Effects of Eicosapentaenoic Acid (EPA) on Browning of Subcutaneous Adipose Tissue in UCP1 Knockout Male Mice. *Int. J. Mol. Sci.* **2023**, *24*, 8708. [CrossRef]
152. Miller, E.K.; Pahlavani, M.; Ramalingam, L.; Scoggin, S.; Moustaid-Moussa, N. Uncoupling Protein 1-Independent Effects of Eicosapentaenoic Acid in Brown Adipose Tissue of Diet-Induced Obese Female Mice. *J. Nutr. Biochem.* **2021**, *98*, 108819. [CrossRef]
153. Pahlavani, M.; Razafimanjato, F.; Ramalingam, L.; Kalupahana, N.S.; Moussa, H.; Scoggin, S.; Moustaid-Moussa, N. Eicosapentaenoic Acid Regulates Brown Adipose Tissue Metabolism in High-Fat-Fed Mice and in Clonal Brown Adipocytes. *J. Nutr. Biochem.* **2017**, *39*, 101–109. [CrossRef] [PubMed]
154. Wang, S.; Wang, X.; Ye, Z.; Xu, C.; Zhang, M.; Ruan, B.; Wei, M.; Jiang, Y.; Zhang, Y.; Wang, L.; et al. Curcumin Promotes Browning of White Adipose Tissue in a Norepinephrine-Dependent Way. *Biochem. Biophys. Res. Commun.* **2015**, *466*, 247–253. [CrossRef] [PubMed]
155. Shehzad, A.; Ha, T.; Subhan, F.; Lee, Y.S. New Mechanisms and the Anti-Inflammatory Role of Curcumin in Obesity and Obesity-Related Metabolic Diseases. *Eur. J. Nutr.* **2011**, *50*, 151–161. [CrossRef] [PubMed]
156. Lone, J.; Choi, J.H.; Kim, S.W.; Yun, J.W. Curcumin Induces Brown Fat-like Phenotype in 3T3-L1 and Primary White Adipocytes. *J. Nutr. Biochem.* **2016**, *27*, 193–202. [CrossRef] [PubMed]
157. Song, Z.; Revelo, X.; Shao, W.; Tian, L.; Zeng, K.; Lei, H.; Sun, H.; Woo, M.; Winer, D.; Jin, T. Dietary Curcumin Intervention Targets Mouse White Adipose Tissue Inflammation and Brown Adipose Tissue UCP1 Expression. *Obesity* **2018**, *26*, 547–558. [CrossRef] [PubMed]
158. Fedoreyev, S.A.; Pokushalova, T.V.; Veselova, M.V.; Glebko, L.I.; Kulesh, N.I.; Muzarok, T.I.; Seletskaya, L.D.; Bulgakov, V.P.; Zhuravlev, Y.N. Isoflavonoid Production by Callus Cultures of Maackia Amurensis. *Fitoterapia* **2000**, *71*, 365–372. [CrossRef] [PubMed]
159. Dixit, M.; Raghuvanshi, A.; Gupta, C.P.; Kureel, J.; Mansoori, M.N.; Shukla, P.; John, A.A.; Singh, K.; Purohit, D.; Awasthi, P.; et al. Medicarpin, a Natural Pterocarpan, Heals Cortical Bone Defect by Activation of Notch and Wnt Canonical Signaling Pathways. *PLoS ONE* **2015**, *10*, e0144541. [CrossRef]
160. Imran, K.M.; Yoon, D.; Kim, Y. A Pivotal Role of AMPK Signaling in Medicarpin-mediated Formation of Brown and Beige. *BioFactors* **2018**, *44*, 168–179. [CrossRef] [PubMed]
161. Lama, A.; Pirozzi, C.; Severi, I.; Morgese, M.G.; Senzacqua, M.; Annunziata, C.; Comella, F.; Del Piano, F.; Schiavone, S.; Petrosino, S.; et al. Palmitoylethanolamide Dampens Neuroinflammation and Anxiety-like Behavior in Obese Mice. *Brain Behav. Immun.* **2022**, *102*, 110–123. [CrossRef]
162. Sugiura, C.; Zheng, G.; Liu, L.; Sayama, K. Catechins and Caffeine Promote Lipid Metabolism and Heat Production Through the Transformation of Differentiated 3T3-L1 Adipocytes from White to Beige Adipocytes. *J. Food Sci.* **2020**, *85*, 192–200. [CrossRef]
163. Kim, H.J.; Yoon, B.K.; Park, H.; Seok, J.W.; Choi, H.; Yu, J.H.; Choi, Y.; Song, S.J.; Kim, A.; Kim, J. Caffeine Inhibits Adipogenesis through Modulation of Mitotic Clonal Expansion and the AKT/GSK3 Pathway in 3T3-L1 Adipocytes. *BMB Rep.* **2016**, *49*, 111–115. [CrossRef]
164. Velickovic, K.; Wayne, D.; Leija, H.A.L.; Bloor, I.; Morris, D.E.; Law, J.; Budge, H.; Sacks, H.; Symonds, M.E.; Sottile, V. Caffeine Exposure Induces Browning Features in Adipose Tissue in Vitro and in Vivo. *Sci. Rep.* **2019**, *9*, 9104. [CrossRef] [PubMed]
165. Kogure, A.; Sakane, N.; Takakura, Y.; Umekawa, T.; Yoshioka, K.; Nishino, H.; Yamamoto, T.; Kawada, T.; Yoshikawa, T.; Yoshida, T. Effects Of Caffeine On The Uncoupling Protein Family In Obese Yellow Kk Mice. *Clin. Exp. Pharmacol. Physiol.* **2002**, *29*, 391–394. [CrossRef]
166. Fernández-Elías, V.E.; Del Coso, J.; Hamouti, N.; Ortega, J.F.; Muñoz, G.; Muñoz-Guerr, J.; Mora-Rodríguez, R. Ingestion of a Moderately High Caffeine Dose Before Exercise Increases Postexercise Energy Expenditure. *Int. J. Sport. Nutr. Exerc. Metab.* **2015**, *25*, 46–53. [CrossRef] [PubMed]
167. Cheng, L.; Wei, Y.; Peng, L.; Wei, K.; Liu, Z.; Wei, X. State-of-the-Art Review of Theabrownins: From Preparation, Structural Characterization to Health-Promoting Benefits. *Crit. Rev. Food Sci. Nutr.* **2023**, *63*, 1–20. [CrossRef] [PubMed]
168. Peng, C.; Wang, Q.; Liu, H.; Gao, B.; Sheng, J.; Gong, J. Effects of Zijuan Pu-Erh Tea Theabrownin on Metabolites in Hyperlipidemic Rat Feces by Py-GC/MS. *J. Anal. Appl. Pyrolysis* **2013**, *104*, 226–233. [CrossRef]
169. Mitani, T.; Watanabe, S.; Yoshioka, Y.; Katayama, S.; Nakamura, S.; Ashida, H. Theobromine Suppresses Adipogenesis through Enhancement of CCAAT-Enhancer-Binding Protein β Degradation by Adenosine Receptor A1. *Biochim. Et Biophys. Acta (BBA) Mol. Cell Res.* **2017**, *1864*, 2438–2448. [CrossRef]
170. Jang, Y.J.; Koo, H.J.; Sohn, E.-H.; Kang, S.C.; Rhee, D.-K.; Pyo, S. Theobromine Inhibits Differentiation of 3T3-L1 Cells during the Early Stage of Adipogenesis via AMPK and MAPK Signaling Pathways. *Food Funct.* **2015**, *6*, 2365–2374. [CrossRef]
171. Jang, M.H.; Mukherjee, S.; Choi, M.J.; Kang, N.H.; Pham, H.G.; Yun, J.W. Theobromine Alleviates Diet-Induced Obesity in Mice via Phosphodiesterase-4 Inhibition. *Eur. J. Nutr.* **2020**, *59*, 3503–3516. [CrossRef]

172. Tanaka, E.; Mitani, T.; Nakashima, M.; Yonemoto, E.; Fujii, H.; Ashida, H. Theobromine Enhances the Conversion of White Adipocytes into Beige Adipocytes in a PPARγ Activation-Dependent Manner. *J. Nutr. Biochem.* **2022**, *100*, 108898. [CrossRef]
173. Wang, Q.; Hu, G.-L.; Qiu, M.-H.; Cao, J.; Xiong, W.-Y. Coffee, Tea, and Cocoa in Obesity Prevention: Mechanisms of Action and Future Prospects. *Curr. Res. Food Sci.* **2024**, *8*, 100741. [CrossRef] [PubMed]
174. Jin, T.; Zhang, Y.; Botchway, B.O.A.; Huang, M.; Lu, Q.; Liu, X. Quercetin Activates the Sestrin2/AMPK/SIRT1 Axis to Improve Amyotrophic Lateral Sclerosis. *Biomed. Pharmacother.* **2023**, *161*, 114515. [CrossRef] [PubMed]
175. Lee, S.G.; Parks, J.S.; Kang, H.W. Quercetin, a Functional Compound of Onion Peel, Remodels White Adipocytes to Brown-like Adipocytes. *J. Nutr. Biochem.* **2017**, *42*, 62–71. [CrossRef] [PubMed]
176. Granato, M.; Rizzello, C.; Gilardini Montani, M.S.; Cuomo, L.; Vitillo, M.; Santarelli, R.; Gonnella, R.; D'Orazi, G.; Faggioni, A.; Cirone, M. Quercetin Induces Apoptosis and Autophagy in Primary Effusion Lymphoma Cells by Inhibiting PI3K/AKT/MTOR and STAT3 Signaling Pathways. *J. Nutr. Biochem.* **2017**, *41*, 124–136. [CrossRef] [PubMed]
177. Kuipers, E.; Dam, A.; Held, N.; Mol, I.; Houtkooper, R.; Rensen, P.; Boon, M. Quercetin Lowers Plasma Triglycerides Accompanied by White Adipose Tissue Browning in Diet-Induced Obese Mice. *Int. J. Mol. Sci.* **2018**, *19*, 1786. [CrossRef] [PubMed]
178. Zhang, F.; Ai, W.; Hu, X.; Meng, Y.; Yuan, C.; Su, H.; Wang, L.; Zhu, X.; Gao, P.; Shu, G.; et al. Phytol Stimulates the Browning of White Adipocytes through the Activation of AMP-Activated Protein Kinase (AMPK) α in Mice Fed High-Fat Diet. *Food Funct.* **2018**, *9*, 2043–2050. [CrossRef] [PubMed]
179. Combarnous, Y.; Nguyen, T.M.D. Comparative Overview of the Mechanisms of Action of Hormones and Endocrine Disruptor Compounds. *Toxics* **2019**, *7*, 5. [CrossRef] [PubMed]
180. Amato, A.A.; Wheeler, H.B.; Blumberg, B. Obesity and Endocrine-Disrupting Chemicals. *Endocr. Connect.* **2021**, *10*, R87–R105. [CrossRef] [PubMed]
181. Petrakis, D.; Vassilopoulou, L.; Mamoulakis, C.; Psycharakis, C.; Anifantaki, A.; Sifakis, S.; Docea, A.; Tsiaoussis, J.; Makrigiannakis, A.; Tsatsakis, A. Endocrine Disruptors Leading to Obesity and Related Diseases. *Int. J. Environ. Res. Public Health* **2017**, *14*, 1282. [CrossRef]
182. Heindel, J.J. Endocrine Disruptors and the Obesity Epidemic. *Toxicol. Sci.* **2003**, *76*, 247–249. [CrossRef]
183. Grün, F.; Blumberg, B. Perturbed Nuclear Receptor Signaling by Environmental Obesogens as Emerging Factors in the Obesity Crisis. *Rev. Endocr. Metab. Disord.* **2007**, *8*, 161–171. [CrossRef] [PubMed]
184. Newbold, R.R.; Padilla-Banks, E.; Snyder, R.J.; Jefferson, W.N. Developmental Exposure to Estrogenic Compounds and Obesity. *Birth Defects Res. A Clin. Mol. Teratol.* **2005**, *73*, 478–480. [CrossRef] [PubMed]
185. Chen, J.-Q.; Brown, T.R.; Russo, J. Regulation of Energy Metabolism Pathways by Estrogens and Estrogenic Chemicals and Potential Implications in Obesity Associated with Increased Exposure to Endocrine Disruptors. *Biochim. Et Biophys. Acta (BBA) Mol. Cell Res.* **2009**, *1793*, 1128–1143. [CrossRef] [PubMed]
186. Lapid, K.; Lim, A.; Clegg, D.J.; Zeve, D.; Graff, J.M. Oestrogen Signalling in White Adipose Progenitor Cells Inhibits Differentiation into Brown Adipose and Smooth Muscle Cells. *Nat. Commun.* **2014**, *5*, 5196. [CrossRef] [PubMed]
187. Naomi, R.; Yazid, M.D.; Bahari, H.; Keong, Y.Y.; Rajandram, R.; Embong, H.; Teoh, S.H.; Halim, S.; Othman, F. Bisphenol A (BPA) Leading to Obesity and Cardiovascular Complications: A Compilation of Current In Vivo Study. *Int. J. Mol. Sci.* **2022**, *23*, 2969. [CrossRef] [PubMed]
188. Matuszczak, E.; Komarowska, M.D.; Debek, W.; Hermanowicz, A. The Impact of Bisphenol A on Fertility, Reproductive System, and Development: A Review of the Literature. *Int. J. Endocrinol.* **2019**, *2019*, 1–8. [CrossRef] [PubMed]
189. Boucher, J.G.; Boudreau, A.; Atlas, E. Bisphenol A Induces Differentiation of Human Preadipocytes in the Absence of Glucocorticoid and Is Inhibited by an Estrogen-Receptor Antagonist. *Nutr. Diabetes* **2014**, *4*, e102. [CrossRef]
190. Desai, M.; Ferrini, M.G.; Jellyman, J.K.; Han, G.; Ross, M.G. In Vivo and in Vitro Bisphenol A Exposure Effects on Adiposity. *J. Dev. Orig. Health Dis.* **2018**, *9*, 678–687. [CrossRef]
191. González-Casanova, J.E.; Bermúdez, V.; Caro Fuentes, N.J.; Angarita, L.C.; Caicedo, N.H.; Rivas Muñoz, J.; Rojas-Gómez, D.M. New Evidence on BPA's Role in Adipose Tissue Development of Proinflammatory Processes and Its Relationship with Obesity. *Int. J. Mol. Sci.* **2023**, *24*, 8231. [CrossRef]
192. de Aguiar Greca, S.-C.; Kyrou, I.; Pink, R.; Randeva, H.; Grammatopoulos, D.; Silva, E.; Karteris, E. Involvement of the Endocrine-Disrupting Chemical Bisphenol A (BPA) in Human Placentation. *J. Clin. Med.* **2020**, *9*, 405. [CrossRef]
193. Chen, Z.; Zuo, X.; He, D.; Ding, S.; Xu, F.; Yang, H.; Jin, X.; Fan, Y.; Ying, L.; Tian, C.; et al. Long-Term Exposure to a 'Safe' Dose of Bisphenol A Reduced Protein Acetylation in Adult Rat Testes. *Sci. Rep.* **2017**, *7*, 40337. [CrossRef] [PubMed]
194. Oliviero, F.; Marmugi, A.; Viguié, C.; Gayrard, V.; Picard-Hagen, N.; Mselli-Lakhal, L. Are BPA Substitutes as Obesogenic as BPA? *Int. J. Mol. Sci.* **2022**, *23*, 4238. [CrossRef] [PubMed]
195. Zhang, W.; Xia, W.; Liu, W.; Li, X.; Hu, J.; Zhang, B.; Xu, S.; Zhou, Y.; Li, J.; Cai, Z.; et al. Exposure to Bisphenol a Substitutes and Gestational Diabetes Mellitus: A Prospective Cohort Study in China. *Front. Endocrinol.* **2019**, *10*, 262. [CrossRef] [PubMed]
196. Dunder, L. Exposure to Bisphenol A (BPA) and Metabolic Disruption. Ph.D. Thesis, Acta Universitatis Upsaliensis, Uppsala, Sweden, 2021.
197. Wen, X.; Xiao, Y.; Xiao, H.; Tan, X.; Wu, B.; Li, Z.; Wang, R.; Xu, X.; Li, T. Bisphenol S Induces Brown Adipose Tissue Whitening and Aggravates Diet-Induced Obesity in an Estrogen-Dependent Manner. *Cell Rep.* **2023**, *42*, 113504. [CrossRef] [PubMed]

198. Hiromori, Y.; Aoki, A.; Nishikawa, J.; Nagase, H.; Nakanishi, T. Transactivation of the Human Retinoid X Receptor by Organotins: Use of Site-Directed Mutagenesis to Identify Critical Amino Acid Residues for Organotin-Induced Transactivation. *Metallomics* **2015**, *7*, 1180–1188. [CrossRef] [PubMed]
199. Kanayama, T.; Kobayashi, N.; Mamiya, S.; Nakanishi, T.; Nishikawa, J. Organotin Compounds Promote Adipocyte Differentiation as Agonists of the Peroxisome Proliferator-Activated Receptor γ/Retinoid X Receptor Pathway. *Mol. Pharmacol.* **2005**, *67*, 766–774. [CrossRef] [PubMed]
200. Kim, S.; Rabhi, N.; Blum, B.C.; Hekman, R.; Wynne, K.; Emili, A.; Farmer, S.; Schlezinger, J.J. Triphenyl Phosphate Is a Selective PPARγ Modulator That Does Not Induce Brite Adipogenesis in Vitro and in Vivo. *Arch. Toxicol.* **2020**, *94*, 3087–3103. [CrossRef] [PubMed]
201. Kim, S.; Li, A.; Monti, S.; Schlezinger, J.J. Tributyltin Induces a Transcriptional Response without a Brite Adipocyte Signature in Adipocyte Models. *Arch. Toxicol.* **2018**, *92*, 2859–2874. [CrossRef]
202. Merlo, E.; Zimerman, J.; Dos Santos, F.C.F.; Zanol, J.F.; da Costa, C.S.; Carneiro, P.H.; Miranda-Alves, L.; Warner, G.R.; Graceli, J.B. Subacute and Low Dose of Tributyltin Exposure Leads to Brown Adipose Abnormalities in Male Rats. *Toxicol. Lett.* **2023**, *376*, 26–38. [CrossRef]
203. Agency for Toxic Substances and Disease Registry (US). *Toxicological Profile for Di(2-Ethylhexyl)Phthalate (DEHP)*; Agency for Toxic Substances and Disease Registry (US): Atlanta, GA, USA, 2022. Available online: https://www.ncbi.nlm.nih.gov/books/NBK590474/ (accessed on 20 May 2024).
204. Feige, J.N.; Gelman, L.; Rossi, D.; Zoete, V.; Métivier, R.; Tudor, C.; Anghel, S.I.; Grosdidier, A.; Lathion, C.; Engelborghs, Y.; et al. The Endocrine Disruptor Monoethyl-Hexyl-Phthalate Is a Selective Peroxisome Proliferator-Activated Receptor γ Modulator That Promotes Adipogenesis. *J. Biol. Chem.* **2007**, *282*, 19152–19166. [CrossRef]
205. Hurst, C.H.; Waxman, D.J. Activation of PPAR and PPAR by Environmental Phthalate Monoesters. *Toxicol. Sci.* **2003**, *74*, 297–308. [CrossRef]
206. Latini, G.; Scoditti, E.; Verrotti, A.; De Felice, C.; Massaro, M. Peroxisome Proliferator-Activated Receptors as Mediators of Phthalate-Induced Effects in the Male and Female Reproductive Tract: Epidemiological and Experimental Evidence. *PPAR Res.* **2008**, *2008*, 1–13. [CrossRef] [PubMed]
207. Schlezinger, J.J.; Howard, G.J.; Hurst, C.H.; Emberley, J.K.; Waxman, D.J.; Webster, T.; Sherr, D.H. Environmental and Endogenous Peroxisome Proliferator-Activated Receptor γ Agonists Induce Bone Marrow B Cell Growth Arrest and Apoptosis: Interactions between Mono(2-Ethylhexyl)Phthalate, 9- *Cis* -Retinoic Acid, and 15-Deoxy-Δ12,14-Prostaglandin J2. *J. Immunol.* **2004**, *173*, 3165–3177. [CrossRef] [PubMed]
208. Useini, A.; Engelberger, F.; Künze, G.; Sträter, N. Structural Basis of the Activation of PPARγ by the Plasticizer Metabolites MEHP and MINCH. *Environ. Int.* **2023**, *173*, 107822. [CrossRef]
209. Froment, P.; Gizard, F.; Defever, D.; Staels, B.; Dupont, J.; Monget, P. Peroxisome Proliferator-Activated Receptors in Reproductive Tissues: From Gametogenesis to Parturition. *J. Endocrinol.* **2006**, *189*, 199–209. [CrossRef]
210. Francis, C.E.; Allee, L.; Nguyen, H.; Grindstaff, R.D.; Miller, C.N.; Rayalam, S. Endocrine Disrupting Chemicals: Friend or Foe to Brown and Beige Adipose Tissue? *Toxicology* **2021**, *463*, 152972. [CrossRef]
211. Hsu, J.-W.; Nien, C.-Y.; Yeh, S.-C.; Tsai, F.-Y.; Chen, H.-W.; Lee, T.-S.; Chen, S.-L.; Kao, Y.-H.; Tsou, T.-C. Phthalate Exposure Causes Browning-like Effects on Adipocytes in Vitro and in Vivo. *Food Chem. Toxicol.* **2020**, *142*, 111487. [CrossRef]
212. Zhang, Y.; Feng, H.; Tian, A.; Zhang, C.; Song, F.; Zeng, T.; Zhao, X. Long-Term Exposure to Low-Dose Di(2-Ethylhexyl) Phthalate Aggravated High Fat Diet-Induced Obesity in Female Mice. *Ecotoxicol. Environ. Saf.* **2023**, *253*, 114679. [CrossRef] [PubMed]
213. Ferguson, K.K.; Bommarito, P.A.; Arogbokun, O.; Rosen, E.M.; Keil, A.P.; Zhao, S.; Barrett, E.S.; Nguyen, R.H.N.; Bush, N.R.; Trasande, L.; et al. Prenatal Phthalate Exposure and Child Weight and Adiposity from in Utero to 6 Years of Age. *Environ. Health Perspect.* **2022**, *130*, 047006. [CrossRef]
214. Berman, Y.E.; Doherty, D.A.; Main, K.M.; Frederiksen, H.; Hickey, M.; Keelan, J.A.; Newnham, J.P.; Hart, R.J. Associations between Prenatal Exposure to Phthalates and Timing of Menarche and Growth and Adiposity into Adulthood: A Twenty-Years Birth Cohort Study. *Int. J. Environ. Res. Public Health* **2021**, *18*, 4725. [CrossRef]
215. Lv, Z.; Cheng, J.; Huang, S.; Zhang, Y.; Wu, S.; Qiu, Y.; Geng, Y.; Zhang, Q.; Huang, G.; Ma, Q.; et al. DEHP Induces Obesity and Hypothyroidism through Both Central and Peripheral Pathways in C3H/He Mice. *Obesity* **2016**, *24*, 368–378. [CrossRef] [PubMed]
216. Gadupudi, G.; Gourronc, F.A.; Ludewig, G.; Robertson, L.W.; Klingelhutz, A.J. PCB126 Inhibits Adipogenesis of Human Preadipocytes. *Toxicol. Vitr.* **2015**, *29*, 132–141. [CrossRef]
217. Gourronc, F.A.; Perdew, G.H.; Robertson, L.W.; Klingelhutz, A.J. PCB126 Blocks the Thermogenic Beiging Response of Adipocytes. *Environ. Sci. Pollut. Res.* **2020**, *27*, 8897–8904. [CrossRef] [PubMed]
218. Mostafalou, S. Persistent Organic Pollutants and Concern Over the Link with Insulin Resistance Related Metabolic Diseases. In *Reviews of Environmental Contamination and Toxicology*; Springer: Berlin/Heidelberg, Germany, 2016; pp. 69–89.
219. Kim, M.J.; Pelloux, V.; Guyot, E.; Tordjman, J.; Bui, L.-C.; Chevallier, A.; Forest, C.; Benelli, C.; Clément, K.; Barouki, R. Inflammatory Pathway Genes Belong to Major Targets of Persistent Organic Pollutants in Adipose Cells. *Environ. Health Perspect.* **2012**, *120*, 508–514. [CrossRef] [PubMed]

220. Rozman, K.; Strassle, B.; Iatropoulos, M.J. Brown Adipose Tissue Is a Target Tissue in 2,3,7,8-Tetrachlorodibenzo-p-Dioxin (TCDD) Induced Toxicity. In *Toxic Interfaces of Neurones, Smoke and Genes: Proceeding of the European Society of Toxicology Meeting Held in Kuopio, 16–19 June 1985*; Springer: Berlin/Heidelberg, Germany, 1986; pp. 356–360.
221. Joffin, N.; Noirez, P.; Antignac, J.-P.; Kim, M.; Marchand, P.; Falabregue, M.; Le Bizec, B.; Forest, C.; Emond, C.; Barouki, R.; et al. Release and Toxicity of Adipose Tissue-Stored TCDD: Direct Evidence from a Xenografted Fat Model. *Environ. Int.* **2018**, *121*, 1113–1120. [CrossRef] [PubMed]
222. Bhalla, D.; van Noort, V. Molecular Evolution of Aryl Hydrocarbon Receptor Signaling Pathway Genes. *J. Mol. Evol.* **2023**, *91*, 628–646. [CrossRef] [PubMed]
223. Okey, A.B. An Aryl Hydrocarbon Receptor Odyssey to the Shores of Toxicology: The Deichmann Lecture, International Congress of Toxicology-XI. *Toxicol. Sci.* **2007**, *98*, 5–38. [CrossRef]
224. Nukaya, M.; Lin, B.C.; Glover, E.; Moran, S.M.; Kennedy, G.D.; Bradfield, C.A. The Aryl Hydrocarbon Receptor-Interacting Protein (AIP) Is Required for Dioxin-Induced Hepatotoxicity but Not for the Induction of the Cyp1a1 and Cyp1a2 Genes. *J. Biol. Chem.* **2010**, *285*, 35599–35605. [CrossRef]
225. Carver, L.A.; Bradfield, C.A. Ligand-Dependent Interaction of the Aryl Hydrocarbon Receptor with a Novel Immunophilin Homolog In Vivo. *J. Biol. Chem.* **1997**, *272*, 11452–11456. [CrossRef]
226. Whitlock, J.P.; Chichester, C.H.; Bedgood, R.M.; Okino, S.T.; Ko, H.P.; Ma, Q.; Dong, L.; Li, H.; Clarkekatzenberg, R. Induction of Drug-Metabolizing Enzymes by Dioxin. *Drug Metab. Rev.* **1997**, *29*, 1107–1127. [CrossRef]
227. Baba, T.; Mimura, J.; Gradin, K.; Kuroiwa, A.; Watanabe, T.; Matsuda, Y.; Inazawa, J.; Sogawa, K.; Fujii-Kuriyama, Y. Structure and Expression of the Ah Receptor Repressor Gene. *J. Biol. Chem.* **2001**, *276*, 33101–33110. [CrossRef]
228. Jackson, E.; Shoemaker, R.; Larian, N.; Cassis, L. Adipose Tissue as a Site of Toxin Accumulation. In *Comprehensive Physiology*; Wiley: Hoboken, NJ, USA, 2017; pp. 1085–1135.
229. Shimba, S.; Todoroki, K.; Aoyagi, T.; Tezuka, M. Depletion of Arylhydrocarbon Receptor during Adipose Differentiation in 3T3-L1 Cells. *Biochem. Biophys. Res. Commun.* **1998**, *249*, 131–137. [CrossRef] [PubMed]
230. Xu, C.-X.; Wang, C.; Zhang, Z.-M.; Jaeger, C.D.; Krager, S.L.; Bottum, K.M.; Liu, J.; Liao, D.-F.; Tischkau, S.A. Aryl Hydrocarbon Receptor Deficiency Protects Mice from Diet-Induced Adiposity and Metabolic Disorders through Increased Energy Expenditure. *Int. J. Obes.* **2015**, *39*, 1300–1309. [CrossRef] [PubMed]
231. Kerley-Hamilton, J.S.; Trask, H.W.; Ridley, C.J.A.; DuFour, E.; Ringelberg, C.S.; Nurinova, N.; Wong, D.; Moodie, K.L.; Shipman, S.L.; Moore, J.H.; et al. Obesity Is Mediated by Differential Aryl Hydrocarbon Receptor Signaling in Mice Fed a Western Diet. *Environ. Health Perspect.* **2012**, *120*, 1252–1259. [CrossRef]
232. Alexander, D.L.; Ganem, L.G.; Fernandez-Salguero, P.; Gonzalez, F.; Jefcoate, C.R. Aryl-Hydrocarbon Receptor Is an Inhibitory Regulator of Lipid Synthesis and of Commitment to Adipogenesis. *J. Cell Sci.* **1998**, *111*, 3311–3322. [CrossRef]
233. Dou, H.; Duan, Y.; Zhang, X.; Yu, Q.; Di, Q.; Song, Y.; Li, P.; Gong, Y. Aryl Hydrocarbon Receptor (AhR) Regulates Adipocyte Differentiation by Assembling CRL4B Ubiquitin Ligase to Target PPARγ for Proteasomal Degradation. *J. Biol. Chem.* **2019**, *294*, 18504–18515. [CrossRef]
234. Baker, N.A.; Shoemaker, R.; English, V.; Larian, N.; Sunkara, M.; Morris, A.J.; Walker, M.; Yiannikouris, F.; Cassis, L.A. Effects of Adipocyte Aryl Hydrocarbon Receptor Deficiency on PCB-Induced Disruption of Glucose Homeostasis in Lean and Obese Mice. *Environ. Health Perspect.* **2015**, *123*, 944–950. [CrossRef] [PubMed]
235. Haque, N.; Ojo, E.S.; Krager, S.L.; Tischkau, S.A. Deficiency of Adipose Aryl Hydrocarbon Receptor Protects against Diet-Induced Metabolic Dysfunction through Sexually Dimorphic Mechanisms. *Cells* **2023**, *12*, 1748. [CrossRef]
236. Li, S.; Bostick, J.W.; Ye, J.; Qiu, J.; Zhang, B.; Urban, J.F.; Avram, D.; Zhou, L. Aryl Hydrocarbon Receptor Signaling Cell Intrinsically Inhibits Intestinal Group 2 Innate Lymphoid Cell Function. *Immunity* **2018**, *49*, 915–928.e5. [CrossRef]
237. Seymour, E.M.; Bennink, M.R.; Bolling, S.F. Diet-Relevant Phytochemical Intake Affects the Cardiac AhR and Nrf2 Transcriptome and Reduces Heart Failure in Hypertensive Rats. *J. Nutr. Biochem.* **2013**, *24*, 1580–1586. [CrossRef]
238. Korkina, L.; Kostyuk, V.; De Luca, C.; Pastore, S. Plant Phenylpropanoids as Emerging Anti-Inflammatory Agents. *Mini-Rev. Med. Chem.* **2011**, *11*, 823–835. [CrossRef] [PubMed]
239. Puppala, D.; Gairola, C.G.; Swanson, H.I. Identification of Kaempferol as an Inhibitor of Cigarette Smoke-Induced Activation of the Aryl Hydrocarbon Receptor and Cell Transformation. *Carcinogenesis* **2006**, *28*, 639–647. [CrossRef] [PubMed]
240. Gargaro, M.; Epifano, F.; Fiorito, S.; Taddeo, V.A.; Genovese, S.; Pirro, M.; Turco, A.; Puccetti, P.; Schmidt-Weber, C.B.; Fallarino, F. Interaction of 7-Alkoxycoumarins with the Aryl Hydrocarbon Receptor. *J. Nat. Prod.* **2017**, *80*, 1939–1943. [CrossRef] [PubMed]
241. Nakai, R.; Fukuda, S.; Kawase, M.; Yamashita, Y.; Ashida, H. Curcumin and Its Derivatives Inhibit 2,3,7,8,-Tetrachloro-Dibenzo-p -Dioxin-Induced Expression of Drug Metabolizing Enzymes through Aryl Hydrocarbon Receptor-Mediated Pathway. *Biosci. Biotechnol. Biochem.* **2018**, *82*, 616–628. [CrossRef] [PubMed]
242. Ciolino, H.P.; Daschner, P.J.; Wang, T.T.Y.; Yeh, G.C. Effect of Curcumin on the Aryl Hydrocarbon Receptor and Cytochrome P450 1A1 in MCF-7 Human Breast Carcinoma Cells. *Biochem. Pharmacol.* **1998**, *56*, 197–206. [CrossRef] [PubMed]
243. Cheng, J.; Wang, S.; Lv, S.-Q.; Song, Y.; Guo, N.-H. Resveratrol Inhibits AhR/Notch Axis and Reverses Th17/Treg Imbalance in Purpura by Activating Foxp3. *Toxicol. Res.* **2023**, *12*, 381–391. [CrossRef] [PubMed]
244. Beedanagari, S.R.; Bebenek, I.; Bui, P.; Hankinson, O. Resveratrol Inhibits Dioxin-Induced Expression of Human CYP1A1 and CYP1B1 by Inhibiting Recruitment of the Aryl Hydrocarbon Receptor Complex and RNA Polymerase II to the Regulatory Regions of the Corresponding Genes. *Toxicol. Sci.* **2009**, *110*, 61–67. [CrossRef]

245. Ciolino, H.P.; Daschner, P.J.; Yeh, G.C. Resveratrol Inhibits Transcription of CYP1A1 in Vitro by Preventing Activation of the Aryl Hydrocarbon Receptor. *Cancer Res.* **1998**, *58*, 5707–5712. [PubMed]
246. Satake, K.; Ishii, T.; Morikawa, T.; Sakamoto, T.; Nishii, Y. Quercetin Reduces the Development of 2,3,7,8-Tetrachlorodibenzo-p-Dioxin-Induced Cleft Palate in Mice by Suppressing CYP1A1 via the Aryl Hydrocarbon Receptor. *Nutrients* **2022**, *14*, 2448. [CrossRef]
247. Ondrová, K.; Zůvalová, I.; Vyhlídalová, B.; Krasulová, K.; Miková, E.; Vrzal, R.; Nádvorník, P.; Nepal, B.; Kortagere, S.; Kopečná, M.; et al. Monoterpenoid Aryl Hydrocarbon Receptor Allosteric Antagonists Protect against Ultraviolet Skin Damage in Female Mice. *Nat. Commun.* **2023**, *14*, 2728. [CrossRef]
248. Kim, S.-H.; Henry, E.C.; Kim, D.-K.; Kim, Y.-H.; Shin, K.J.; Han, M.S.; Lee, T.G.; Kang, J.-K.; Gasiewicz, T.A.; Ryu, S.H.; et al. Novel Compound 2-Methyl-2 H-Pyrazole-3-Carboxylic Acid (2-Methyl-4-o-Tolylazo-Phenyl)-Amide (CH-223191) Prevents 2,3,7,8-TCDD-Induced Toxicity by Antagonizing the Aryl Hydrocarbon Receptor. *Mol. Pharmacol.* **2006**, *69*, 1871–1878. [CrossRef] [PubMed]
249. Murray, I.A.; Flaveny, C.A.; DiNatale, B.C.; Chairo, C.R.; Schroeder, J.C.; Kusnadi, A.; Perdew, G.H. Antagonism of Aryl Hydrocarbon Receptor Signaling by 6,2′,4′-Trimethoxyflavone. *J. Pharmacol. Exp. Ther.* **2010**, *332*, 135–144. [CrossRef] [PubMed]
250. Smith, K.J.; Murray, I.A.; Tanos, R.; Tellew, J.; Boitano, A.E.; Bisson, W.H.; Kolluri, S.K.; Cooke, M.P.; Perdew, G.H. Identification of a High-Affinity Ligand That Exhibits Complete Aryl Hydrocarbon Receptor Antagonism. *J. Pharmacol. Exp. Ther.* **2011**, *338*, 318–327. [CrossRef] [PubMed]
251. Dumbrava, E.E.; Cecchini, M.; Zugazagoitia, J.; Lopez, J.S.; Jäger, D.; Oliva, M.; Ochsenreither, S.; Gambardella, V.; Chung, K.Y.; Longo, F.; et al. Initial Results from a First-in-Human, Phase I Study of Immunomodulatory Aryl Hydrocarbon Receptor (AhR) Inhibitor BAY2416964 in Patients with Advanced Solid Tumors. *J. Clin. Oncol.* **2023**, *41*, 2502. [CrossRef]
252. Mckean, M.; Aggen, D.H.; Lakhani, N.J.; Bashir, B.; Luke, J.J.; Hoffman-Censits, J.H.; Alhalabi, O.; Bowman, I.A.; Guancial, E.A.; Tan, A.; et al. TPS3169 Poster Session Phase 1a/b Open-Label Study of IK-175, an Oral AHR Inhibitor, Alone and in Combination with Nivolumab in Patients with Locally Advanced or Metastatic Solid Tumors and Urothelial Carcinoma. *J. Clin. Oncol.* **2022**, *40*, TPS3169. [CrossRef]
253. Takeda, Y.; Dai, P. A Developed Serum-Free Medium and an Optimized Chemical Cocktail for Direct Conversion of Human Dermal Fibroblasts into Brown Adipocytes. *Sci. Rep.* **2020**, *10*, 3775. [CrossRef] [PubMed]
254. Chen, S.; Bastarrachea, R.A.; Shen, J.-S.; Laviada-Nagel, A.; Rodriguez-Ayala, E.; Nava-Gonzalez, E.J.; Huang, P.; DeFronzo, R.A.; Kent, J.W.; Grayburn, P.A. Ectopic BAT MUCP-1 Overexpression in SKM by Delivering a BMP7/PRDM16/PGC-1a Gene Cocktail or Single PRMD16 Using Non-Viral UTMD Gene Therapy. *Gene Ther.* **2018**, *25*, 497–509. [CrossRef] [PubMed]
255. Bates, R.; Huang, W.; Cao, L. Adipose Tissue: An Emerging Target for Adeno-Associated Viral Vectors. *Mol. Ther. Methods Clin. Dev.* **2020**, *19*, 236–249. [CrossRef]
256. Descamps, D.; Benihoud, K. Two Key Challenges for Effective Adenovirus-Mediated Liver Gene Therapy:Innate Immune Responses and Hepatocyte-Specific Transduction. *Curr. Gene Ther.* **2009**, *9*, 115–127. [CrossRef]
257. Shirley, J.L.; de Jong, Y.P.; Terhorst, C.; Herzog, R.W. Immune Responses to Viral Gene Therapy Vectors. *Mol. Ther.* **2020**, *28*, 709–722. [CrossRef]
258. Balkow, A.; Hoffmann, L.S.; Klepac, K.; Glöde, A.; Gnad, T.; Zimmermann, K.; Pfeifer, A. Direct Lentivirus Injection for Fast and Efficient Gene Transfer into Brown and Beige Adipose Tissue. *J. Biol. Methods* **2016**, *3*, e48. [CrossRef] [PubMed]
259. Tseng, Y.-H.; Kokkotou, E.; Schulz, T.J.; Huang, T.L.; Winnay, J.N.; Taniguchi, C.M.; Tran, T.T.; Suzuki, R.; Espinoza, D.O.; Yamamoto, Y.; et al. New Role of Bone Morphogenetic Protein 7 in Brown Adipogenesis and Energy Expenditure. *Nature* **2008**, *454*, 1000–1004. [CrossRef]
260. Schlimgen, R.; Howard, J.; Wooley, D.; Thompson, M.; Baden, L.R.; Yang, O.O.; Christiani, D.C.; Mostoslavsky, G.; Diamond, D.V.; Duane, E.G.; et al. Risks Associated With Lentiviral Vector Exposures and Prevention Strategies. *J. Occup. Environ. Med.* **2016**, *58*, 1159–1166. [CrossRef] [PubMed]
261. Kvaratskhelia, M.; Sharma, A.; Larue, R.C.; Serrao, E.; Engelman, A. Molecular Mechanisms of Retroviral Integration Site Selection. *Nucleic Acids Res.* **2014**, *42*, 10209–10225. [CrossRef] [PubMed]
262. Casana, E.; Jimenez, V.; Jambrina, C.; Sacristan, V.; Muñoz, S.; Rodo, J.; Grass, I.; Garcia, M.; Mallol, C.; León, X.; et al. AAV-Mediated BMP7 Gene Therapy Counteracts Insulin Resistance and Obesity. *Mol. Ther. Methods Clin. Dev.* **2022**, *25*, 190–204. [CrossRef]
263. Sommer, N.; Roumane, A.; Han, W.; Delibegović, M.; Rochford, J.J.; Mcilroy, G.D. Gene Therapy Restores Adipose Tissue and Metabolic Health in a Pre-Clinical Mouse Model of Lipodystrophy. *Mol. Ther. Methods Clin. Dev.* **2022**, *27*, 206–216. [CrossRef] [PubMed]
264. O'Neill, S.M.; Hinkle, C.; Chen, S.-J.; Sandhu, A.; Hovhannisyan, R.; Stephan, S.; Lagor, W.R.; Ahima, R.S.; Johnston, J.C.; Reilly, M.P. Targeting Adipose Tissue via Systemic Gene Therapy. *Gene Ther.* **2014**, *21*, 653–661. [CrossRef]
265. Casana, E.; Jimenez, V.; Sacristan, V.; Muñoz, S.; Jambrina, C.; Rodó, J.; Garcia, M.; Mallol, C.; León, X.; Franckhauser, S.; et al. BMP7 Overexpression in Adipose Tissue Induces White Adipogenesis and Improves Insulin Sensitivity in Ob/Ob Mice. *Int. J. Obes.* **2021**, *45*, 449–460. [CrossRef]
266. Anderson, J.M.; Boardman, A.A.; Bates, R.; Zou, X.; Huang, W.; Cao, L. Hypothalamic TrkB.FL Overexpression Improves Metabolic Outcomes in the BTBR Mouse Model of Autism. *PLoS ONE* **2023**, *18*, e0282566. [CrossRef]

267. Huang, W.; Liu, X.; Queen, N.J.; Cao, L. Targeting Visceral Fat by Intraperitoneal Delivery of Novel AAV Serotype Vector Restricting Off-Target Transduction in Liver. *Mol. Ther. Methods Clin. Dev.* **2017**, *6*, 68–78. [CrossRef]
268. Mizukami, H.; Mimuro, J.; Ogura, T.; Okada, T.; Urabe, M.; Kume, A.; Sakata, Y.; Ozawa, K. Adipose Tissue as a Novel Target for In Vivo Gene Transfer by Adeno-Associated Viral Vectors. *Hum. Gene Ther.* **2006**, *17*, 921–928. [CrossRef] [PubMed]
269. Jimenez, V.; Muñoz, S.; Casana, E.; Mallol, C.; Elias, I.; Jambrina, C.; Ribera, A.; Ferre, T.; Franckhauser, S.; Bosch, F. In Vivo Adeno-Associated Viral Vector–Mediated Genetic Engineering of White and Brown Adipose Tissue in Adult Mice. *Diabetes* **2013**, *62*, 4012–4022. [CrossRef] [PubMed]
270. Kharitonenkov, A.; DiMarchi, R. Fibroblast Growth Factor 21 Night Watch: Advances and Uncertainties in the Field. *J. Intern. Med.* **2017**, *281*, 233–246. [CrossRef] [PubMed]
271. Jimenez, V.; Jambrina, C.; Casana, E.; Sacristan, V.; Muñoz, S.; Darriba, S.; Rodó, J.; Mallol, C.; Garcia, M.; León, X.; et al. FGF21 Gene Therapy as Treatment for Obesity and Insulin Resistance. *EMBO Mol. Med.* **2018**, *10*, e8791. [CrossRef] [PubMed]
272. Carreira, A.C.; Zambuzzi, W.F.; Rossi, M.C.; Astorino Filho, R.; Sogayar, M.C.; Granjeiro, J.M. Bone Morphogenetic Proteins: Promising Molecules for Bone Healing, Bioengineering, and Regenerative Medicine. *Vitam. Horm.* **2015**, *99*, 293–322. [CrossRef] [PubMed]
273. Yoshizawa, T.; Sato, Y.; Sobuz, S.U.; Mizumoto, T.; Tsuyama, T.; Karim, M.F.; Miyata, K.; Tasaki, M.; Yamazaki, M.; Kariba, Y.; et al. SIRT7 Suppresses Energy Expenditure and Thermogenesis by Regulating Brown Adipose Tissue Functions in Mice. *Nat. Commun.* **2022**, *13*, 7439. [CrossRef] [PubMed]
274. Dumesic, P.A.; Wilensky, S.E.; Bose, S.; Van Vranken, J.G.; Gygi, S.P.; Spiegelman, B.M. RBM43 Links Adipose Inflammation and Energy Expenditure through Translational Regulation of PGC1α. *bioRxiv* **2023**. [CrossRef] [PubMed]
275. Cho, Y.K.; Son, Y.; Saha, A.; Kim, D.; Choi, C.; Kim, M.; Park, J.-H.; Im, H.; Han, J.; Kim, K.; et al. STK3/STK4 Signalling in Adipocytes Regulates Mitophagy and Energy Expenditure. *Nat. Metab.* **2021**, *3*, 428–441. [CrossRef]
276. Qiao, A.; Ma, W.; Deng, J.; Zhou, J.; Han, C.; Zhang, E.; Boriboun, C.; Xu, S.; Zhang, C.; Jie, C.; et al. Ablation of Sam68 in Adult Mice Increases Thermogenesis and Energy Expenditure. *FASEB J.* **2021**, *35*. [CrossRef]
277. Huang, L.; Liu, P.; Yang, Q.; Wang, Y. The KRAB Domain-Containing Protein ZFP961 Represses Adipose Thermogenesis and Energy Expenditure through Interaction with PPARα. *Adv. Sci.* **2022**, *9*, 2102949. [CrossRef]
278. Maurya, S.; Sarangi, P.; Jayandharan, G.R. Safety of Adeno-Associated Virus-Based Vector-Mediated Gene Therapy—Impact of Vector Dose. *Cancer Gene Ther.* **2022**, *29*, 1305–1306. [CrossRef] [PubMed]
279. Ertl, H.C.J. Mitigating Serious Adverse Events in Gene Therapy with AAV Vectors: Vector Dose and Immunosuppression. *Drugs* **2023**, *83*, 287–298. [CrossRef] [PubMed]
280. Malogolovkin, A.; Egorov, A.D.; Karabelsky, A.; Ivanov, R.A.; Verkhusha, V.V. Optogenetic Technologies in Translational Cancer Research. *Biotechnol. Adv.* **2022**, *60*, 108005. [CrossRef] [PubMed]

MDPI AG
Grosspeteranlage 5
4052 Basel
Switzerland
Tel.: +41 61 683 77 34

Pharmaceuticals Editorial Office
E-mail: pharmaceuticals@mdpi.com
www.mdpi.com/journal/pharmaceuticals

www.ingramcontent.com/pod-product-compliance
Lightning Source LLC
Chambersburg PA
CBHW040815250926
51850CB00007BA/1176
* 9 7 8 3 7 2 5 8 6 8 0 2 5 *